Biological and Clinical Progress in Breast Cancer

Biological and Clinical Progress in Breast Cancer

Editor: Ava Santiago

FOSTER
ACADEMICS

www.fosteracademics.com

www.fosteracademics.com

FOSTER ACADEMICS

Cataloging-in-publication Data

Biological and clinical progress in breast cancer / edited by Ava Santiago.
p. cm.
Includes bibliographical references and index.
ISBN 978-1-64646-596-5
1. Breast--Cancer. 2. Breast--Cancer--Molecular aspects.
3. Breast--Cancer--Pathophysiology. 4. Breast--Cancer--Treatment.
I. Santiago, Ava.
RC280.B8 B56 2023
616.994 49--dc23

Foster Academics,
118-35 Queens Blvd., Suite 400,
Forest Hills, NY 11375, USA

ISBN 978-1-64646-596-5 (Hardback)

Contents

Preface

Every book is initially just a concept; it takes months of research and hard work to give it the final shape in which the readers receive it. In its early stages, this book also went through rigorous reviewing. The notable contributions made by experts from across the globe were first molded into patterned chapters and then arranged in a sensibly sequential manner to bring out the best results.

Breast cancer is a type of cancer that starts from the breast cells. Some of its common symptoms are formation of lump in the breast, dimpling of breast skin, and changes in the size and appearance of the breast. There are many different types of breast cancer such as ductal carcinoma in situ, invasive lobular carcinoma, angiosarcoma, Paget's disease of the breast and inflammatory breast cancer. Factors such as obesity, lack of physical exercise, alcoholism, hormone replacement therapy during menopause, and ionizing radiation may result in the development of breast cancer. It can be diagnosed with the help of biopsy. The treatment of breast cancer involves performing surgery, prescribing medications, and therapies such as chemotherapy or radiation therapy. A number of latest researches have been included in this book to keep the readers updated with the latest concepts related to the biological and clinical progress in breast cancer. It is an excellent resource guide for oncologists as well as students.

It has been my immense pleasure to be a part of this project and to contribute my years of learning in such a meaningful form. I would like to take this opportunity to thank all the people who have been associated with the completion of this book at any step.

Editor

1

Histamine and Breast Cancer: A New Role for a well known Amine

Graciela Cricco[1], Nora Mohamad[1], María Soledad Sáez[1], Eduardo Valli[1,2], Elena Rivera[1] and Gabriela Martín[1,2]
[1]*Laboratory of Radioisotopes, School of Pharmacy and Biochemistry, University of Buenos Aires*
[2]*Scientific and Technical Research National Council (CONICET) Argentina*

1. Introduction

Metastases are the most devastating aspect of cancer since most deaths from cancer are related to them. The ability of tumors to invade the neighboring extracellular matrix, which is primarily accompanied by augmented matrix metalloproteinases (MMPs) production and cell migration, is critical for metastases.

After surgical removal of primary breast tumors, malignant cells may still remain and radiotherapy is an efficient modality to reduce the risk of local recurrence. However, proliferative, invasive, and metastatic capacities can be increased in the surviving tumor cells of irradiated breast and other neoplasias (Baluna et al, 2006; Tsukamoto et al, 2007; Tsutsumi et al, 2009). To improve the efficacy of radiotherapy, this phenomenon must be further studied to elaborate therapeutic modalities to prevent radiation enhancement of cancer cell invasion.

Histamine is an endogenous biogenic amine extensively distributed throughout the organism which exerts multiple functions in physiologic and pathophysiological processes by stimulation of four G-protein coupled receptors (H1, H2, H3 and H4 histamine receptors) with different tissue expression patterns and functions. It is well known that diverse tumoral tissues and cell lines express the different histamine receptors through which histamine brings about its effects on cell proliferation, differentiation, survival and death. A great deal of evidence shows a relevant role of histamine in tumor progression, however controversial results are published depending on the cell type and the histamine receptor subtype that is activated (Blaya et al, 2010; Francis et al, 2009; Parsons & Ganellin, 2006; Soule et al, 2010). It has also been determined that numerous tumour tissues and cell lines express L-histidine decarboxylase, the histamine-synthesizing enzyme, and contain high levels of endogenous histamine which released to the extracellular media may exert its effects via a paracrine or autocrine regulation (Falus et al, 2001; Pós et al, 2004; Rivera et al, 2000). Additionally some effects on tumor growth may be mediated by histamine regulation of angiogenesis and immunity (Lázár-Molnár et al, 2002; Tomita et al, 2003).

Our research team has demonstrated the expression of histamine membrane receptors and their association to different signalling pathways in breast cancer biopsies and a large number of transformed cell lines, being our works the first ones to report the presence of H3 and H4 receptors linked to cell proliferation in breast and pancreatic cancer cell lines. We determined that histamine can modulate not only cell proliferation but differentiation, apoptosis and secretion of different growth factors (Cricco et al, 2006, 2008; Medina et al, 2006, 2008, 2009; Rivera et al, 2000, 2004). We have demonstrated that the highly invasive and metastatic breast cancer cell line MDA-MB 231 expresses the four known types of histamine receptors through which histamine differentially regulates cell proliferation in a dose dependent way. At concentrations over 10 μM a significant decrease in clonogenic growth was observed, while at concentrations lower than 0.5 μM proliferation was increased. The negative effect on proliferation was associated with the induction of arrest in G2/M phase of cell cycle, differentiation and a significant augmentation of apoptotic death (Medina et al, 2006).

Histamine and antihistamines have a modulatory effect on epithelial and endothelial cell adhesion and on the expression of different MMPs (Asano et al, 2004; Ciprandi et al, 2003; Gschwandtner et al, 2008). It has also been described a stimulatory action on migration of fibroblasts, haematopoyetic and immune cells, mainly via H4 receptors (Gschwandtner et al, 2010; Kohyama et al, 2010). However most of these reports refer to normal cells, existing less information regarding to tumor cells. Recently we have demonstrated the ability of HA to modulate MMPs, tissue inhibitors of matrix metalloproteinases (TIMPs) and cell adhesion in the breast cancer cell lines HBL-100 and MDA-MB 231 (Genre et al, 2009). We have also determined the upregulation of MMP2 and cell migration in the pancreatic carcinoma cell line PANC-1 by histamine (Cricco et al, 2006).

Reactive oxygen species (ROS) such as superoxide anion and hydrogen peroxide (H2O2) are continuously produced as by-products of aerobic metabolism primarily in the mitochondria and other cellular sources. In addition, external agents like ultraviolet radiation and ionizing radiation also increase intracellular ROS levels. Under physiologic conditions cells are protected against oxidative stress by an interacting network of antioxidant enzymes like superoxide dismutases, catalase and glutathion peroxidase. Though ROS may induce cellular damage when there is an imbalance between their generation and scavenging, numerous studies support the role of ROS as essential participants in cell signaling depending on their concentration, timing and location (Thannickal and Fanburg, 2000).

The aim of the present study was to investigate the role of HA and HA receptors activation in early cellular events involved in metastatic capacity, such as expression and activity of matrix metalloproteinases MMP2 and MMP9, cell migration and invasion in MDA-MB 231 cells. Since ionizing radiation may affect metastatic competence depending upon cell type and irradiation characteristics, and given that histamine increases MDA-MB 231 cells intrinsic sensibility to ionizing radiation by downregulating catalase activity and enhancing H2O2 intracellular levels at the same doses that inhibit cell proliferation (Medina et al, 2006), the possible interaction between histamine treatment and irradiation was also evaluated. The identification of drugs that can both regulate tumor cell survival and metastatic ability will help to delineate more effective strategies for therapeutic intervention in malignant diseases.

2. Effects of histamine and histamine receptor agonists upon matrix metalloproteinases MMP2 and MMP9

MMP2 and MMP9, also called gelatinase A and gelatinase B respectively, belong to a large family of zinc-dependent endopeptidases formed by more than 20 members which participate in the proteolysis of basement membrane and extracellular matrix proteins, collagen and fibronectin. MMPs are involved in normal tissue remodeling events like wound healing, bone resorption and mammary involution. Their anomalous expression is associated to various pathological processes including inflammation and cancer (Freije et al, 2003). MMPs are secreted in a latent zymogen form (proenzyme). The inactive enzyme conformation is maintained due to thiol interactions between cysteine residues in the prodomain and the zinc atom present in the catalytic site of all MMPs. *In vitro*, MMPs activation can occur when the prodomain is cleaved by other proteases or when the zinc-cysteine bound is interrupted (Van Wart & Birkedal-Hansen, 1990).

Regulation of MMPs occurs on three levels: alteration of gene expression, activation of latent zymogens and inhibition by TIMPs. This regulation is tightly controlled in normal states while it is altered during tumor cell progression, being a critical step for cancer invasion and metastases (Chakraborti et al, 2003). Initially, it was believed that the major role of MMPs in metastases was to facilitate the breakdown of physical barriers. At present, it is widely accepted that MMPs may have a more complex role making important contributions at other steps in the metastatic process (Chabottaux & Noel, 2007). *In vitro* and *in vivo* studies demonstrate an entire correlation between MMP2, MMP9 and TIMPs expression and metastasis (Baum et al, 2007; Chambers & Matrisian, 1997; Duffy et al, 2008; John & Tuszynski, 2001; Wroblewski et al, 2002). Accordingly, MMP2 and MMP9 have been associated with breast cancer development and tumor progression (Köhrmann et al, 2009). An elevated activity of gelatinases in plasma and sera of patients with breast cancer confirms the role of these enzymes in the development of such tumors though clinical correlation with parameters like tumor grade and stage, size and lymph node involvement is still fragmentary (Decokc et al 2005; La Rocca et al, 2004; Stankovic et al, 2010).

In a previous work we determined a dissimilar role of histamine in the modulation of gelatinolytic activities and cell adhesion in mammary cell lines with different tumorigenic capacity (Genre et al, 2009), To further investigate histamine action and also histamine receptors implicated in breast cancer invasiveness we conducted *in vitro* experiments employing different doses of histamine and histamine receptor agonists and antagonists (listed in Table 1) in MDA-MB 231 cell line (ATCC HTB-26). Cells were cultured in RPMI supplemented with 10% fetal bovine serum, L-glutamine (0.3 g/L) and gentamicin (0.04 g/L) under standard conditions of 5% CO_2 and temperature of 37°C.

Ligand	Characteristic	References
2-(3-trifluoromethylphenil)histamine dimaleate (Sigma Aldrich)	H1 histamine receptor agonist	Leschke et al (1995). Synthesis and histamine H1 receptor agonist activity of a series of 2-phenylhistamines, 2-heteroarylhistamines, and analogues. *J Med Chem*, Vol. 38, No8, (April 1995), pp. 1287-1294, ISSN 0022-2623
Amthamine dihydrobromide (Tocris)	H2 histamine receptor agonist	Eriks el al (1992). Histamine H2 -receptor agonists -synthesis, in vitro pharmacology, and qualitative structure activity relationships of substituted 4-(2-Aminoethyl)thiazoles and 5-(2-Aminoethyl)thiazoles. *J Med Chem*, Vol. 35, No17, (August 1992), pp. 3239-3246, ISSN:0022-2623

Table 1. Histamine receptor agonists and antagonists employed in this study. (Continued)

Ligand	Characteristic	References
R(alpha) methylhistamine dihydrobromide (Tocris)	H3 histamine receptor agonist	Leurs el al (1995). The medicinal chemistry and therapeutic potential of ligands for the histamine H3 receptor. *Prog Drug Res,* Vol. 45, pp.107-165, ISSN 0071-786X
VUF 8430 dihydrobromide (Tocris)	H4 histamine receptor agonist	Lim et al (2006). Discovery of S-(2-guanidylethyl)-isothiourea (VUF 8430) as a potent nonimidazole histamine H4 receptor agonist. *J Med Chem,* Vol.49, No.23, (November 2006), pp. 6650-6651, ISSN 0022-2623
Clobenpropit dihydrobromide (Tocris)	H4 histamine receptor agonist and H3 histamine receptor antagonist	Liu et al (2001). Cloning and pharmacological characterization of a fourth histamine receptor (H_4) expressed in bone marrow. *Mol Pharmacol,* Vol.59, No3, (March 2001), pp 420-426, ISSN 0026-895X
Ranitidine hydrochloride (Sigma Aldrich)	H2 histamine receptor antagonist	Brittain & Daly (1981) A review of the animal pharmacology of ranitidine -a new, selective histamine H_2-antagonist. *Scand J Gastroenterol, Suppl,* Vol.69, (June 1981), pp. 1-9, ISSN 0085-5928
JNJ7777120 (Johnson & Johnson)	H4 histamine receptor antagonist	Jablanowski et al (2003). The first potent and selective non-imidazole human histamine H_4 receptor antagonists. *J Med Chem,* Vol. 6, No19, (September 2003), pp. 3957-3960. Sep 11;46(19):3957-60, ISSN 0022-2623

Table 1. Histamine receptor agonists and antagonists employed in this study.

2.1 Evaluation of matrix metalloproteinases activity

MMP2 and MMP9 gelatinolytic activity was evaluated by zymography, a powerful electrophoretic technique for identifying proteolytic activity of enzymes separated in polyacrylamide gels under nonreducing conditions. Cells were cultured in serum-free RPMI medium for 24h in absence or presence of treatments. Conditioned media mixed with non-reducing buffer were electrophoresed in 7% SDS-polyacrylamide gel containing 1% of gelatin. Gels were then rinsed, incubated (48h at 37°C) and subsequently stained (0.1% Coomasie Brilliant Blue). Activity of lytic bands was determined by densitometry (Image J 1.42q, NIH, US).

There was a biphasic effect when cells were cultured with histamine concentrations varying from 0.1 μM to 20 μM. A significant increase in the activity of MMP2 and MMP9 pro and active forms was observed with 0.5 μM histamine (low dose) while a dramatic reduction in the activity of MMP2 and MMP9 (pro and active forms) occurred with histamine over 10 μM (high doses) as shown in Figure 1.

Testing H1, H2, H3 and H4 histamine receptor agonists we could observe that activities of both MMPs were differentially modulated. 10 μM H2 agonist amthamine evoked the reduction in lytic bands induced by high doses of histamine while 10 μM H4 agonists VUF 8430 and clobenpropit produced a significant rise of MMP2 and MMP9 activities as low doses of histamine did (Figure 2). The increase and decrease in gelatinolytic activities produced by histamine were blocked by the specific H4 antagonist JNJ7777120 (10 μM) and H2 antagonist ranitidine (10 μM) respectively (data not shown). In addition, no significant changes in both activities were determined employing H1 and H3 histamine agonists so that they were no longer tested in current assays.

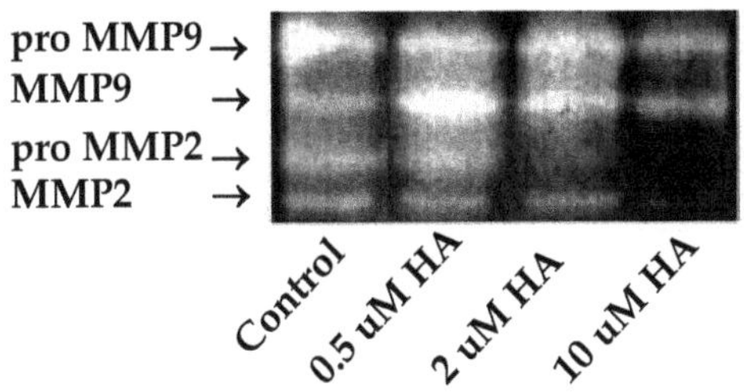

Fig. 1. Effect of histamine on MMP2 and MMP9 gelatinolytic activity. Activity was evaluated by zymography after 24h of treatment with different concentrations of histamine in serum free RPMI medium. The figure shows a representative gel.

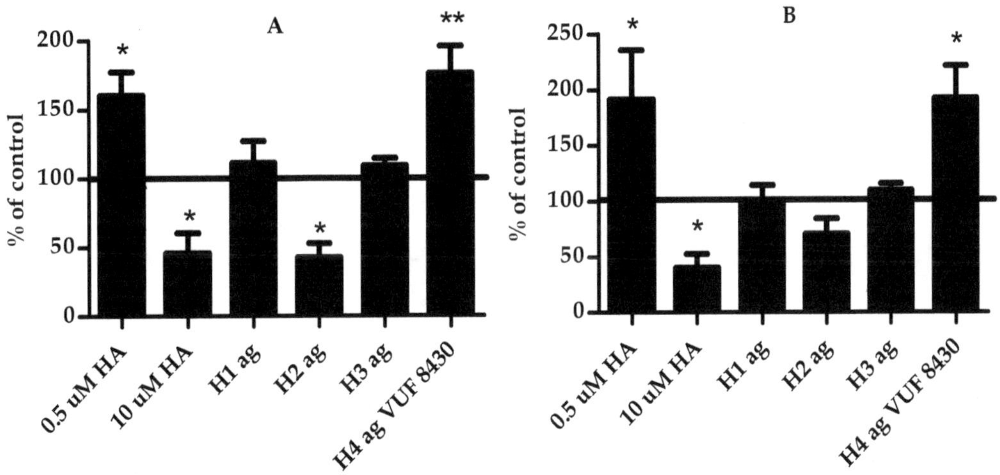

Fig. 2. Effect of histamine and histamine receptor agonists on MMPs gelatinolytic activity. A: MMP2 zymography. B: MMP9 zymography. Activity of lytic bands for each treatment was determined by densitometry and normalized to control values. Bars show the means ± SEM of three experiments run in triplicates. *$p<0.05$ and **$p<0.01$ vs control. One way Anova, Dunnet post test.

2.2 Determination of MMP2 and MMP9 mRNA steady state levels

MMP2 and MMP9 mRNA steady state levels were evaluated in cell cultures after 24h treatments using RT-PCR. Total RNA was extracted with Trizol®. Retrotranscription was carried out with MMLV enzyme. DNA was amplifyed by PCR and products were run in 2% agarose gels containing ethidium bromide. Semiquantification using GAPDH as housekeeping gene was performed with the Image J 1.42q (NIH, US) software.

	Primer sequence 5´-3´	PCR product size (bp)
MMP2	*s* ACC CAT TTA CAC CTA CAC CAA G *a* GTA TAC CGC ATC AAT CTT TTC CG	306
MMP9	*s* CCC ATT TCG ACG ATG AC *a* GGC ACT GAG GAA GAA TGA TCT AAG	639
GAPDH	s GCA GGG GGG AGC CAA AAG GG *a* TGC CAG CCC CAG CGT CAA AG	566

Table 2. Sequence of primers used in PCR reactions.

A significant reduction of mRNA steady states levels of both MMPs was observed when MDA-MB 231 cells were treated with histamine concentrations over 10 μM in agreement to our previous report (Genre et al, 2009), being this effect reproduced by 10 μM amthamine. On the other hand, there was an important increase in mRNA expression when these cells received 0.5 μM HA (low dose of HA) or H4 agonist VUF 8430 (Figure 3). Similar results were obtained employing the H4 agonist clobenpropit.

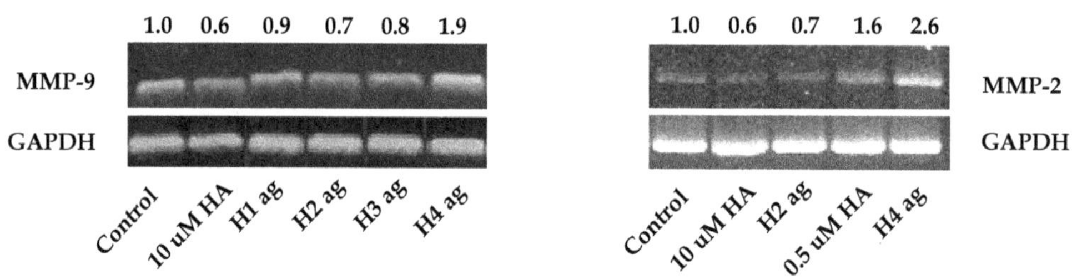

Fig. 3. mRNA expression of MMPs in MDA-MB231 cells. MMP2 and MMP9 mRNA steady state levels were determined by RT-PCR after 24h treatment with histamine and histamine receptor agonists. Figure shows representative gels for PCR products. The numbers above represent for each treatment the relative expression to controls of MMPs normalized to GAPDH.

2.3 Immunodetection of MMP2 and MMP9

Protein expression determination was performed by immunocytochemistry. MDA-MB 231 cells were grown on coverglasses and after 24h treatment cells were fixed, permeabilized and endogenous peroxidase was inhibited. Cells were incubated for 18h at 4°C with anti-MMP9 Ab (1/50, Calbiochem) or anti-MMP2 Ab (1/50, Cell Signalling) and for 2h with horse radish peroxidase conjugated anti-rabbit IgG (1/100, Sigma-Aldrich). This was followed by diaminobencidine and hematoxylin staining and observation by optical microscope.

Immunocytochemical staining supported the results of RT-PCR. A higher cytoplasmatic expression of MMP9 was seen when cells were treated with 0.5 μM histamine or H4 agonists. In turn a lower expression of MMP9 was detected in the presence of 10 μM histamine or H2 agonist (Figure 4). Similar results were obtained for MMP2 (data not shown).

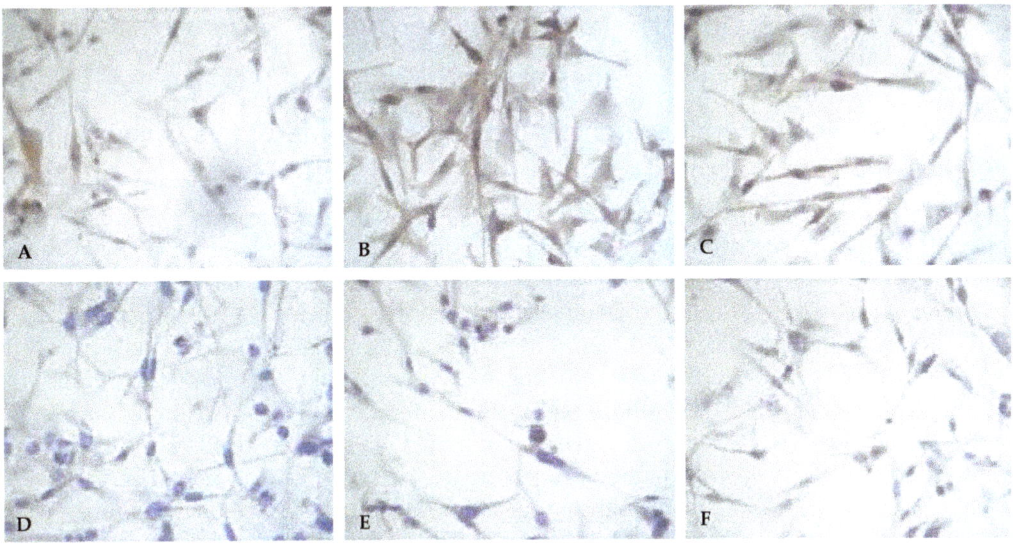

Fig. 4. Action of histamine and histamine receptor agonists on MMP2 and MMP9 protein expression in MDA-MB 231 cells. Expression was evaluated by immunocytochemistry. A: control, B: 0.5 μM HA, C: H4 agonist VUF 8340, D: negative control, E: 10 μM HA, F: H2 agonist. Photographs correspond to MMP9 expression. 400x magnification. Similar results were obtained for MMP2 expression.

Our research indicates that the mRNA and protein expression patterns of MMP2 and MMP9 were dose-dependently modified by HA through H2 and H4 receptors in MDA-MB 231 cells. Additionally, changes in gelatinolytic activity of MMP2 and MMP9 were registered in parallel to these results suggesting that an increment in protein expression may account for the increase in gelatinolytic activity.

These data constitute the first report about histamine-induced MMPs enhancement through H4 receptors in breast tumor cells. Most of *in vitro* reports upon histamine and MMPs modulation are related to inflammatory and allergic processes via H1 and H2 receptors and more recently via H4 receptors. Asano and coworkers showed that fexofenadine hydrochloride, a selective H1 receptor antagonist, may inhibit mRNA and protein expression of MMP2 and MMP9 in nasal fibroblasts and thereby possibly reduce the severity of allergic rhinitis, characterized by remodeling of the nasal wall and eosinophil and mast cell infiltration (Asano et al, 2004). It has been reported the histamine-induced production of MMP2 through H1 and H2 receptors in microvascular endothelial cells is associated to angiogenic processes (Doyle & Haas, 2009). An increase in mRNA level, protein expression and gelatinolytic activity of MMP9 is observed in human keratinocytes via H1 receptors stimulation in skin remodelling and fibrosis (Gschwandtner et al, 2008). Moreover, the *in vitro* production of other MMPs as MMP3, MMP8 and MMP13 is stimulated by histamine in human articular chondrocytes and rheumatoid synovial fibroblasts (Tetlow & Woolley, 2002; 2004). Modulation of mRNA for MMP1 by histamine has also been described in human corneal epithelial cells (Sharif et al, 1998). Regarding tumor cells, we have reported that histamine is able to reduce cell adhesion and to enhance the gelatinolytic activity of MMP2 in the pancreatic cancer cell line PANC-1 (Cricco et al, 2006). Furthermore, tranilast an antiallergic compound used clinically to control atopic and fibrotic disorders exerts its action by reducing the expression and activity of MMP2 in human malignant glioma cells (Platten et al, 2001).

3. Histamine and histamine agonists modulate MDA-MB 231 cells migration and invasion

In view of current results on MMP2 and MMP9 expression and activity we explored the migratory capacity of MDA-MB 231 mammary cells. Directed migration is an essential component of cell invasion during tumor progression and metastasis. The migratory response of MDA-MB 231 cells to histamine and histamine agonists was investigated using a 24-well transwell unit with polyethylene terephthalate (PET) membranes having a pore size of 8.0 μm (BD Falcon, Basel, Switzerland). For invasion assay the upper part of the transwell was coated with Matrigel®, a synthetic basement membrane (BD Biosciences, Bedford, MA). A fixed number of cells (1.10^4/chamber) was plated on the transwell. The medium in compartments of the lower chambers contained 2% FBS plus treatments. Inserts were incubated for 6 h at 37°C. Non migrating cells on the upper surface of membranes were gently scrubbed with a cotton swab. Cells migrated or invading the lower surface of the membrane were fixed with methanol, and stained with hematoxilin. Ten random fields were counted under a light microscope at 50x magnification.

Histamine exerted a dual action on the migratory behavior of cells. It is improved by doses of histamine lower than 1 μM and reduced by concentrations over 10 μM (Figure 5). The stimulatory response disclosed by histamine was evoked by the H4 agonists and prevented by the specific H4 antagonist. On the other hand, histamine-induced inhibitory effect on cell motility was mimicked by the H2 agonist while relapsed by ranitidine. H1 agonist and H3 agonist did not modify cell migration; consequently they were not longer tested.

In addition similar results were displayed by histamine and histamine agonists when invasiveness was evaluated, as depicted in Figure 6. These results are in full concordance with those obtained for MMPs, reinforcing the idea that histamine may have a key role as mediator of MDA-MB 231 cells invasive ability.

A body of evidence shows a chemotactic response of inflammatory and immune cells to histamine. Because of its preferential expression in immunocompetent cells, the H4 receptor is closely related with the regulatory functions of histamine during the immune response. It has been published that histamine mediates chemotaxis via the H4 receptor in mast cells, in human monocyte-derived dendritic cells and in eosinophils, related to immune and inflammatory disorders (Baumer et al, 2008; Gutzmer et al, 2005; Hofstra et al, 2003; Ling et al, 2004; Thurmond et al, 2004). Barnad et al (2007) proved that exposure to histamine cause eosinophils to migrate from the bloodstream to the inflammatory focus into tissues, inducing actin polymerization through the H4 receptor. Histamine also activates signaling pathways typical of chemotaxis inducing migratory responses in T lymphocytes, via the H4 receptor (Truta-Feles K et al, 2010). Besides this chemotactic action in immune cells it has also been reported that histamine promotes invasiveness specifically through activation of H1 receptor in human cytotrophoblasts required to initiate blastocyst implantation (Liu et al, 2004).

Regarding tumor cells it has been reported that histamine acts as a chemoattractant for human carcinoma and melanoma cells via H1 receptor stimulation (Blaya et al, 2010; Tilly et al, 1990). Accordingly, the antiallergic compound tranilast inhibits cell migration and invasion in human malignant glioma cells blocking H1 receptors (Platten et al, 2001). A divergent response (stimulatory or inhibitory) on the migration rate of SW756 cervical carcinoma cells has been disclosed by histamine acting on H1 receptor or H4 receptor, respectively (Rudolph et al, 2008). However, as far as we know, our work is the first report about histamine-modulated migration and invasion through H4 and H2 receptors in breast tumor cells.

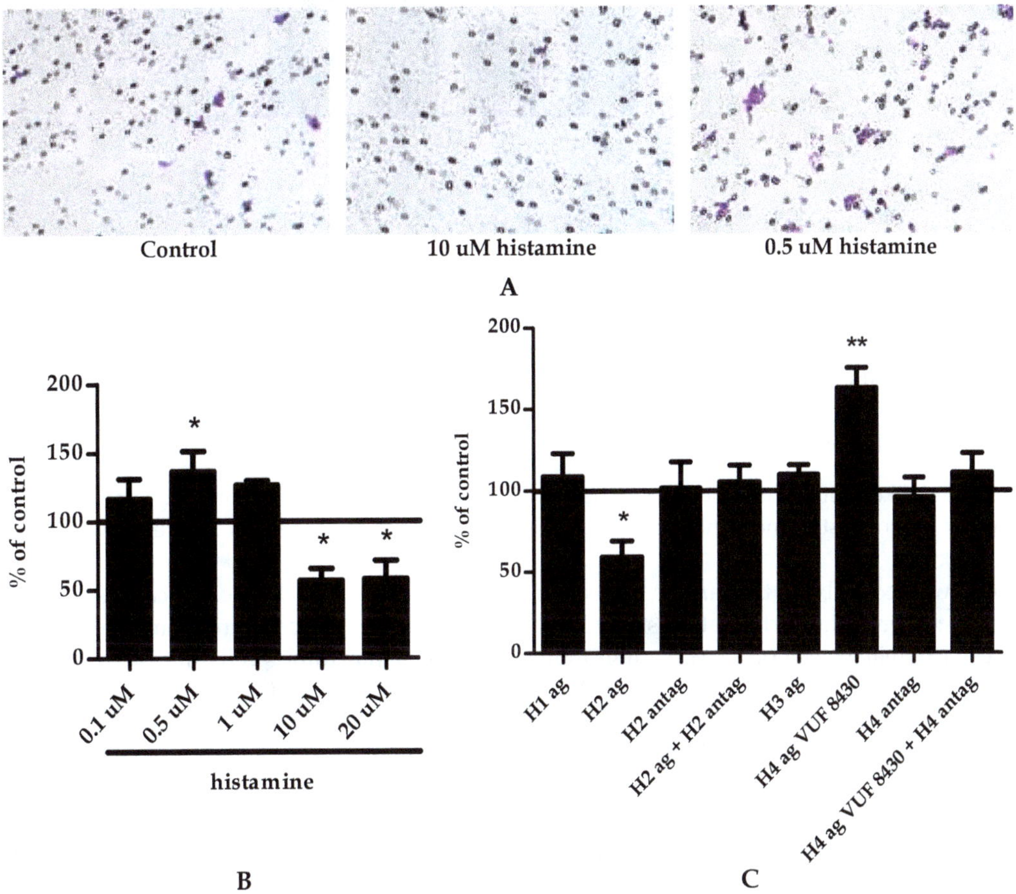

Fig. 5. Histamine induced migration of MDA-MB 231 cells. Migration was evaluated by using transwell units with 8 μm pore size PET membranes. A: Photographs are representative of random fields observed at 50x magnification. B-C: Bars show the means ± SEM of three experiments run in duplicates. Results are expressed for each treatment as the number of cells on the lower side of membranes normalized to control values. B: Concentration-response curve of histamine. C: Effect of histamine receptor agonists and antagonists on cell migration. $^{*}p<0.05$ and $^{**}p<0.01$ vs control. One way ANOVA, Dunnet post test.

4. H202 involvement in histamine actions

Many cell surface receptors produce transient levels of ROS (specifically H2O2) when are activated by peptide growth factors, cytokines and ligands of G protein-coupled receptors

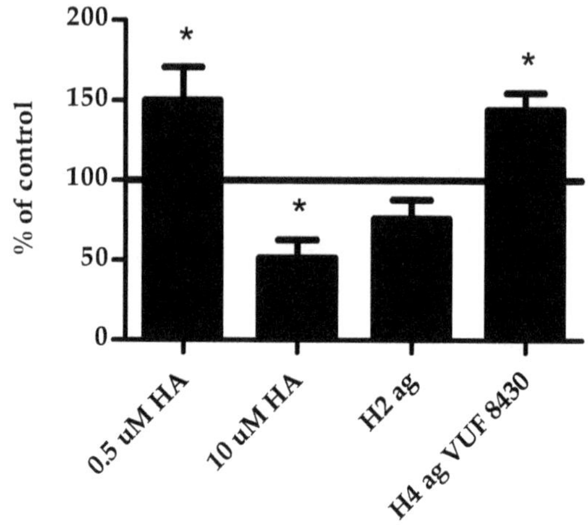

Fig. 6. Effect of histamine and histamine receptor agonists on cell invasion. Invasion was evaluated by using transwell units with 8 μm pore size PET membranes coated with Matrigel®. Bars show the means ± SEM of three experiments run in duplicates. Results are expressed for each treatment as the number of cells invading the lower side of membranes normalized to control values. *$p<0.05$ vs control. One way Anova, Dunnet post test.

(GPCRs) like histamine receptors (Rhee et al, 2000). In a previous work we reported that high doses of histamine enhance H2O2 intracellular levels in MDA-MB 231 cells (Medina et al, 2006).

ROS will contribute to various aspects of malignant tumors, including carcinogenesis, aberrant growth and metastasis which is a complex process including epithelial-mesenchymal transition (EMT), migration, invasion of the tumor cells and angiogenesis around the tumor lesion (Pani et al, 2009). Significant amounts of ROS are able to kill cancer cells through their oxidative action. At lower concentrations, however, ROS work as second messengers in signal transduction, and activate a variety of proteins or upregulate their transcription. The ROS-regulated genes relevant to EMT and metastasis include EGF, EGFR, VEGF, E-cadherin, integrin and MMPs (Nishikawa 2008; Wu, 2006).

In order to explore the effect of ROS on cellular events related to invasiveness of MDA-MB 231 cells we conducted the following experiments.

4.1 Measurement of ROS levels

The fluorescent dye dichlorofluorescein diacetate (DFH-DA) is an important tool to indicate oxidations in cells and is one of a very few markers available for measuring intracellular ROS levels in live cells. DFH-DA is a non polar and non fluorescent compound that freely diffuses through cell membranes. Once it enters the cells, its ester moiety is cleaved by intracellular esterases, and then DFH is retained in the cells. Oxidation of DFH by ROS yields a fluorescent species that can be detected by flow cytometry.

In order to investigate the effect of ROS on cellular events related to invasiveness we measured the steady state levels of ROS employing 5 μM DFH-DA dye in MDA-MB 231 cells after 1h treatment with histamine, histamine agonists and antagonists. Exogenous catalase (125 IU/mL) was added 15 minutes before treatments to metabolize intracellular H2O2 levels.

Histamine augmented intracellular steady state of ROS levels in a dose-dependent manner (Tabla 3). Histamine in low concentration and 10 μM H4 agonists increased intracellular ROS levels up to 135%, while high doses of histamine and 10 μM H2 agonists augmented them up to 190%. When exogenous catalase was added to histamine-treated cells there was a significant reduction of ROS levels almost to control value confirming that intracellular H2O2 was the major species involved since H2O2 is the only substrate for catalase.

Treatment	mean fluorescence (% respect of control values)
0.5 μM HA	123 ± 5
5 μM HA	140 ± 8*
20 μM HA	184 ± 10**
H4 agonist	135 ± 9*
H2 agonist	190 ± 15**
catalase	83 ± 6
catalase + 10 μM HA	120 ± 7
catalase + 0.5 μM HA	105 ± 6

Table 3. Effect of histamine, histamine receptor agonists and catalase on ROS levels in MDA-MB 231 cells. ROS levels were assessed by flow cytometry using DFH-DA, a specific fluorescent dye, and mean fluorescence values for each treatment were normalized to controls. Table show the means ± SEM of three experiments run in duplicates *$p<0.05$ and **$p<0.01$ vs control. One way Anova, Dunnet post test.

4.2 Gelatinolytic activity is modified by endogenous and exogenous H2O2 levels

MDA-MB 231 cells were treated with different concentrations of exogenous H2O2 and assayed by zymography. A biphasic response of MMP2 and MMP9 was observed depending on the H2O2 concentration added, as shown in Figure 7. Results indicate that different thresholds of H2O2 may be required for enhancing or inhibiting MMPs activities.

A link between ROS and MMPs has been widely discussed. Evidence supports that activation of proenzymes (MMP1, MMP2, MMP7 and MMP9) is regulated by ROS through interactions with thiol groups (Nelson & Melendez, 2004). It has been reported that higher doses of H2O2 may alter signal transduction pathways leading to protein degradation (Rhee et al, 2003). Our data are in agreement with Rajagopalan and coworkers who demonstrated ROS-induced activation of MMP2 at low doses of exogenous H2O2 (4 μM) and inactivation at higher doses (10–50 μM) in macrophage-derived foam cells when they studied the stability of atherosclerotic plaques (Rajagopalan et al, 1996). Suppression of MMP2 activity by H2O2 in a dose- and time-dependent manner was also observed during acute ulceration being reverted by antioxidants (Ganguly et al, 2006). However, most of reports inform about a positive modulation of MMP2 and MMP9 in response to oxidative stress in different tissues and cell lines including mammary cells (Mori et al, 2004).

Addition of exogenous catalase to tumor mammary cells half an hour before treatments was able to impede both the increase and decrease in gelatinolytic activities disclosed by histamine and histamine agonists confirming that intracellular H2O2 levels were involved in the modulation of enzymatic activity of both MMPs (Figure 8).

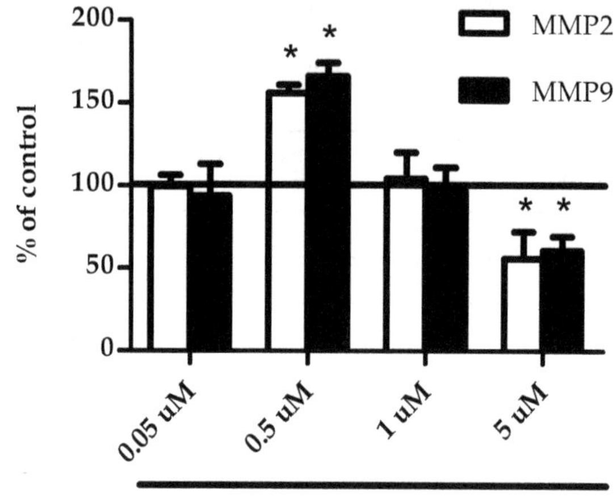

Fig. 7. Action of exogenous H2O2 on MMP2 and MMP9 gelatinolytic activity. Concentration-response curve obtained by zymography. Activity of lytic bands for each treatment was determined by densitometry and normalized to control values. Bars show the means ± SEM of three experiments run in triplicates *p<0.05 vs control. Two way Anova, Bonferroni post test.

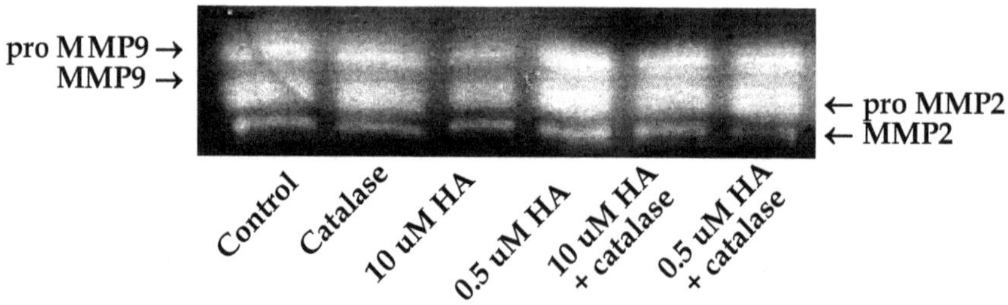

Fig. 8. Effect of catalase on histamine-regulated gelatinolytic activity of MMP2 and MMP9. Activity was evaluated by zymography after 24 h of treatment in serum free RPMI medium. Figure shows a representative gel.

4.3 Cell migration is influenced by H2O2 levels

In order to correlate H2O2 levels with the migratory capacity in MDA-MB 231 cells, we assayed different H2O2 concentrations using transwells. Cell migration was modified by exogenous H2O2 in a dose dependent manner (Figure 9A). It was significantly stimulated by low doses while inhibited by high ones. Considering that histamine and histamine agonists differentially modulate intracellular H2O2 as shown in table 3, our research suggests that the magnitude of these rises in histamine-treated cells may therefore be essential for the migratory and invasive behavior. This possibility is supported by the results obtained when exogenous catalase (125 IU/mL) was added to cell cultures (Figure 9B).

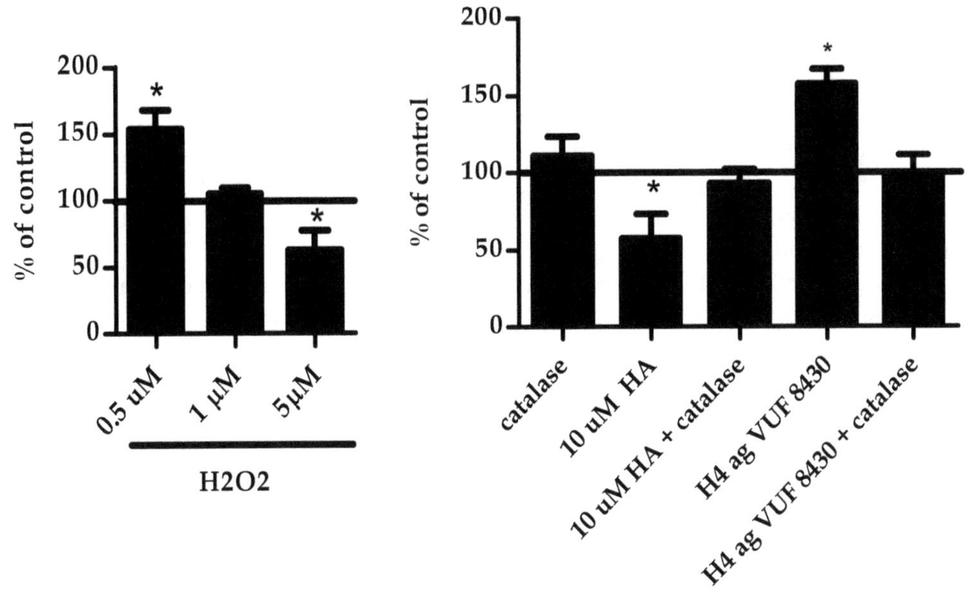

A B

Fig. 9. Effect of H2O2 on migration of MDA-MB 231 cells. Migration was evaluated by using transwell units with 8 um pore size PET membranes. Bars show the means ± SEM of three experiments run in duplicates. Results are expressed for each treatment as the number of cells counted on the lower side of membranes normalized to control values. A: Concentration-response curve for exogenous H2O2. B: Effect of catalase on histamine induced-cell migration. *$p<0.05$ vs control. One way ANOVA, Dunnet post test.

Overall, our data strongly support the hypothesis that ROS are involved in histamine-induced modulation of MMP2 and MMP9, which are assumed to play a critical role in tumor invasion. Divergent migration and invasion responses (stimulatory or inhibitory) to histamine may be due to changes in the cellular redox balance through H2 and H4 receptor activation as in the case of MMPs. Likely, when H2O2 is produced at high concentrations in MDA-MB 231 cells, it may be capable to affect enzymatic activities by altering signaling pathways and even cause cellular damage. Many elements in the process leading to cell migration are considered to be redox-sensitive (Pani et al, 2009; Svineng et al, 2008). ROS modify the activity of several key enzymes, resulting in the reorganization of actin cytoskeleton, adhesion and stimulation of migration. There is evidence that ROS can regulate such critical target molecules as PKC, MAPK, PI3K, tyrosine phospatases, PTEN, Src and focal adhesion kinase (FAK) (Rhee et al, 2000, 2003).

Preliminary results obtained in our laboratory show an increase in c-Src phosphorylation in the presence of low doses of histamine or H2O2 exogenously added suggesting a possible role of this kinase in MDA-MB 231 cells migration induced by histamine (data not shown).

4.4 Determination of catalase activity

We have previously reported that histamine in a high concentration inhibits catatase activity in MDA-MB 231 cells (Medina et al, 2006). To further correlate catalase activity with the intracellular H2O2 levels generated by histamine and histamine agonists treatments, we measured the endogenous enzymatic activity spectrophotometrically. Briefly, cells were treated for 24h, scrapped and collected in potassium phosphate buffer 50 mM pH 7.0. This was followed by sonic disruption. Protein concentration was determined by Bradford assay. Catalase activity was determined using whole cell homogenates by measuring the exponential decay of 20 mM H2O2 ($\Delta\varepsilon_{240}$ = 43.6 M^{-1} cm^{-1}) at 25°C monitored at 240 nm. Specific activity was expressed as the number of catalase units per mg of protein. One catalase unit is defined as the amount of catalase that breaks 1 μmol of H2O2 down per minute, at 25°C and pH 7.

There was a reduction of the enzymatic activity when cells were cultured in the presence of 0.5 μM histamine or H4 agonists, being this reduction more significant at higher doses of histamine or with H2 agonists (Figure 10). Data indicate that the modulation of catalase activity in our experimental conditions is critical in the control of endogenous H2O2 levels which in turn trigger different biological responses. In this sense, other authors have demonstrated in colon and liver tumor cells that high basal levels of ROS are mainly controlled by catalase (Laurent et al, 2005). Expression of catalase is known to be regulated at message, protein and activity levels. Soluble factors from tumor cells as TNF alpha have been suggested to be repressors of catalase expression, and cell signaling molecules as PKA, PKC and Casein Kinase II have been reported to elevate catalase activity *in vitro* (Nishikawa 2002; Reimer el 1994; Yano & Yano, 2002). Histamine could act at any of these levels (Baker et al, 2002; Igaz et al, 2001; Leurs et al, 2009; Steffel el al, 2006)

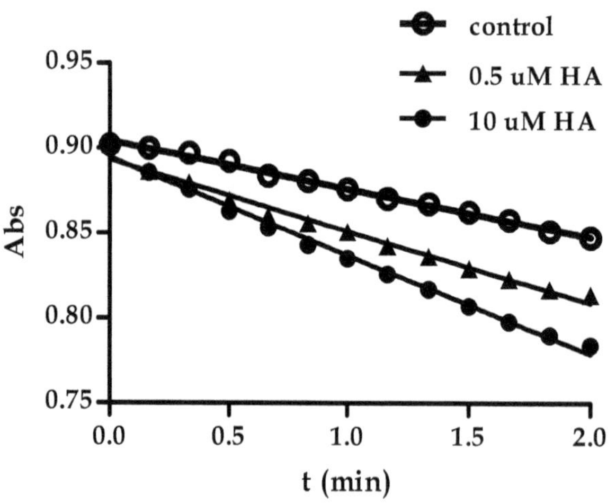

Treatment	Catalase activity (IU/mg protein)
control	10.8 ± 0.9
0.5 μM HA	8.5 ± 0.8*
10 μM HA	5.4 ± 0.6*
H2 agonist	6.2 ± 0.7*
H4 agonist	8.1 ± 0.9*

Fig. 10. Effect of histamine and histamine receptor agonists on catalase activity. Activity was evaluated spectrophotometrically by measuring the extinction of the H202, the substrate of catalase enzyme. Slopes of straight lines fit by linear regression represent the rate of extinction and are correlated with enzymatic activity. Embedded table shows catalase activities for histamine and histamine receptor agonists. Results are expressed as means ± SEM of two experiments run in duplicates. *$p<0.05$ vs control. One way Anova. Dunnet post test.

5. Ionizing radiation enhances the activity of MMPs and cell migration – Interaction between histamine and ionizing radiation

The mechanisms that control the therapeutic efficacy of radiotherapy have classically focused on the ability of ionizing radiation to kill cancer cells while sparing normal tissues. Radiation therapy after surgery consists typically of irradiation of the breast with 50-60 gray, delivered over 6 weeks in 2 gray fractions. Fractionation allows time to normal cells to recover, to tumor cells to reenter to radio-sensitive phase of the cell cycle and to hypoxic tumor areas to re-oxygenate and as a result become more responsive to ionizing radiation.

Sensitivity of tumor cells to ionizing radiation is crucial to outline the probability of local control and finally of cure of cancers by radiotherapy. Many factors are involved in affecting susceptibility of tumor cells to ionizing radiation and the generation of ROS as a result of photon irradiation accounts for approximately 75% of radiation-induced damage. ROS production occurs within seconds of starting radiation treatment and this initial redox perturbation has important implications in terms of the final cellular response to ionizing radiation.

As already mentioned we have previously demonstrated that histamine is able to increment MDA-MB 231 cells intrinsic radiosensitivity by downregulating catalase activity and increasing H2O2 intracellular levels at the same doses that inhibits cell proliferation. Recently we have established a radioprotective role of histamine on bone marrow against cellular damage induced by ionizing radiation (Medina et al, 2010). We have also proved that histamine prevents radiation-induced toxicity on small intestine by modulating the antioxidant enzymes expression and by suppressing apoptosis and increasing proliferation of damaged intestinal mucosa (Medina et al, 2007). Intracellular ROS concentration is critical for cell growth and survival; in normal cells ROS levels are kept low, but quite the opposite in tumor cells high levels of ROS close to the threshold of cytotoxicity are related to cell proliferation. Thus drugs that modulate antioxidant enzymes may differentially affect normal and neoplastic cells growth and death. In view of these antecedents, we proposed to study the interaction between histamine and ionizing radiation on the proinvasive ability of this cell line. MDA-MB 231 cells were gamma irradiated with a 2 gray dose using an IBL 437C, H type irradiator in presence or absence of histamine or histamine agonists. After irradiation culture media were conditioned for 24 h and then zymographies were carried out; migration assays were immediately performed. Ionizing radiation increased ROS levels in irradiated control cells and a rise in MMPs activity and cell migration was also found compared to non irradiated control cells (Figure 11). This effect observed on cellular events related to MDA-MB 231 invasiveness was counteracted when irradiated cells were treated with high doses of histamine or with H2 agonist, which may be due to the largest amount of ROS generated in these conditions.

The effects of irradiation on malignant biological behaviors of cells surviving irradiation have been reported for a variety of tumor cells. Many of these reports provide evidence that irradiated tumor cells acquire malignant potency through increased motility and invasiveness, up-regulation of MMPs, as well as an enhanced capacity for adhesion. The activation of different signal transduction cascades including stress kinases, the PI3K/Akt/NF-kB pathway or the c-Src is implicated in these radiation-induced responses. The same signaling mechanisms are engaged in ROS mediated actions on invasive capacity (Cheng el al, 2006; Hwang et al, 2006; Jung et al, 2007; Wild-Bold el al 2006). Current studies

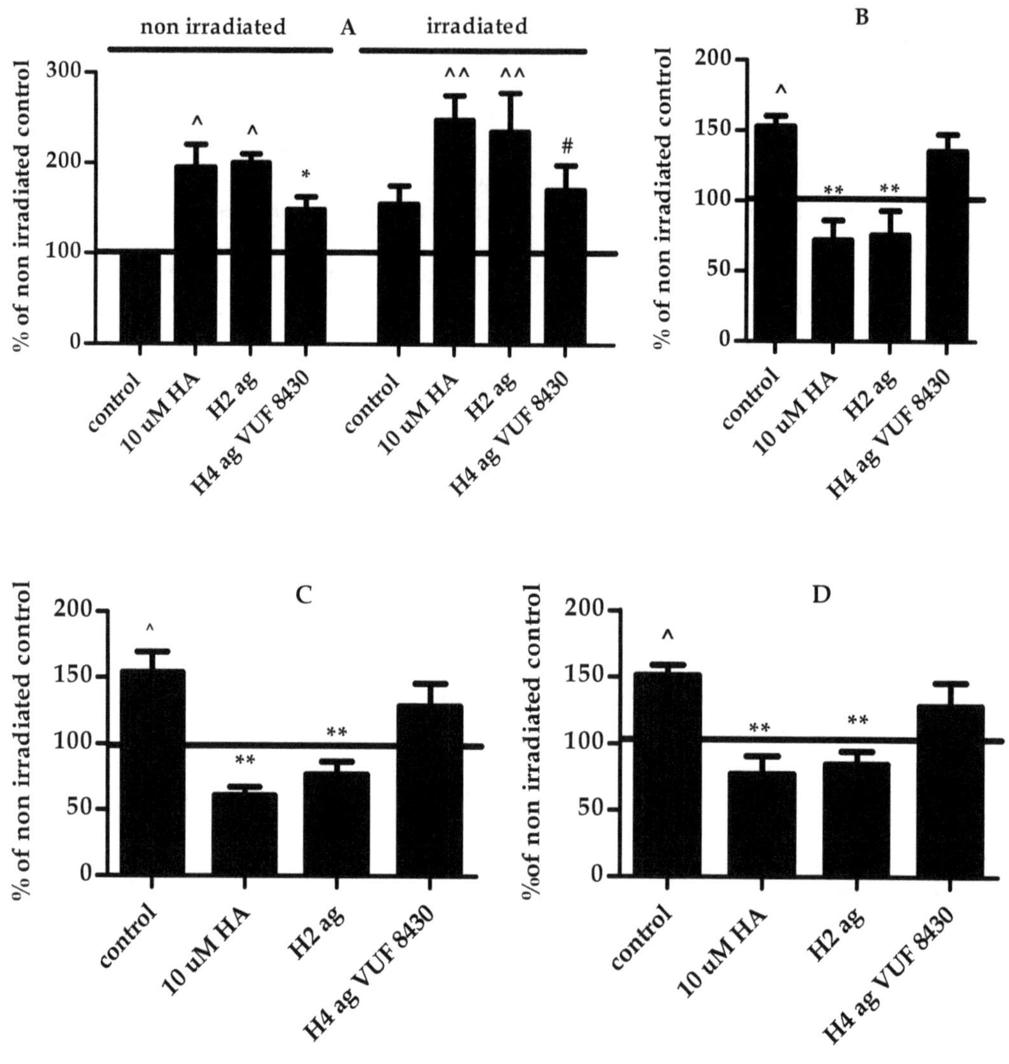

Fig. 11. Effect of ionizing radiation on MDA-MB 231 cells. A: ROS levels induced by histamine and histamine receptor agonists. B: Effect of histamine and histamine receptor agonists on cell migration of irradiated cells. C: Effect of histamine and histamine receptor agonists on MMP2 gelatinolytic activity of irradiated cells. D: Effect of histamine and histamine receptor agonists on MMP9 gelatinolytic activity of irradiated cells. Bars represent the means ± SEM of at least three experiments run in duplicates ^ $p<0.05$ and ^^$p<0.01$ vs non irradiated control, *$p<0.05$ vs 10 μM HA and vs control, **$p<0.01$ vs control, # $p<0.05$ vs 10 μM HA. Two way Anova, Bonferroni post test.

in our laboratory are intended to confirm the crucial role of distinct levels of ROS generated in the opposite responses of MDA-MB 231 cells to different histamine concentrations and ionizing radiation, and to identify the signaling pathways concerned.

6. Conclusions

Understanding the molecular mechanisms of metastases is one of the most relevant issues in cancer research. New growths (metastases) at distant sites from the primary tumor require a number of steps to be completed successfully. Tumor cells must bind to one or more components of the basement membrane or extracellular matrix, degrade them to migrate, intravasate in blood and lymphatic vessels and finally extravasate to be seeded at distant locations. MMP2 and MMP9 are mainly involved in these processes, being abundantly expressed in various malignant tumors.

In the last decade a subcutaneous formulation of histamine dihydrochloride has been used as an adjuvant with interleukin-2 therapy for the potential treatment of metastatic melanoma, acute myelogenous leukemia and renal cell carcinoma, mainly based upon its action on immunity (Perz & Ho, 2008). Our research provides novel evidence for a possible use of histamine as a pharmacological agent with low side effects that targets oncogenic pathways which may regulate breast tumor cell proliferation and/or survival and simultaneously may control invasion and metastasis.

Radiotherapy is a highly effective modality for locoregional treatment of breast tumors and other cancers. Despite the fact that it has been classically considered to exert its therapeutic effect by killing tumor cells, clinical and experimental evidence indicates that results extend beyond cancer cell death pointing out that ionizing radiation might promote a metastatic behavior of cancer cells. Our current results also open a perspective for the potential use of histamine to improve radiotherapy efficacy not only increasing intrinsic radiosensitivity of breast tumor cells specifically, but wielding an effect on the possible development of radio-induced metastases.

In view that a shift in the paradigm from a population-based to a personalized patient-based treatment emerges as a near step in cancer therapy correlating molecular expression signatures with treatment outcomes, the determination of histamine receptors in patient tumors seems feasible and may help design more effective therapies.

7. Acknowledgements

This work was supported by grants from the University of Buenos Aires (UBACYT B029), from the National Agency for Scientific and Technological Promotion (PICT 01022) and from the EU-FP7 COST Action BM0806 (Recent advances in histamine receptor H4R research). We thank Dr Nicholas Carruthers from Johnson & Johnson for the H4 antagonist JNJ7777120.

8. References

Asano, K., Kanai, K. & Suzaki, H. (2004). Suppressive activity of fexofenadine hydrochloride on metalloproteinase production from nasal fibroblasts in vitro. *Clin Exp Allergy*, Vol.34, No.12, (December 2004), pp 1890-1898, ISSN 0954-7894

Bakker, R., Timmerman, H. & Leurs, R. (2002). Histamine receptors: specific ligands, receptor biochemistry, and signal transduction. *Clin Allergy Immunol*, Vol.17, (2002) pp 27-64, ISSN 1075-7910

Baluna, R., Eng, T. & Thomas, C. (2006). Adhesion molecules in radiotherapy. *Radiat Res*, Vol.166, No.6, (December 2006), pp 819-831, ISSN 0033-7587

Barnard R., Barnard, A., Salmon, G., Wai, L. & Sreckovic, S. (2008). Histamine-Induced Actin Polymerization in Human Eosinophils: An Imaging Approach for Histamine H4 Receptor. *Cytometry A.*, Vol.73, No.4, (April 2008), pp 299-304, ISSN 1552-4930

Baum, O., Hlushchuk, R., Forster, A., Greiner, R., Clézardin, P., Zhao, Y., Djonov, V & Gruber, G. (2007). Increased invasive potential and up-regulation of MMP-2 in MDA-MB-231 breast cancer cells expressing the beta3 integrin subunit. *Int J Oncol*, Vol.30, No.2, (February 2007), pp 325-332, ISSN 1019-6439

Bäumer, W., Wendorff, S., Gutzmer, R., Werfel, T., Dijkstra, D., Chazot, P., Stark, H. & Kietzmann, M. (2008). Histamine H4 receptors modulate dendritic cell migration through skin--immunomodulatory role of histamine. *Allergy*, Vol.63, No.10, (October 2008), pp 1387-1394, ISSN 1398-9995

Blaya, B., Nicolau-Galmés, F., Jangi, S., Ortega-Martínez, I., Alonso-Tejerina, E., Burgos-Bretones, J., Pérez-Yarza, G., Asumendi, A. & Boyano, M. (2010). Histamine and histamine receptor antagonists in cancer biology. *Inflamm Allergy Drug Targets*, Vol.9, No.3, (July 2010), pp 146-157, ISSN 1871-5281

Ciprandi, G., Tosca, M., Cosentino, C., Riccio, A., Passalacqua, G. & Canonica, G. (2003). Effects of fexofenadine and other antihistamines on components of the allergic response: adhesion molecules. *J Allergy Clin Immunol*, Vol.112, No.4 Suppl, (October 2003), pp S78-82, ISSN 0091-6749

Chakraborti, S., Mandal, M., Das, S., Mandal, A. & Chakraborti, T. (2003). Regulation of matrix metalloproteinases: an overview. *Mol Cell Biochem,* Vol.253, No.1-2, (November 2003), pp 269-285, ISSN 0300-8177

Chambers, A. & Matrisian, L. (1997). Changing views of the role of matrix metalloproteinases in metastasis. *J Natl Cancer Inst,* Vol. 3, No.89(17), (September 1997), pp 1260-1270, Review, ISSN 0027-8874

Cheng, J., Chou, C., Kuo, M. & Hsieh, C. (2006). Radiation-enhanced hepatocellular carcinoma cell invasion with MMP-9 expression through PI3K/Akt/NF-jB signal transduction pathway. *Oncogene,* Vol.25, No.53, (November 2006), pp 7009–7018, ISSN 0950-9232

Cricco, G., Núñez, M., Medina, V., Garbarino, G., Mohamad, N., Gutiérrez, A., Cocca, C., Bergoc, R., Rivera, E. & Martín, G. (2006). Histamine modulates cellular events involved in tumour invasiveness in pancreatic carcinoma cells. *Inflamm Res*, Vol.55, Suppl 1, (April 2006), pp S83-S84, ISSN 1023-3830

Cricco, G., Martín, G., Medina, V., Núñez, M., Mohamad, N., Croci, M., Crescenti, E., Bergoc, R. & Rivera, E. (2006) Histamine inhibits cell proliferation and modulates the expression of Bcl-2 family proteins via the H2 receptor in human pancreatic cancer cells. *Anticancer Res*, Vol.26, No.6B, (November-December 2006), pp 4443-4450, ISSN 0250-7005

Cricco, G., Mohamad, N., Sambuco, L., Genre, F., Croci, M., Gutiérrez, A., Medina, V., Bergoc, R., Rivera, E. & Martín, G. (2008). Histamine regulates pancreatic carcinoma cell growth through H3 and H4 receptors.G. *Inflamm Res.* Vol.57, Suppl 1, (March 2008), pp S23-S24, ISNN 1023-3830

Decock, J., Hendrickx, W., Wildiers, H., Christiaens, M., Neven, P., Drijkoningen, M. & Paridaens, R. (2005). Plasma gelatinase levels in patients with primary breast cancer in relation to axillary lymph node status, Her2/neu expression and other clinicopathological variables. *Clinical Exp Metastasis,* Vol.22, No.6, (October 2005), pp 495-502, ISSN 0262-0898

Doyle, J. & Haas, T. (2009). Differential role of beta-catenin in VEGF and histamine-induced MMP-2 production in microvascular endothelial cells. *J Cell Biochem,* Vol.15, No.107(2), (May 2009) pp 272-83, ISSN 0730-2312

Duffy, M., McGowan, P. & Gallagher, W. (2008). Cancer invasion and metastasis: changing views. *J Pathol.* Vol.214, No.3, (February 2008), pp 283-293, ISSN 0022-3417

Falus, A., Hegyesi, H., Lázár-Molnár, E., Pós, Z., László, V. & Darvas, Z. (2001). .Paracrine and autocrine interactions in melanoma: histamine is a relevant player in local regulation. *Trends Immunol,* Vol.22, No.12, (December 2001), pp 648-652, ISSN 1471-4906

Francis, H., Onori, P., Gaudio, E., Franchitto, A., DeMorrow, S., Venter, J., Kopriva, S., Carpino, G., Mancinelli, R., White, M., Meng, F., Vetuschi, A., Sferra, R. & Alpini. (2009). H3 histamine receptor-mediated activation of protein kinase Calpha inhibits the growth of cholangiocarcinoma in vitro and in vivo. *Mol Cancer Res,*Vol.7, No.10, (October 2009), pp 1704-1713, ISSN 1541-7786

Freije, J., Balbín, M., Pendás, A., Sánchez, L., Puente, X. & López-Otín, C. (2003). Matrix metalloproteinases and tumor progression. *Adv Exp Med Biol,* Vol.532, (2003), pp 91-107, ISSN 0065-2598

Ganguly, K., Kundu, P., Banerjee, A., Reiter, R. & Swarnakar, S. (2006). Hydrogen peroxide-mediated downregulation of matrix metalloprotease-2 in indomethacin-induced acute gastric ulceration is blocked by melatonin and other antioxidants. *Free Radic Biol Med,* Vol.41, No.6, (September 2006), pp 911-925, ISSN 0891-5849

Genre, F., Valli, E., Medina, V., Gutiérrez, A., Sambuco, L., Rivera, E., Cricco, G. & Martín, G. (2009). Effect of histamine on the expression of metalloproteinases and cell adhesion in breast cancer cell lines. *Inflamm Res,*Vol.58, Suppl 1, (April 2009), 55-56, ISSN 1023-3830

Gschwandtner, M., Purwar, R., Wittmann, M., Bäumer, W., Kietzmann, M., Werfel, T. & Gutzmer, R. (2008). Histamine upregulates keratinocyte MMP-9 production via the histamine H1 receptor. *J Invest Dermatol,* Vol.128, No.12, (December 2008), pp 2783-2791, ISSN 0022-202X

Gschwandtner, M., Rossbach, K., Dijkstra, D., BäμMer, W., Kietzmann, M., Stark, H., Werfel, T. & Gutzmer, R. (2010). Murine and human Langerhans cells express a functional histamine H4 receptor: modulation of cell migration and function. *Allergy,* Vol.65, No.7, (July 2010), pp 840-849, ISSN 0105-4538

Gutzmer, R., Diestel, C., Mommert, S., Köther, B., Stark, H., Wittmann, M. & Werfel, T. (2005). Histamine H4 receptor stimulation suppresses IL-12p70 production and mediates chemotaxis in human monocyte-derived dendritic cells. *J Immunol,* Vol.174, No.9, (May 2005), pp 5224-5232, ISSN 0022-1767

Hwang, S., Jung, J., Jeong, J., Kim, Y., Oh, E., Kim, T., Kim, J., Cho, K. & Han, I. (2006). Dominant-negative Rac increases both inherent and ionizing radiation-induced cell migration in C6 rat glioma cells. *Int J Cancer,* Vol. 118, No.8, (April 2006), pp 2056-2063, ISSN 0020-7136

Hofstra, C., Desai, P., Thurmond, R. & Fung-Leung, W. (2003). Histamine H4 receptor mediates chemotaxis and calcium mobilization of mast cells. *J Pharmacol Exp Ther*, Vol.305, No.3, (June 2003), pp1212-1221, ISSN 0022-3565

Igaz, P., Novák, I., Lázaár, E., Horváth, B., Héninger, E. & Falus A. (2001). Bidirectional communication between histamine and cytokines. *Inflamm Res,* Vol.50, No.3, (March 2001), pp 123-128, Review, ISSN 1023-3830

John, A. & Tuszynski, G. (2001). The role of matrix metalloproteinases in tumor angiogenesis and tumor metastasis. *Pathol Oncol Res,* Vol.7, No.1, (February 2001), pp 14-23, ISSN 1219-4956

Jung, J., Hwang, S., Hwang, J., Oh, E., Park, S. & Han, I. (2007). Ionising radiation induces changes associated with epithelial-mesenchymal transdifferentiation and increased cell motility of A549 lung epithelial cells. *Eur J Cancer*, Vol.43, No.7, (May 2007), pp 1214-1224, ISSN 1359-6349

Kattan, Z., Minig, V., Leroy, P., Dauça, M. & Becuwe P. (2008). Role of manganese superoxide dismutase on growth and invasive properties of human estrogen-independent breast cancer cells. *Breast Cancer Res Treat,* Vol.108, No.2, (March 2008), pp 203-215, ISSN 0167-6806

Köhrmann, A., Kammerer, U., Kapp, M., Dietl, J. & Anacker J. (2009). Expression of matrix metalloproteinases (MMPs) in primary human breast cancer and breast cancer cell lines: New findings and review of the literature. *BMC Cancer,* Vol.9, No.188, (June 2009), ISSN 1471-2407

Kohyama, T., Yamauchi, Y., Takizawa, H., Kamitani, S., Kawasaki, S. & Nagase, T. (2010). Histamine stimulates human lung fibroblast migration. *Mol Cell Biochem,* Vol 337. No.1-2, (April 2010), pp 77-81, ISSN 0300-8177

La Rocca, G., Pucci-Minafra, I., Marrazzo, A., Taormina, P. & Minafra, S. (2004). Zymographic detection and clinical correlations of MMP-2 and MMP-9 in breast cancer sera. *British J Cancer, Vol.*90, No.7, (April 2004), 1414–1421, ISSN 0007-0920

Laurent, A., Nicco, C., Chéreau, C., Goulvestre, C., Alexandre, J., Alves, A., Lévy, E., Goldwasser, F., Panis, Y., Soubrane , O., Weill, B. & Batteux, F. (2005). Controlling tumor growth by modulating endogenous production of reactive oxygen species. Cancer Res, Vol.65, No.3, (February 2005), pp 948-956, ISSN 0008-5472

Lázár-Molnár, E., Hegyesi, H., Pállinger, E., Kovács, P., Tóth, S., Fitzsimons, C., Cricco, G., Martin, G., Bergoc, R., Darvas, Z., Rivera, E. & Falus A. (2002). Inhibition of human primary melanoma cell proliferation by histamine is enhanced by interleukin-6. *Eur J Clin Invest,* Vol.32, No.10, (October 2002), pp 743-749, ISSN 0014-2972

Leurs, R., Chazot, P., Shenton, F., Lim, H. & de Esch, I. (2009). Molecular and biochemical pharmacology of the histamine H4 receptor. *Br J Pharmacol,* Vol.157, No.1, (May 2009), pp 14-23, ISSN 0007-1188

Ling, P., Ngo, K., Nguyen, S., Thurmond, R., Edwards, J., Karlsson, L. & Fung-Leung, W. (2004). Histamine H4 receptor mediates eosinophil chemotaxis with cell shape change and adhesion molecule upregulation. *Br J Pharmacol.* Vol.142, No.1, (May 2004), pp 161-171, ISSN 0007-1188

Liu, Z., Kilburn, B., Leach, R., Romero, R., Paria, B. & Armant, D. (2004). Histamine enhances cytotrophoblast invasion by inducing intracellular calcium transients through the histamine type-1 receptor. *Mol Reprod Dev,* Vol.68, No3, (July 2004), pp 345-353, ISSN 1040-452X

McArdle, F., Pattwell, D., Vasilaki, A., McArdle, A. & Jackson, M. (2005). Intracellular generation of reactive oxygen species by contracting skeletal muscle cells. *Free Radic Biol Med,* Vol.39, No.5, (September 2005), pp 651-657, ISSN 0891-5849

Medina, V., Cricco, G., Nuñez, M., Martín, G., Mohamad, N., Correa-Fiz, F., Sanchez-Jimenez, F., Bergoc, R. & Rivera, E. (2006). Histamine-mediated signaling processes in human malignant mammary cells. *Cancer Biol Ther,* Vol.5, No.11, (Nov 2006), p 1462-1471, ISSN 1538-4047

Medina, V., Croci, M., Mohamad, N., Massari, N., Garbarino, G., Cricco, G., Núñez, M., Martín, G., Crescenti, E., Bergoc, R. & Rivera, E. (2007). Mechanisms underlying the radioprotective effect of histamine on small intestine. *Int J Radiat Biol,*Vol.83, No.10, (October 2007), pp 653-63, ISSN 0955-3002

Medina, V., Croci, M., Crescenti, E., Mohamad, N., Sanchez-Jiménez, F., Massari, N., Nuñez, M., Cricco, G., Martin, G., Bergoc, R. & Rivera, E. (2008). The role of histamine in human mammary carcinogenesis: H3 and H4 receptors as potential therapeutic targets for breast cancer treatment. *Cancer Biol Ther,* Vol.7, No.1, (January 2008), pp 28-35, ISNN 1538-4047

Medina, V., Massari, N., Cricco, G., Martín, G., Bergoc, R. & Rivera, E. (2009). Involvement of hydrogen peroxide in histamine-induced modulation of WM35 human malignant melanoma cell proliferation. *Free Radic Biol Med.* Vol.46, No.11, (June 2009), pp 1510-1515, ISSN 0891-5849

Medina, V., Croci, M., Carabajal, E., Bergoc, R. & Rivera, E. (2010). Histamine protects bone marrow against cellular damage induced by ionising radiation.*Int J Radiat Biol,* Vol.86, No.4, (April 2010), pp 283-290, ISSN 0955-3002

Mori, K., Shibanuma, M. & Nose, K. (2004). Invasive potential induced under long-term oxidative stress in mammary epithelial cells. *Cancer Res,* Vol.64, No.20, (October 2004), pp 7464-72, ISSN 0008-5472

Murthy, S., Ryan, A., He, C., Mallampalli, R. & Carter, A. (2010). Rac1-mediated mitochondrial H2O2 generation regulates MMP-9 gene expression in macrophages via inhibition of SP-1 and AP-1. *J Biol Chem,* Vol.285, No.32, (August 2010), pp 25062-25073, ISSN 0021-9258

Nelson, K. & Melendez, J. (2004). Mitochondrial redox control of matrix metalloproteinases. *Free Radic Biol Med,*Vol. 37, No.6, (September 2004), pp 768-84, ISSN 0891-5849

Nishikawa, M. (2008). Reactive oxygen species in tumor metastasis. *Cancer Lett,* Vol.266, No.1, (July 2008), pp 53-59, ISSN 0304-3835

Pani, G., Giannoni, E., Galeotti, T. & Chiarugi, P. (2009). Redox-Based Escape Mechanism from Death: The Cancer Lesson. *Antioxidants & Redox Signaling,* Vol.11, No.11, (November 2009), pp 2791-2806, ISSN 1523-0864

Parsons, M. & Ganellin, C. Histamine and its receptors. (2006). *Br J Pharmacol,* Vol.147, Suppl.1, (Jan 2006), pp S127-S135, ISSN 0007-1188

Perz, J. & Ho, A. (2008).Histamine dihydrochloride for the treatment of acute myeloid leukemia, malignant melanoma and renal cell carcinoma. *Future Oncol*, Vol.4, No.2, (April 2008), pp 169-177, ISSN 1479-6694

Platten, M., Wild-Bode, C., Wick, W., Leitlein, J., Dichgans, J. & Weller, M. (2001). N-[3,4-dimethoxycinnamoyl]-anthranilic acid (tranilast) inhibits transforming growth factor-beta relesase and reduces migration and invasiveness of human malignant glioma cells. *Int J Cancer*, Vol.93, No.1, (July 2001), pp 53-61, ISSN 0020-7136

Pos, Z., Hegyesi, H. & Rivera, E. (2004). Histamine and cell proliferation, In: *Histamine biology and medical aspects,* A. Falus (Ed), 199-225, SpringMed Publishing Ltd, ISBN 3-8055-7715-X, Budapest, Hungary

Rajagopalan, S., Meng, X., Ramasamy, S., Harrison, G. &. Galis, Z. (1996). Reactive Oxygen Species Produced by Macrophage-derived Foam Cells Regulate the Activity of Vascular Matrix Metalloproteinases In Vitro Implications for Atherosclerotic Plaque Stability. *J Clin Invest*, Vol.98, No.11, (December 1996), pp 2572–2579, ISSN 0021-9738

Reimer, D., Bailley, J. & Singh, S. (1994). Complete cDNA and 5' genomic sequences and multilevel regulation of the mouse catalase gene. *Genomics*, Vol.21, No.2, (May 1994), pp 325-336, ISSN 0888-7543

Rhee, S., Bae, Y., Lee, S. & Kwon, J. (2000). Hydrogen Peroxide: A Key Messenger That Modulates Protein Phosphorylation Through Cysteine Oxidation, 10.10.2010, Available from htpp//www.stke.org/cgi/content/full/OC_sigtrans;2000/53/pe1

Rhee, S., Chang, T., Bae, Y., Lee, S. & Kang, S. (2003). Cellular regulation by hydrogen peroxide. *J Am Soc Nephrol,* Vol.14, No.8 Suppl 3, (August 2003), pp S211-215, ISSN 1046-6673

Rivera, E., Cricco, G., Engel, N., Fitzsimons, C., Martín, G. & Bergoc, R. (2000). Histamine as an autocrine growth factor: an unusual role for a widespread mediator. *Semin Cancer Biol,* Vol.10, No.1, (February 2000), pp 15-23, ISSN 1044-579X

Rudolph, M., Boza, Y., Yefi, R., Luza, S., Andrews, E., Penissi, A., Garrido, P. & Rojas, I. (2008). The influence of mast cell mediators on migration of SW756 cervical carcinoma cells. *J Pharmacol Sci,* Vol.106, No.2, (February 2008), pp 208-218, ISSN 1347-8613

Sharif, N., Wiernas, T., Howe, W., Griffin, B., Offord, E. & Pfeifer, A. (1998). Human corneal epithelial cell functional responses to inflammatory agents and their antagonists. *Invest Ophthalmol Vis Sci.* Vol.39, No13, (December 1998), pp 2562-2571, ISSN 1552-5783

Soule, B., Simone, N., DeGraff ,W., Choudhuri, R., Cook, J. & Mitchell J. (2010). Loratadine dysregulates cell cycle progression and enhances the effect of radiation in human tumor cell lines. *J Radiat Oncol,* Vol.5, No8, (February 2010), ISSN 0360-3016

Stankovic, S., Konjevic, G., Gopcevic, K., Jovic, V., Inic, M. & Jurisic, V. (2010)., Activity of MMP-2 and MMP-9 in sera of breast cancer patients. *Pathol Res Pract*, Vol.206, No.4, (April 2010), pp 241-247, ISSN 0344-0338

Steffel, J., Arnet, C., Akhmedov, A., Iseli, S., Lüscher, T. & Tanner FC. (2006). Histamine differentially interacts with tumor necrosis factor-alpha and thrombin in endothelial tissue factor induction: the role of c-Jun NH2-terminal kinase. *J Thromb Haemost*, Vol.4, No.11, (November 2006), pp 2452-2460, ISSN 1538-7933

Svineng, G., Ravuri, C., Rikardsen O., Huseby, N. & Winberg, J. (2008). The role of reactive oxygen species in integrin and matrix metalloproteinase expression and function. *Connect Tissue Res.* Vol.49, No.3, (2008), pp 197-202, ISSN 0300-8207

Tetlow, L. & Woolley, D. (2002). Histamine stimulates matrix metalloproteinase-3 and -13 production by human articular chondrocytes in vitro. *Ann Rheum Dis,* Vol.61, No8, (August 2002), pp 737-740, ISSN 1468-2060

Tetlow, L. & Woolley, D. (2004). Effect of histamine on the production of matrix metalloproteinases-1, -3, -8 and -13, and TNFalpha and PGE(2) by human articular chondrocytes and synovial fibroblasts in vitro: a comparative study. *Virchows Arch.* Vol.445, No5, (November 2004), pp 485-490, ISSN 1432-2307

Thannickal, V. & Fanburg, B. (2000). Reactive oxygen species in cell signaling. *Am J Physiol Lung Cell Mol Physiol,* Vol.279, No.6, (December 2000), pp L1005-L1028, ISSN 1040-0605

Thurmond, R., Desai, P., Dunford, P., Fung-Leung, W., Hofstra, C., Jiang, W., Nguyen, S., Riley, J., Sun, S., Williams, K., Edwards, J. & Karlsson, L. (2004). A potent and selective histamine H4 receptor antagonist with anti-inflammatory properties . *J Pharmacol Exp Ther.*; Vol.309, No.1, (April 2004), pp 404-413, ISSN 0022-3565

Tilly, B., Tertoolen, L., Remorie, R., Ladoux, A., Verlaan, I., de Laat, S. & Moolenaar, W. (1990). Histamine as a growth factor and chemoattractant for human carcinoma and melanoma cells: action through Ca2(+)-mobilizing H1 receptors. *J Cell Biol,* Vol.110, No.4, (April 1990), pp 1211-1215, ISSN 0021-9525

Tomita, K., Izumi, K. & Okabe, S. (2003). Roxatidine- and cimetidine-induced angiogenesis inhibition suppresses growth of colon cancer implants in syngeneic mice. *J Pharmacol Sci,* Vol.93, No.3, (November 2003), pp 321-30, ISSN 1347-8613

Truta-Feles, K., Lagadari, M., Lehmann, K., Berod, L., Cubillos, S., Piehler, S., Herouy, Y., Barz, D., Kamradt, T., Maghazachi, A. & Norgauer, J. (2010). Histamine modulates γδ-T lymphocyte migration and cytotoxicity, via Gi and Gs protein-coupled signalling pathways. *Br J Pharmacol,* Vol.161, No.6, (November 2010), pp 1291-1300, ISSN 0007-1188

Tsukamoto, H., Shibata, K., Kajiyama, H., Terauchi, M., Nawa, A. & Kikkawa, F. (2007). Irradiation-induced epithelial-mesenchymal transition (EMT) related to invasive potential in endometrial carcinoma cells. *Gynecol Oncol,* Vol.107,No.3, (December 2007), pp 500-504, ISSN 0090-8258

Tsutsumi, K., Tsuda, M., Yazawa, N., Nakamura, H., Ishihara, S., Haga, H., Yasuda, M., Yamazaki, R., Shirato, H., Kawaguchi, H., Nishioka, T. & Ohba, Y. (2009). Increased motility and invasiveness in tumor cells that survive 10 Gy irradiation. *Cell Struct Funct,* Vol.34, No.2, (July 2009), pp 89-96, ISSN 0386-7196

Van Wart, H. & Birkedal-Hansen, H. (1990). The cysteine switch: a principle of regulation of metalloproteinase activity with potential applicability to the entire matrix metalloproteinase gene family. *Proc Natl Acad Sci USA,* Vol.87, No.14, (July 1990), pp 5578–5582, ISSN 0027-8424

Wroblewski, L., Pritchard, D., Carter, S. &, Varro A. (2002). Gastrin-stimulated gastric epithelial cell invasion: the role and mechanism of increased matrix metalloproteinase 9 expression. *Biochem J*, Vol.365, Pt 3, (August 2002), pp 873-879, ISSN 0264-6021

Wild-Bode, C., Weller, M., Rimner, A., Dichgans, J. & Wick, W. (2001). Sublethal Irradiation Promotes Migration and Invasiveness of Glioma Cells: Implications for Radiotherapy of Human Glioblastoma. *Cancer Res*, Vol.61, No. 6, (March 2001), pp 2744-2750, ISSN 0008-5472

Wu, W. (2006). The signaling mechanism of ROS in tumor progression. *Cancer Metastasis Rev*. Vol.25, No.4, (December 2006), pp 695-705, ISSN 0167-7659

Yano, S. & Yano, N. (2002). Regulation of catalase enzyme activity by cell signaling molecules. *Mol Cell Biochem*, Vol.240, No1-2, (November 2002), pp 119-130, ISNN 0300-8177

2

Differences in Membrane Composition and Organization of Crucial Molecules Define the Invasive Properties of MCF-7 Breast Cancer Cells

Van slambrouck Séverine and Steelant Wim
New Mexico Institute of Mining and Technology,
St. Thomas University,
USA

1. Introduction

Breast cancer is the leading cause of cancer deaths among women in the United States and Europe [Jemal et al., 2011]. Most of these women die from their metastases, also known as the spread of primary breast cancer cells, to distant organs such as lung, brain and bone [Mehrotra et al., 2004]. Metastatic development comprises a complex series of linked, sequential steps. These steps include disconnection of intercellular adhesions and separation of single cells within a primary tumour, interaction with the surrounding extracellular matrix, local migration and invasion, followed by intravasation, transit through blood vessels and extravasation at distant organs, where they establish secondary tumours or metastases. In other words, the most lethal aspects of breast cancer are the processes of tumour cell migration and invasion, both prerequisites for the formation of metastases [Yilmaz & Christofori, 2010]. At present, however, the mechanisms responsible for the acquisition of invasive and metastatic potential of tumour cells are poorly understood. Thus, a better understanding of the biology and molecular interactions that regulate and coordinate the steps of tumour cell migration and invasion, is required to effectively treat metastatic breast cancer and control the devastating nature of breast cancer. It is widely accepted that cancer cells, capable of initiating metastases acquire specific features and exert activities that are not shared with the primary tumour cells [Liotta & Kohn, 2001]. Over the past years, a number of particular complex invasion-associated cellular activities have been recognized and characterized, including variations in expression levels of cell-cell and cell-matrix adhesion molecules and proteases that degrade the surrounding extracellular matrix, along with changes in expression or activity levels of a variety of cellular proteins in multiple branched signalling pathways [Mareel & Leroy, 2003]. Additionally, previous studies have highlighted the importance of aberrant glycosylation as a crucial event in the induction of invasion and metastasis [Hakomori, 2002], including altered glycosylation of cell-surface glycoproteins [Kim & Varki, 1997] and GSLs (glycosphingolipids) [Hakomori, 1998]. GSLs are common components of cell membranes. In malignant cells, they have been identified as tumour-associated antigens as defined by specific monoclonal antibodies [Hakomori, 1996]. Essentially all GSLs, in tumour and normal cells, can cluster and assemble with specific membrane proteins and signal transducers. Of importance is that clustering of particular GSLs may affect cellular activities associated with tumour cell migration and invasion, since they are recognized to mediate cell-cell and cell-matrix adhesion and initiate signal transduction, induced by stimulation of GSLs [Hakomori et al., 1998]. Roles for GSLs in invasion were demonstrated recently for GM3 (monosialoganglioside 3) in mouse melanoma B16 cells [Iwabuchi et al., 1998; Iwabuchi et al., 1998] and in human bladder KK47 cells [Mitsuzuka et al., 2005], for GM1 in mouse Lewis lung cancer cells [Zhang et al., 2006], for DSGG (diasyl-GalNAcLc4) in renal cell carcinoma [Satoh et al., 2000; Ito et al., 2001] and for GD3 (disialoganglioside 3) in melanoma cells [Hamamura et al., 2005]. The glycosphingolipid, MSGb5 (monosialyl-Gb5), also known as SSEA-4 (stage-specific embryonic antigen-4) [Kannagi et al., 1983], is found maximally expressed in human renal cell carcinomas and correlates with metastases [Saito et al., 1991; Saito et al., 1997]. The molecular mechanisms regulating synthesis of MSGb5 have been studied previously [Saito et al., 2003]; however, no clear functional role of MSGb5 in the invasive and metastatic behaviour of tumour cells has been demonstrated. In this chapter, we present data on a functional role of the glycosphingolipid MSGb5 in the human mammary carcinoma variant cell line MCF-7/AZ, showing increased invasiveness and motility in response to stimulation of MSGb5 by its monoclonal antibody RM1 or through induced clustering of MSGb5 by ET-18-OMe. ET-18-OMe is a synthetic ether lipid analogue shown to induce loss of cell-cell adhesion and to stimulate invasion of MCF-7/AZ breast cancer cells [Steelant et al., 2001] and was used as a molecular probe in the presented study.

2. TLC patterns of GSLs from cell extracts of MCF-7AZ and MCF-7/6 cells

The major GSLs identified in the two human breast cancer cell lines, MCF-7/AZ and MCF-7/6, were characterized as: globo-series Gb3, Gb4, MsGb5 and ganglio-series structure GM2, by TLC developed in a solvent system of chloroform/methanol/aqueous $CaCl_2$ and visualized with orcinol staining (Figure 1) [Saito et al., 1971]. Lacto-series structures were presumably below the detection limit.

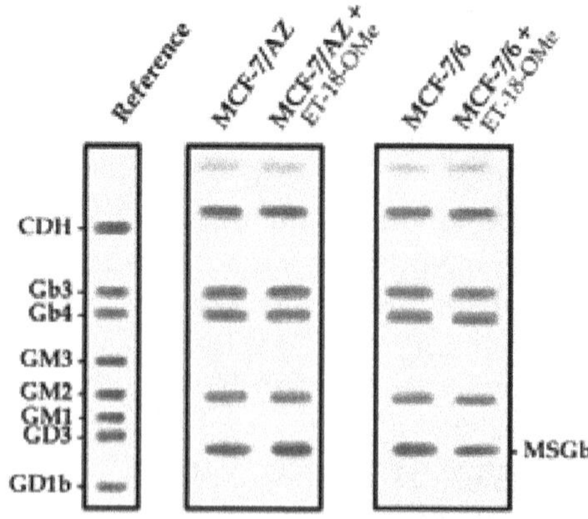

Fig. 1. TLC pattern of GSLs from whole cell extracts of MCF-7/AZ and MCF-7/6 cells with or without ET-18-OMe. GSLs were extracted from cells of the same protein weight, spotted onto TLC plates, developed in a solvent system of chloroform/methanol/0.2% aqueous $CaCl_2$, visualized by spraying with 0.5% orcinol in 2M sulfuric acid. CDH (lactosylceramide), Gb3, Gb4, MSGb5, GM3, GM1, GD3 and GD1b were used as reference markers.

All identified GSLs were present in the insoluble low-density fractions, as prepared after elimination of sucrose by dialysis and detected by TLC immunostaining with specific monoclonal antibodies (mouse IgM 1A4 to Gb3, mouse IgM 9G7 to Gb4, mouse IgM SSEA-3 to Gb5, mouse IgM RM1 to MSGb5, mouse IgM MBr1 to globo-H (α1→2 fucosyl-Gb5), mouse IgM MK1-8 to GM2, mouse IgG_3 DH2 to GM3 and mouse IgM 5F3 to disialyl-Gb5) [Kannagi & Hakomori, 2001; Ito et al., 2001] (Figure 2). The cell variants in this study lack the abundant presence of GM3 and GM1 as was reported by Nohara et al. (1998) in MCF-7 cells, but show a comparable expression pattern for Gb3 and other globo-series structures similar to Gb5 and globo-H. Furthermore, we found that treatment with the ether lipid ET-18-OMe did not alter the expression levels of GSLs present in these cell lines.

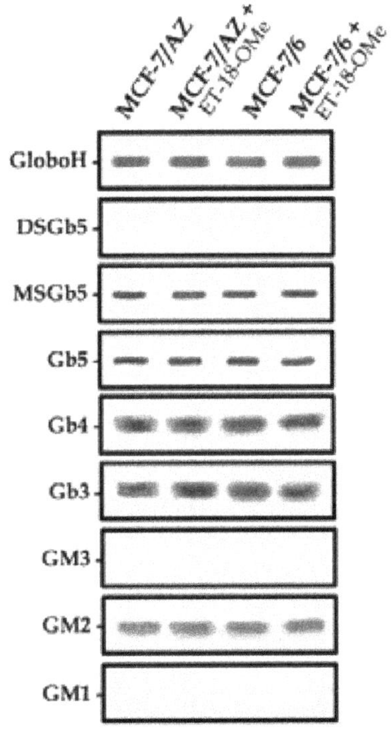

Fig. 2. TLC pattern of GSLs in low-density fractions of MCF-7/AZ and MCF-7/6 cells with or without ET-18-OMe. GSL fractions were prepared after elimination of sucrose by dialysis using C_{18} columns. Immunostaining of various GLS structures present in the low-density fractions were detected by using nine antibodies directed against the respective structures.

3. RM1 and ET-18-OMe stimulate motility and invasion through clustering of MsGb5 in MCF-7/AZ cells

The two human breast cancer cell variants, MCF-7/AZ and MCF-7/6, are non-invasive into a collagen type I gel-layer as determined by a method using specific assembly [Bracke et al., 1999] and the motility of the two variants as revealed by wound migration assay is basically the same. When MCF-7/AZ cells were treated with monoclonal anti-MSGb5 antibody RM1 or with ET-18-OMe, their invasiveness into collagen I layer was greatly enhanced, while no such effect could be observed on MCF-7/6 cells. Control IgM antibodies from normal mouse serum and antibodies to other GSLs (anti-globo-H MBr-1, anti-Gb3 1A4, anti-Gb5 SSEA-3, anti-GM2 MK1-8) [Steelant et al., 2002], did not increase invasiveness of either cell variant (Figure 3).

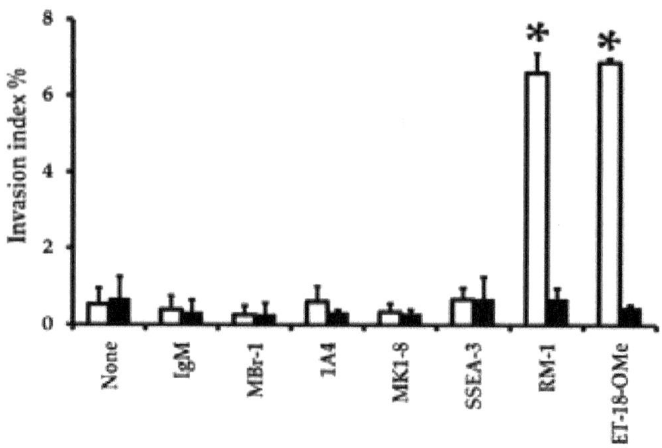

Fig. 3. Invasiveness of MCF-7/AZ cells and MCF-7/6 cells. Effect of mouse IgM or antibodies against Globo-H (MBr-1), Gb3 (1A4), Gb5 (SSEA-3), GM2 (MK1-8), MSGb5 (RM1) and ET-18-OMe on invasion into collagen type I of MCF-7/AZ cells (open columns) and MCF-7/6 cells (black columns). The invasion index expresses the percentage of cells invading into collagen type I over the total number of cells after 24 h. Results are means + S.D., * indicate statistical difference from control conditions, untreated MCF-7/AZ and MCF-7/6 cells, $p < 0.05$.

The motility of MCF-7/AZ cells was also enhanced upon treatment with anti-MSGb5 monoclonal antibody RM1, and again similar treatment did not influence the migratory capacity of the other variant cell line, MCF-7/6 (Figure 4).

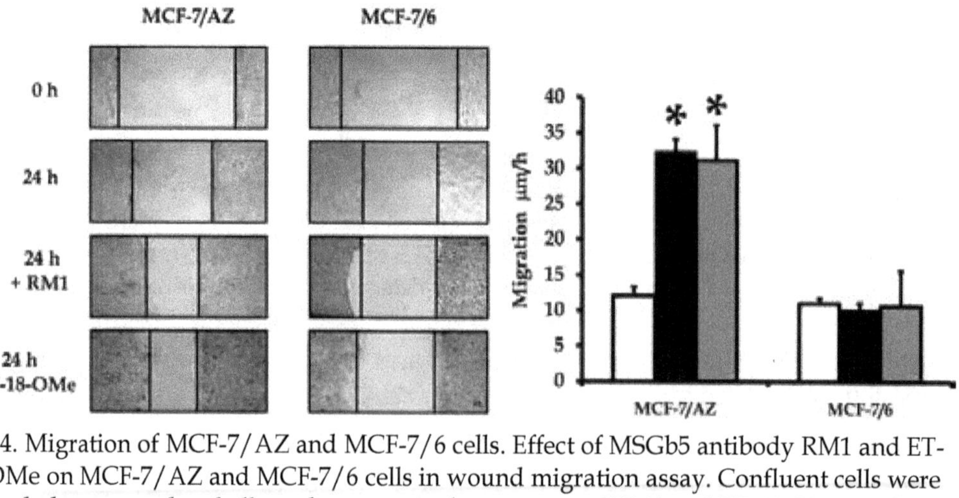

Fig. 4. Migration of MCF-7/AZ and MCF-7/6 cells. Effect of MSGb5 antibody RM1 and ET-18-OMe on MCF-7/AZ and MCF-7/6 cells in wound migration assay. Confluent cells were wounded, measured and allowed to grow in the presence of RM1 and ET-18-OMe. Scale bar = 250 µm. After 24 h, the distances over which the cells migrated were measured and results are expressed as migratory velocity (µm/h). *, indicate statistical difference from untreated MCF-7/AZ and MCF-7/6 cells ($p<0.05$).

Although both cell lines displayed no differences in their GSL composition upon treatment with ET-18-OMe, the possibility arose that changes in organization and clustering of GSLs could be responsible for the observed biological activity and this presumably through assembly with and activation of associated signal transducers. Such an activation model was reported for disialylgalactosylgloboside, DSGG, in the renal cell carcinoma cell line TOS-1 [Satoh et al., 2000] and for GM3 in B16 melanoma cells [Iwabuchi et al., 1998; Iwabuchi et al., 1998]. Alterations in the organization pattern of MSGb5 were observed by immunofluoresescence and confocal microscopy (Figure 5). MSGb5 was detected in both variant cell lines MCF-7/AZ and MCF-7/6, which was consistent with the TLC data. Fluorescence examination of MCF-7/AZ cells treated with ET-18-OMe revealed clustering of MSGb5 at the membrane within minutes. Clustering of MSGb5 in MCF-7/6 cells was not observed (data not shown), nor clustering of other GSLs, for example Gb3 and Gb5 in MCF-7/AZ cells after ET-18-OMe treatment.

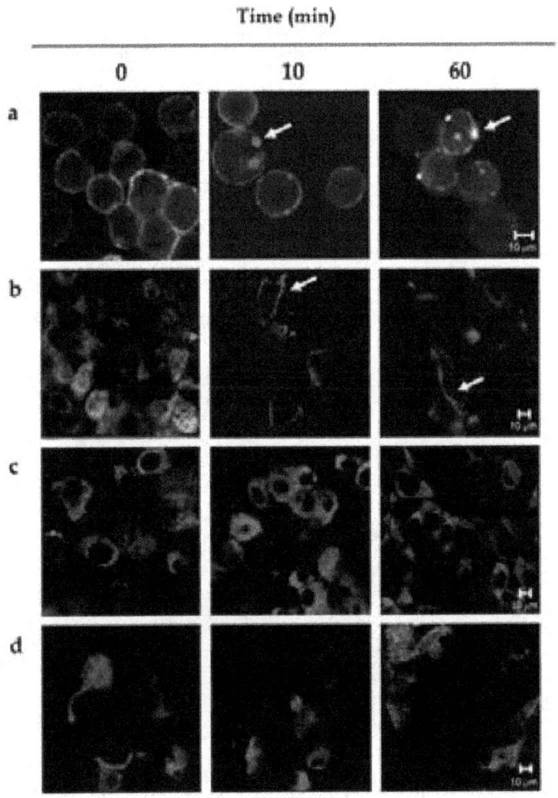

Fig. 5. Clustering of MSGb5 in MCF-7/AZ cells. The organizational pattern of MSGb5 by fluorescence(a) and confocal microscopy(b). Cells in suspension (a) or grown on glass coverslips (b-d), and analysed using antibodies against MSGb5, Gb3 and Gb5 and detected with FITC-labeled anti-mouse antibody. (a) and (b) show the homogenous organization of MSGb5, in untreated MCF-7/AZ cells; arrows indicate clustering of MSGb5 on the membrane of MCF-7/AZ cells after 10 and 60 min ET-18-OMe treatment. Organizational pattern of Gb3 (c) and Gb5 (d) by confocal microscopy, by using antibodies 1A4 against Gb3 and SSEA-3 against Gb5, followed by FITC-labeled mouse antibodies. Scale bar = 10 μm.

4. Src, the FAK-src signalling complex and the activation of the downstream pathway mediating invasion and motility in MCF-7/AZ cells

Several studies provide evidence that the non-receptor tyrosine kinase, src, is implicated in cancer progression of several cancer types. Changes in its expression and tyrosine phosphorylation correlate with the acquisition of an invasive cell phenotype [Guarino, 2010]. The motility and invasion promoting effects of RM1 and ET-18-OMe on MCF-7/AZ cells in our studies suggested that RM1 and ET-18-OMe initiate signalling pathways in MCF-7/AZ cells but not in MCF-7/6 cells. The possible involvement of src kinase in the signalling pathway leading to enhanced migration and invasion could be demonstrated by pretreating MCF-7/AZ cells with PP1, a pharmacological inhibitor of src kinase activity in the collagen I and wound migration assays (Figure 6).

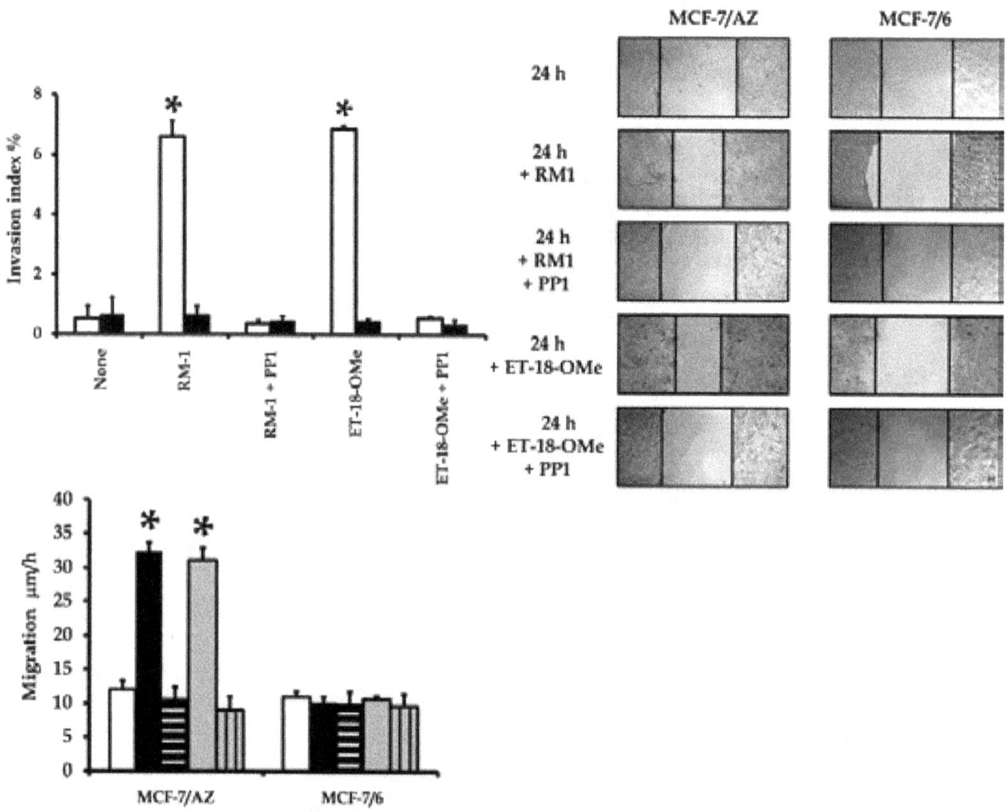

Fig. 6. Invasion and migration of MCF-7/AZ and MCF-7/6 cells. Effect of pharmacological inhibitor PP1 on RM1 or ET-18-OMe-mediated enhanced invasiveness (left panel) and migration of MCF-7/AZ cells (Right panel). Left: Invasion into collagen type I of MCF-7/AZ (open columns) and MCF-7/6 cells (black columns). The invasion index expresses the percentage of cells invading into collagen type I over the total number of cells. Right: Wound migration assay of MCF-7/AZ and MCF-7/6 cells. Scale bar = 250 µm. After 24 h, the distances over which the cells migrated were measured and results are expressed as migratory velocity (µm/h). *, indicate statistical difference from untreated MCF-7/AZ and MCF-7/6 cells ($p<0.05$).

Accordingly, western blotting results revealed that src kinase activity in MCF-7/AZ cells was greatly increased within minutes of RM1 or ET-18-OMe treatment, and abolished by pretreatment with PP1, while there was no such activation of src by both treatments in MCF-7/6 cells. In addition, expression levels of src were left unaltered (Figure 7).

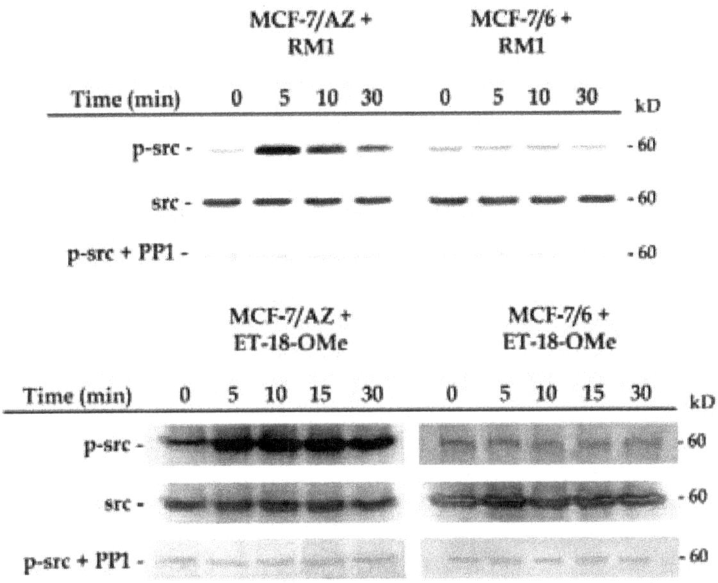

Fig. 7. Expression levels of phosphorylated src (Tyr416) upon RM1, RM1 + PP1, ET-18-OMe and ET-18-OMe + PP1 treatment in MCF-7/AZ and MCF-7/6 cells. Cells of 70% confluency were treated for indicated times, and lysed. Cell lysates, containing 30 μg of proteins, were analysed by SDS-PAGE (7.5% gels) and immunoblotted with antibody against src (Tyr416). The membrane was stripped at 50°C for 30 min in stripping buffer (100 mM 2-mercapto-ethanol, 2% (w/v) SDS, 62.5 mM Tris-HCl (pH 6.8)) and reblotted with anti-src antibody, for src total expression levels and equal loading.

These results clearly demonstrated a prominent role for src in motility and invasion induced by RM1 and ET-18-OMe. A possible mechanism by which src further promotes invasive behavior is through formation of a transient complex with focal adhesion kinase (FAK) [Hauck et al., 2002; Hsia et al., 2003]. FAK is another non-receptor tyrosine kinase recognized in cancer progression since it is found upregulated in malignant human tumour samples [Chatzizacharias et al., 2008]. Correspondingly, in our western blotting studies, RM1 and ET-18-OMe treatment increased the activity of FAK at tyrosine residue 397 (FAK Tyr397), the major autophosphorylation site [Parsons, 2003], in MCF-7/AZ cells and this also within minutes of treatment, while chemical levels of FAK remained unchanged (Figure 8). Similar treatment of MCF-7/6 cells did not change the activation of FAK Tyr397.

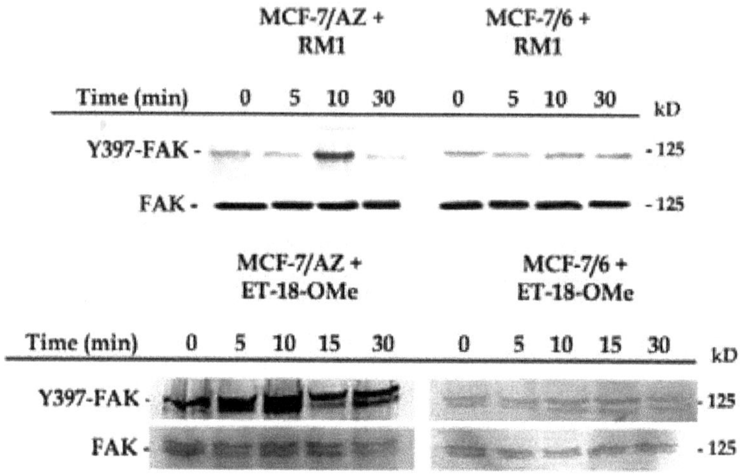

Fig. 8. Expression levels of phosphorylated FAK (Tyr397) upon RM1 and ET-18- OMe treatment in MCF-7/AZ and MCF-7/6 cells. Cells of 70% confluency were treated for indicated times, and lysed. Cell lysates, containing 30 μg of proteins, were analysed by SDS-PAGE (7.5% gels) and immunoblotted with antibody against FAK (Tyr397). The membrane was stripped and reblotted with anti-FAK, for FAK total expression levels and equal loading.

FAK plays an important role in relaying signals to intracellular targets, such as src, generated by cellular adhesion molecules and other cell surface molecules when they interact with the surrounding extracellular matrix [Parsons, 2003; Mitra et al., 2005]. The activation of FAK results in increased phosphorylation at Tyr397, the major autophosphorylation site, and subsequently in the recruitment and binding of src through its SH2 domain and further stabilization of the src-FAK interaction by src's SH3 domain [Thomas et al., 1998]. The formation of this transient bipartite kinase complex disrupts an inhibitory intramolecular interaction, resulting in increased activity of src [Schaller et al., 1994; Xing et al., 1994]. The specific organization plays a crucial role in src-dependent and mediated phosphorylation of other tyrosine residues on FAK within the kinase domain activation loop (Tyr576 and Tyr577) and at the C-terminal domain residues, Tyr861 and Tyr925 [Calalb et al., 1995; Calalb et al., 1996; Schlaepfer et al., 1996]. Interesting is that the activated FAK (Tyr397)-src signalling complex allows the activation of multiple different downstream pathways depending on which specific tyrosine residue on FAK is activated [Brunton et al., 2005]. As shown in scheme 1, the activated FAK-src complex can result in the activation of the mitogen-activated protein kinase (MAPK)-cascade through FAK Tyr925 [Schlaepfer et al. 1998], p130Cas via FAK Tyr861 [Lim et al., 2004] or paxillin by FAK Tyr576 [Calalb et al., 1995]. These three signalling pathways downstream of the FAK-src signalling complex, all lead to increased release of matrix metalloproteinase-2 (MMP-2) and MMP-9, the major proteinases responsible for the degradation of collagen type I [Kurata et al., 2000; Liu et al., 2000; Hsia et al., 2003; Brabek et al., 2004; Brabek et al., 2005; Bjorklund & Koivunen, 2005].

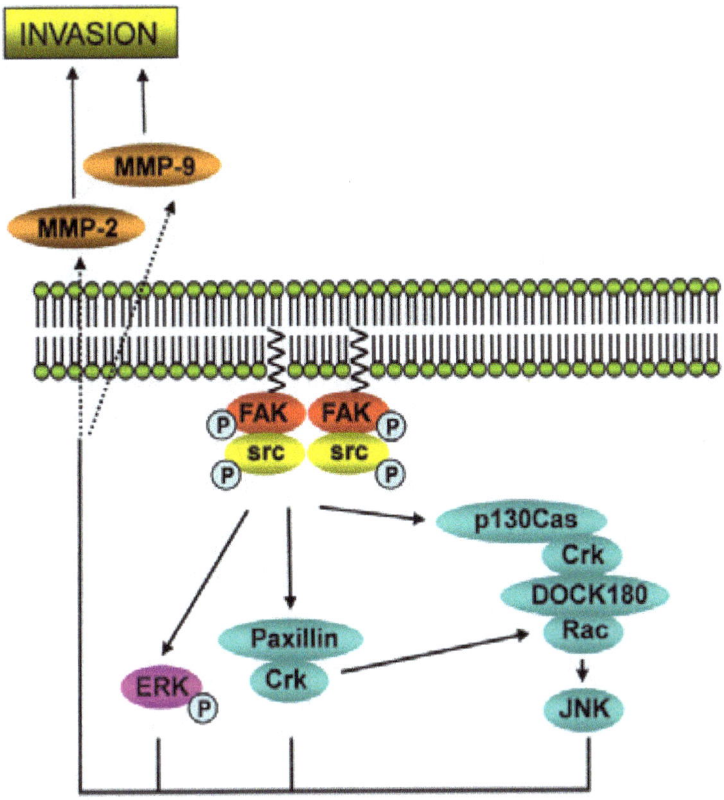

Scheme 1. Possible pathways downstream of the transient FAK-src complex leading to increased expression of MMPs, facilitating invasion into collagen type I layer.

Our results support that ET-18-OMe treatment results in the formation of a temporary FAK-src complex through FAK (Tyr397) activation and the subsequent src-dependent phosphorylation of FAK on Tyr925, since pretreatment of MCF-7/AZ cells with PP1, blocked the activation of src (Figure 7) and FAK Tyr925, while the activation of FAK at Tyr397 was only partially reduced (Figure 9). These results also point out that ET-18-OMe-mediated activation and autophosphorylation of FAK at Tyr397 is upstream and required for the activation of src and that src activity is responsible for the activation of the additional tyrosine residue 925 of FAK but not of FAK Tyr576 and 861 (Figure 9). Furthermore, we provide evidence linking FAK Tyr925 phosphorylation to the activation of the MAPK-pathway, since treatment of MCF-7/AZ cells with ET-18-OMe resulted in the downstream activation of extracellular signal-regulated kinase 1 and 2 (ERK1/2) and PP1 blocked the enhanced activation. In addition, we demonstrated that p130Cas and paxillin, which are known substrates of src associated with phosphorylation of FAK on Tyr861 and 576 respectively [Lim et al., 2004; Calalb et al., 1995], are not involved in the ET-18-OMe-induced effect and confirmed the lack of phosphorylation at FAK Tyr861 and 576 (Figure 10).

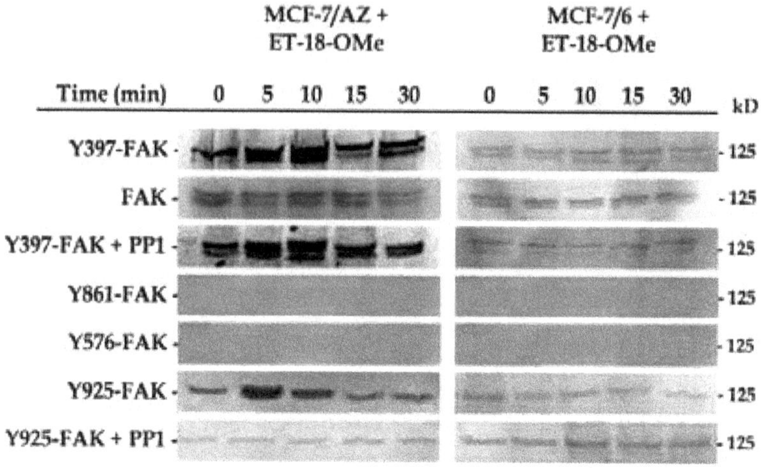

Fig. 9. Expression levels of FAK (Tyr397, Tyr925) upon ET-18-OMe and ET-18-OMe + PP1 treatment in MCF-7/AZ and MCF-7/6 cells. Cells of 70% confluency were treated for indicated times, and lysed. Cell lysates, containing 30 μg of proteins, were analysed by SDS-PAGE (7.5% gels) and immunoblotted with antibodies against FAK (Tyr397, Tyr576, Tyr861 and Tyr925). The membranes were stripped and reblotted with anti-FAK, for FAK total expression levels and equal loading.

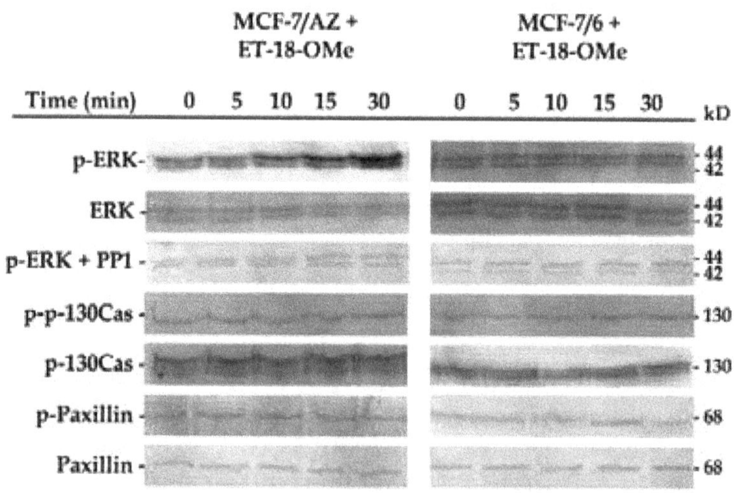

Fig. 10. Expression levels of ERK (Thr202/Tyr204) upon ET-18-OMe and ET-18-OMe + PP1 treatment in MCF-7/AZ and MCF-7/6 cells. Cells of 70% confluency were treated for indicated times, and lysed. Cell lysates, containing 30 μg of proteins, were analysed by SDS-PAGE (7.5% gels) and immunoblotted with antibodies against ERK (Thr202/Tyr204), p130Cas (Tyr410) and paxillin (Ser178). The membranes were stripped and reblotted with anti-ERK, anti-p130Cas and paxillin for total ERK, p130Cas and paxillin expression levels and equal loading.

5. MSGb5 activates the FAK-src signalling complex

Tumour cell invasion includes alterations of expression levels of integrin receptors. Integrin receptors are important upstream regulators of intracellular and downstream signalling events associated with cancer cell invasion. This family of heterodimeric α/β subunit receptors, expressed on every cell type, is capable of interacting with specific ligands in the surrounding extracellular matrix. Binding to these components results in clustering of integrin receptors in the plasmamembrane and recruitment and association of signalling proteins with integrin cytoplasmic domains to initiate downstream signalling events [Schwartz, 2001]. Since src and FAK are recognized as two critical mediators of integrin signalling, we addressed the question whether particular integrins were implicated in ET-18-OMe-induced activation of FAK and src and invasiveness of MCF-7/AZ cells. The integrin receptors α1β1 and α2β1 are the major receptors binding to collagen type I in the extracellular matrix [Gullberg et al., 1992]. Given that RM1 and ET-18-OMe induce invasiveness of MCF-7/AZ cells in collagen type I layer, we examined the expression levels of integrin subunits α1, β1 and α2 upon treatment with ET-18-OMe by Western blotting. Expression of the α1 and β1 subunits were found decreased over time in MCF-7/AZ cells, and no changes of either integrin subunit was observed in the variant cell line (Figure 11), whereas the integrin α2 subunit was not detectable in both cell lines (data not shown).

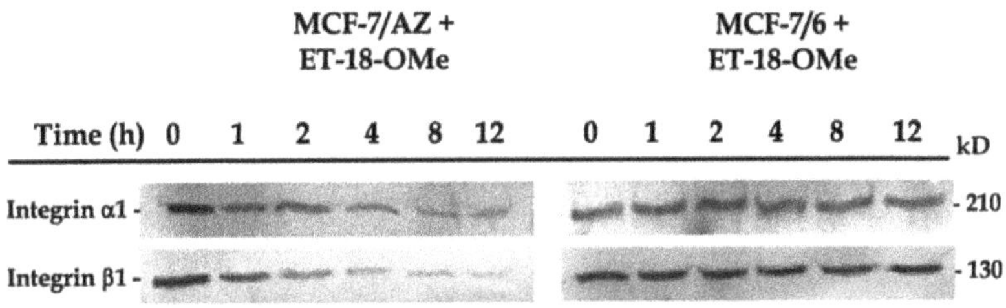

Fig. 11. Expression of integrin subunits α1 and β1 in MCF-7/AZ and MCF-7/6 cells upon ET-18-OMe treatment. Cells of 70% confluency were treated for indicated times, and lysed. Cell lysates, containing 30 μg of proteins, were analysed by SDS-PAGE (7.5% gels) and immunoblotted with antibodies against the integrin α1 and β1 subunit.

Since activation of integrin-dependent signalling occurs via clustering of integrin receptors and association with FAK signalling elements to the cytoplasmic tails of the receptor [Miyamoto et al., 1995], organizational patterns of the α1 and β1 subunits and co-clustering with signalling molecules FAK and src, upon ET-18-OMe treatment were examined by fluorescence microscopy and co-immunoprecipitation experiments. The microscopy data revealed that ET-18-OMe did not change the organization of the respective integrin subunits and the fact that signalling molecules FAK and src could not be detected in the immunoprecipitates of either integrin subunits confirmed that integrin receptors α1β1 and α2β1 were not of crucial importance in the activation of downstream signalling events in MCF-7/AZ cells mediated by ET-18-OMe or RM1 (data not shown). This was in sharp contrast with data reported by other investigators [Schaller et al., 1995]. However, the recognition that glycosphingolipids may influence cellular phenotype by clustering and assembly with signal transducing molecules, let us to explore the possible involvement of the glycosphingolipid MSGb5 in initiating the signalling events in MCF-7/AZ cells upon

RM1 or ET-18-OMe treatment. This idea was supported by two of our observations namely that RM1 and ET-18-OMe treatment resulted in clustering of MSGb5 in MCF-7/AZ cells and that similar treatment profoundly affected the cellular activities associated with the migratory and invasive capacity of MCF-7/AZ cells. A close connection between MSGb5 and signalling molecules was shown by co-immunoprecipitation experiments, in which aliquots of cell lysates were immunoprecipitated by incubation with anti-MSGb5 antibody and captured with protein G-Sepharose beads. The signalling molecules, FAK and src as well as their activated forms, src (Tyr416) and FAK (Tyr397), were detected in MSGb5 immunoprecipitates prepared from MCF-7/AZ cells treated with ET-18-OMe for indicated time points, and the obtained results were in line with the earlier performed kinase experiments. In MCF-7/6 cells, FAK and src were found associated with MSGb5, and as expected no kinase activity was observed upon ET-18-OMe treatment (Figure 12). The involvement of other glycosphingolipids could be excluded since no clustering and no association between FAK and src with Gb3, Gb5 or GM2 (data not shown) could be found in MCF-7/AZ cells. Equal levels of MSGb5 were detected in the immunoprecipitates of both cell lines.

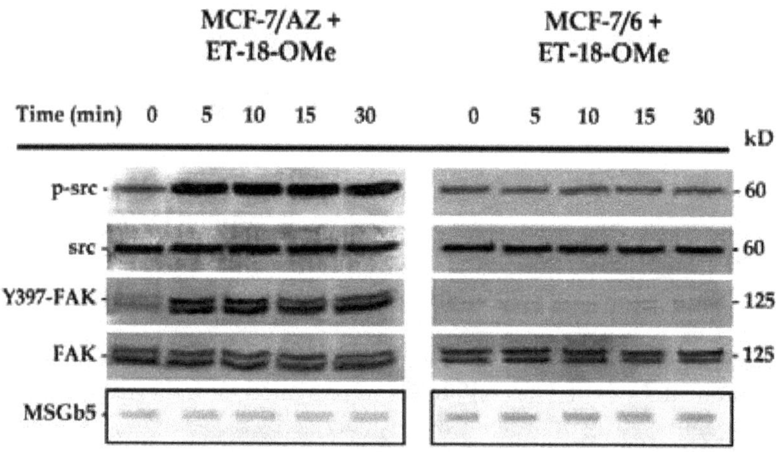

Fig. 12. MSGb5 associates with src (Tyr416) and FAK (Tyr397) in MCF-7/AZ cells after ET-18-OMe treatment. MSGb5 was immunoprecipitated from whole cell lysates with mouse IgG_3 anti-MSGb5 antibody. Aliquots of immunoprecipitates were electrophoresed, transferred and immunoblotted, with anti-src (Tyr416), anti-src, anti-FAK (Tyr397) and anti-FAK. MSGb5 content in the different immunoprecipitates was determined by TLC.

6. Concept of "Glycosynapse"

Glycosphingolipids are highly expressed during defined stages of development and after oncogenic transformation and are referred to as stage-specific embryonic antigen and tumour-associated antigens respectively [Hakomori, 1998]. Most studies, however, use the presence of GSLs as markers of low-density membrane fractions and are neither focused on their structural variety nor their possible functional roles. In this chapter, we present data supporting a functional role for MSGb5 in migration and invasion of MCF-7/AZ cells upon stimulation with RM1 or treatment with ET-18-OMe, resulting in MSGb5 clustering and activation of associated signalling molecules. These observations can be placed in the concept of the 'glycosynapse' [Hakomori, 2002]. This term defines glycosylation-dependent adhesion and signalling, mediated via glycosylepitopes of GSLs in microenvironments where tumour cells interface with other tumour cells, host cells or the surrounding matrix, in analogy to the 'immune synapse' which on its turn controls functional adhesion and signalling between immunocytes [Ilangumaran et al., 2000]. In addition to glycosylation-dependent adhesion of GSLs between interfacing glycosynapses, conversion of phenotypes is highly controlled by the presence, interactions and organization of other crucial molecules in the glycosynapse, such as growth factor receptors, integrin receptors, tetraspanins, mucins and gangliosides [Hakomori & Handa, 2002]. Furthermore, this new concept has been extended to phenotypic conversion induced through the deletion or addition of a single component, resulting in a disorganized glycosynapse framework and initiating altered signalling events [Mitsuzuka et al., 2005]. We can relate our observations to the latter revised glycosynapse concept and more specifically to the formation of a disorganized glycosynapse framework. We conclude that phenotypic conversion from non-invasive to invasive MCF-7/AZ breast cancer cells is induced by: (i) an aberrant MSGb5 pattern; (ii) loss of integrin receptor subunits $\alpha 1$ and $\beta 1$; and (iii) high tetraspanin CD9 expression levels [Steelant et al., 2002], all of which are responsible for the formation of disorganized glycosynapse framework interfaces, thereby inducing activation of FAK, src and downstream ERK, with consequent enhanced secretion and activity of MMP-2 and MMP-9, and thus leading to invasion.

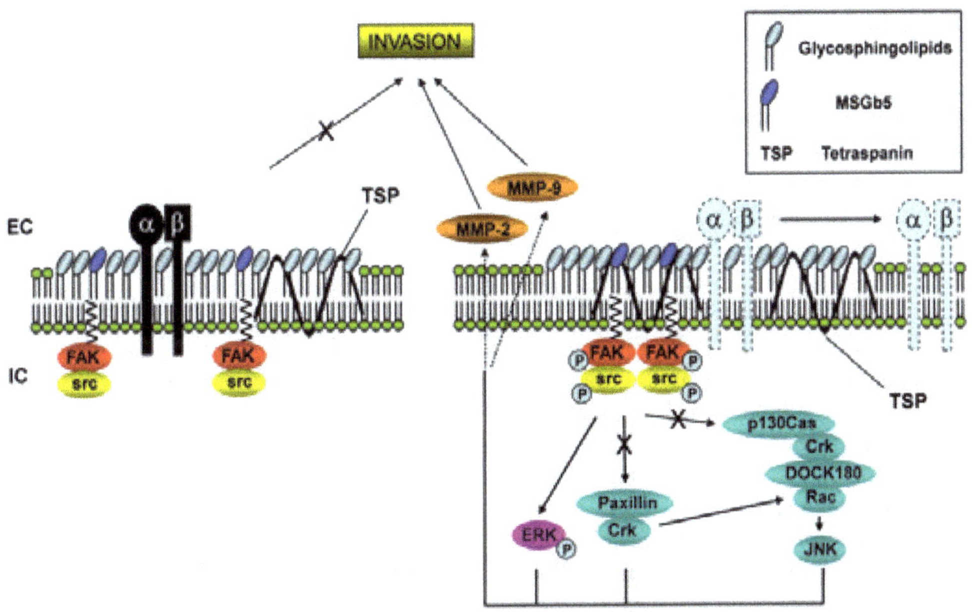

Scheme 2. Cancer cell invasion revised. In non-invasive MCF-7/AZ cells integrin subunits α1 and β1 form a stable complex with tetraspanin CD9 and GLSs, associated with non-active signalling molecules, FAK and src. In invasive MCF-7/AZ cells clustering of MSGb5 and loss of integrin subunits α1 and β1 disorganize the glycosynapse framework, resulting in activation of downstream signalling to invasion. EC, extracellular; IC, intracellular; TSP, tetraspanin.

7. Conclusion

In conclusion, our studies are an extension of previous work on the glycosynapse [Hakomori, 2002], re-formulating the classic concept of integrin-dependent invasion of tumour cells and providing evidence that phenotypic conversion can be explained by differences in composition and organization of crucial molecules in the glycosynapse. At present, only a few studies have appeared that focus, in particular, on GM3 [Mitsuzuka et al., 2005, Toledo et al., 2005]. The present study reveals a novel insight into the composition and organization of the glycosynapses in MCF-7/AZ breast cancer cells, which explain phenotypic changes. Further studies along this line are necessary to understand the complex interplay of distinct molecules in invasion, as well as other basic cellular mechanisms, and their implications on disease processes, which will be expected to lead to novel therapeutic approaches.

8. Acknowledgements

These studies were supported by the Belgian Federation Against Cancer, the US National Institutes of Health [RR-16480] under the BRIN/INBRE program of the National Center for Research Resources and the New Mexico Tech startup funds and the New Mexico Department of Veteran Services.

9. References

Bjorklund, M. & Koivunen, E. (2005) Gelatinase-mediated migration and invasion of cancer cells. *Biochimica et Biophysica Acta*, 1755, 1, 37-69.

Brabek, J.; Constancio, S.S.; Shin, N.Y.; Pozzi, A.; Weaver, A.M. & Hanks, S.K. (2004). CAS promotes invasiveness of Src-transformed cells. *Oncogene*, 23, 44, 7406–7415.

Brabek, J.; Constancio, S.S.; Siesser, P.F.; Shin, N.Y.; Pozzi, A. & Hanks, S.K. (2005). Crk-associated substrate tyrosine phosphorylation sites are critical for invasion and metastasis of SRC-transformed cells. *Molecular Cancer Research*, 3, 6, 307–315.

Bracke, M.E.; Boterberg, T.; Bruyneel, E.A. & Mareel, M.M. (2001). Collagen invasion assay. In: *Metastasis Research Protocols*, Brooks, S. & Schumacher, U. (eds.) , Humana Press, Totowa, pp. 81–89,

Brunton, V.G.; Avizienyte, E.; Fincham, V.J.; Serrels, B.; Metcalf, C.A. 3rd; Sawyer, T.K. & Frame, M.C. (2005). Identification of Src-specific phosphorylation site on focal adhesion kinase: dissection of the role of Src SH2 and catalytic functions and their consequences for tumor cell behaviour. *Cancer Research*, 65, 4, 1335–1342.

Calalb, M.B.; Polte, T.R. & Hanks, S.K. (1995). Tyrosine phosphorylation of focal adhesion kinase at sites in the catalytic domain regulates kinase activity: a role for Src family kinases. *Molecular and Cellular Biology*, 15, 2, 954-963.

Calalb, M.B.; Zhang, X.; Polte, T.R. & Hanks, S.K. (1996). Focal adhesion kinase tyrosine-861 is a major site of phosphorylation by Src. *Biochemical and Biophysical Research Communications*, 228, 3, 662-668.

Chatzizacharias, N.A.; Kouraklis , G.P. & Theocharis, S.E. (2008). Clinical significance of FAK expression in human neoplasia. *Histology and Histopathology*, 23, 5, 629-650.

Guarino, M. (2010). Src signaling in cancer cell invasion. *Journal of Cellular Physiology*, 223, 1, 14-26.

Gullberg, D., Gehlsen, K.R., Turner, D.C., Ahlén, K., Zijenah, L.S., Barnes, M.J. & Rubin, K. (1992). Analysis of alpha 1 beta 1, alpha2 beta 1 and alpha3 beta 1 integrins in cell-collagen interactions: identification of conformation dependent aplha1 beta 1 binding sites in collagen type I. *EMBO Journal*, 11, 11, 3863-3873.

Hakomori, S. (1996). Tumor malignancy defined by aberrant glycosylation and sphingo(glycol)lipid metabolism. *Cancer Research*, 56, 23, 5309-5318.

Hakomori, S. (1998). Cancer-associated glycosphingolipid antigens: their structure, organization, and function. *Acta Anatomica*, 161, 1-4, 79–90.

Hakomori, S.; Yamamura, S. & Handa, A.K. (1998). Signal transduction through glyco(sphingo)lipids: introduction and recent studies on glyco(sphingo)lipid-enriched microdomains. *Annals of the New York Academy of Sciences*, 845, 1–10.

Hakomori, S. (2002). Glycosylation defining cancer malignancy: new wine in an old bottle. *Proceedings of the National Academy of Sciences of the United States of America*, 99, 6, 10231–10233.

Hakomori, S. & Handa, K. (2002). Glycosphingolipid-dependent cross-talk between glycosynapses interfacing tumor cells with their host cells: essential basis to define tumor malignancy. *FEBS Letters*, 531, 1, 88–92.

Hakomori, S. (2002) The glycosynapse. *Proceedings of the National Academy of Sciences of the United States of America*, 99, 1, 225–232.

Hamamura, K.; Furakawa, K.; Hayashi, T.; Hattori, T.; Nakano, J.; Nakashima, H.; Okuda, T.; Mizutani, H.; Hattori, H.; Ueda, M.; Urano, T.; Lloyd, K.O. & Furakawa, K. (2005). Ganglioside GD3 promotes cell growth and invasion through p130Cas and paxillin in malignant melanoma cells. *Proceedings of the National Academy of Sciences of the United States of America*, 102, 31, 11041–11046.

Hauck, C.R.; Hsia, D.A.; Puente, X.S.; Cheresh, D.A. & Schlaepfer, D.D. (2002). FRNK blocks v-Src-stimulated invasion and experimental metastases without effects on cell motility or growth. *EMBO Journal*, 21, 23, 6289–6302.

Hsia, D.A.; Mitra, S.K.; Hauck, C.R.; Streblow, D.N.; Nelson, J. A.; Ilic, D.; Huang, S.; Li, E.; Nemerow, G.R.; Leng, J.; Spencer, K.S.; Cheresh, D.A. & Schlaepfer, D.D. (2003). Differential regulation of cell motility and invasion by FAK. *The Journal of Cell Biology*, 160, 5, 753–767.

Ilangumaran, S.; He, H.T. & Hoessli, D.C. (2000). Microdomains in lymphocyte signalling: beyond GPI-anchored proteins. *Immunology Today*, 21, 1, 2-7.

Ito, A.; Saito, S.; Masuko, T.; Oh-eda, M.; Matsuura, T.; Satoh, M.; Nejad, F.M.; Enomoto, T.; Orikasa, S. & Hakomori, S. I. (2001). Monoclonal antibody (5F3) defining renal cell carcinoma-associated antigen disialosyl globopentaosylceramide (V3NeuAcIV6NeuAcGb5), and distribution pattern of the antigen in tumor and normal tissues. *Glycoconjugate Journal*, 18, 6, 475–485.

Ito, A.; Levery, S.B.; Saito, S.; Satoh, M. & Hakomori, S. (2001). A novel ganglioside isolated from renal cell carcinoma. *Journal of Biological Chemistry*, 276, 20, 16695–16703.

Iwabuchi, K.; Yamamura, S.; Prinetti, A.; Handa, K. & Hakomori, S. (1998). GM3-enriched microdomain involved in cell adhesion and signal transduction through carbohydrate-carbohydrate interaction in mouse melanoma B16 cells. *Journal of Biological Chemistry*, 273, 15, 9130–9138.

Iwabuchi, K.; Handa, K. & Hakomori, S. (1998). Separation of "glycosphingolipid signaling domain" from caveolin-containing membrane fraction in mouse melanoma B16 cells and its role in cell adhesion coupled with signaling. *Journal of Biological Chemistry*, 273, 50, 33766–33773.

Jemal, A.; Bray, F., Center, M.M.; Ferlay, J.; Ward, E. & Forman, D. (2011). Global cancer statistics. *CA: a Cancer Journal for Clinicians*, 61, 2, 69-90.

Kannagi, R.; Cohran, N.A.; Ishigami, F.; Hakomori, S.; Andrews, P.W.; Knowles, B.B. & Solter, D. (1983). Stage-specific embryonic antigens (SSEA-3 and -4) are epitopes of a unique globo-series ganglioside isolated from human teratocarcinoma cells. *EMBO Journal*, 2, 12, 2355–2361.

Kannagi, R. & Hakomori, S. (2001). A guide to monoclonal antibodies directed to glycotopes. *Advances in Experimental Medicine and Biology*, 491, 587–630.

Kim, Y.J. & Varki, A. (1997). Perspectives on the significance of altered glycosylation of glycoproteins in cancer. *Glycoconjugate Journal*, 14, 5, 569–576.

Kurata, H.; Thant, A.A.; Matsuo, S.; Senga, T.; Okazaki, K.; Hotta, N. & Hamaguchi, M. (2000). Constitutive activation of MAP kinase kinase (MEK1) is critical and sufficient for the activation of MMP-2. *Experimental Cell Research*, 254, 1, 180–188.

Liotta, L. & Kohn, E. (2001). The microenvironment of the tumor-host interface. *Nature*, 411, 6835, 375-379.

Lim, Y.; Han, I.; Jeon, J.; Park, H.; Bahk, Y.Y. & Oh E.S. (2004). Phosphorylation of focal adhesion kinase at tyrosine 861 is crucial for Ras transformation of fibroblasts. *Journal of Biological Chemistry*, 279, 28, 29060-29065.

Liu, E.; Thant, A.A.; Kikkawa, F.; Kurata, H.; Tanaka, S.; Nawa, A.; Mizutani, S.; Matsuda, S.; Hanafusa, H. & Hamaguchi, M. (2000). The Ras-mitogen-activated protein kinase pathway is critical for the activation of matrix metalloproteinase secretion and the invasiveness in v-crk-transformed 3Y1. *Cancer Research*, 60, 9, 2361–2364.

Mareel, M. & Leroy, A. (2003). Clinical, cellular, and molecular aspects of cancer invasion. *Physiological Reviews*, 83, 2, 337–376.

Mehrotra J.; Vali, M.; McVeigh, M.; Kominsky, S.L.; Fackler, M.J.; Lahti-Domenici, J.; Polyak, K.; Sacchi, N.; Garrett-Mayer, E.; Argani, P. & Sukumar, S. (2004). Very high frequency of hypermethylated genes in breast cancer metastasis to the bone, brain and lung. *Clinical Cancer Research*, 10, 9, 3104-3109.

Mitra, S.K., Hanson, D.A. & Schlaepfer, D.D. (2005). Focal adhesion kinase: in command and control of cell motility. *Nature Reviews. Molecular Cell Biology*, 6, 1, 56-62.

Mitsuzuka, K.; Handa, K.; Satoh, M.; Arai, Y. & Hakomori, S. (2005). A specific microdomain ("glycosynapse 3") controls phenotypic conversion and reversion of bladder cancer cells through GM3-mediated interaction of $a3\beta1$ integrin with CD9. *Journal of Biological Chemistry*, 280, 42, 35545–35553.

Miyamoto, S.; Teramoto, H.; Coso, O.A.; Gutkind, J.S.; Burbelo, P.D.; Akiyama, S.K. & Yamada, K.M. (1995). Integrin function: molecular hierarchies of cytoskeletal and signaling molecules. *Journal of Cell Biology*, 131, 3, 791-805, 1995.

Nohara, K.; Wang, F. & Spiegel, S. (1998). Glycosphingolipid composition of MDA-MB-231 and MCF-7 human breast cancer cell lines. *Breast Cancer Research and Treatment*, 48, 2, 149–157.

Parsons, J. T. (2003). Focal adhesion kinase: the first ten years. *Journal of Cell Science*, 116, 8, 1409-1416.

Saito, S.; Orikasa, S.; Ohyama, C.; Satoh, M. & Fukushi, Y. (1991). Changes in glycolipids in human renal-cell carcinoma and their clinical significance. *International Journal of Cancer*, 49, 3, 329–334.

Saito, S.; Orikasa, S.; Satoh, M.; Ohyama, C.; Ito, A. & Takahashi, T. (1997). Expression of globo-series gangliosides in human renal cell carcinoma. *Japanese Journal of Cancer Research*, 88, 7, 652–659.

Saito, S.; Aiko, H.; Ito, A.; Ueno, S.,;Wada, T.; Mitsuzuka, K.; Satoh, M.; Arai, Y. & Miyagi, T. (2003). Human α2,3-sialyltransferase (ST3Gal II) is a stage-specific embryonic antigen-4 synthase. *Journal of Biological Chemistry*, 278, 29, 26474–26479.

Saito, T. & Hakomori, S. (1971). Quantitative isolation of total glycosphingolipids from animal cells. *Journal of Lipid Research*, 12, 2, 257–259.

Satoh, M.; Nejad, F.M.; Ohtani, H.; Ito, A.; Ohyama, C.; Saito, S.; Orikasa, S. & Hakomori, S. (2000). Association of renal cell carcinoma antigen, disialylgalactosylgloboside, with c-Src and RhoA in clustered domains at the surface membrane. *International Journal of Oncology*, 16, 3, 529–536.

Schaller, M.D.; Hildebrand, J.D.; Shannon, J.D.; Fox, J.W.; Vines, R.R. & Parsons, J.T. (1994) Autophosphorylation of the focal adhesion kinase, pp125FAK, directs SH2 dependent binding of pp60src. *Molecular and Cellular Biology*, 14, 3, 1680-1688.

Schaller, M.D.; Otey, C.A.; Hildebrand, J.D. & Parsons, J.T. (1995). Focal adhesion kinase and paxillin bind to peptides mimicking beta integrin cytoplasmic domains. *Journal of Cellular Biology*, 130, 5, 1181–1187.

Schlaepfer, D.D. & Hunter T (1996). Evidence for in vivo phosphorylation of the Grb2 SH2-domain binding site on focal adhesion kinase by Src-family protein-tyrosine kinases. *Molecular and Cellular Biology*, 16, 10, 5623-5633.

Schlaepfer, D.D.; Jones, K.C. & Hunter, T. (1998). Multiple Grb2-mediated integrin-stimulated signaling pathways to ERK2/mitogen-activated protein kinase: summation of both c-Src- and focal adhesion kinase-initiated tyrosine phosphorylation events. *Molecular and Cellular Biology*, 18, 5, 2571–2585.

Schwartz, M.A. (2001). Integrin signaling revisited. *Trends in Cell Biology*, 11, 12, 466-470.

Steelant, W.F.; Goeman, J.L.; Philippe, J.; Oomen, L.C.; Hilkens, J.; Krzewinski-Recchi, M.-A.; Huet, G.; Van der Eycken, J.; Delannoy, P.; Bruyneel, E.A. & Mareel, M.M. (2001). Alkyl-lysophospholipid 1-O-octadecyl-2-O-methyl-glycerophosphocholine induces invasion through episialin-mediated neutralization of E-cadherin in human mammary MCF-7 cells in vitro. *International Journal of Cancer*, 92, 4, 527–536.

Steelant, W.F.; Kawakami, Y.; Ito, A.; Handa, A.K.; Bruyneel, E.A.; Mareel, M. & Hakomori, S. (2002). Monosialyl-Gb5 organized with cSrc and FAK in GEM of human breast carcinoma MCF-7 cells defines their invasive properties. *FEBS Letters*, 531, 1, 93–98.

Thomas, J. W.; Ellis, B.; Boerner, R.J.; Knight, W.B.; White, G.C. 2nd & Schaller, M.D. (1998) SH2- and SH3-mediated interactions between focal adhesion kinase and Src. *Journal of Biological Chemistry*, 273, 1, 577-583.

Toledo, M.S.; Suzuki, E.; Handa, K. & Hakomori, S. (2005). Effect of ganglioside and tetraspanins in microdomains on interaction of integrins with fibroblast growth factor receptor. *Journal of Biological Chemistry*, 280, 16, 16227–16234.

Xing, Z.; Chen, H.C.; Nowlen, J.K.; Taylor, S.J., Shalloway, D. & Guan, J. L. (1994). Direct interaction of v-Src with the focal adhesion kinase mediated by the Src SH2 domain. *Molecular Biology of the Cell*, 5, 4, 413-421.

Yilmaz, M. & Christofori, G. (2010). Mechanisms of motility in metastasizing cells. *Molecular Cancer Research*, 8, 5, 629-642.

Zhang, Q.; Furukawa, K.; Chen, H.H.; Sakakibara, T.; Urano, T. & Furukawa, K. (2006). Metastatic potential of mouse Lewis lung cancer cells is regulated via ganglioside GM1 by modulating matrix metalloprotease-9 localization in lipid rafts. *Journal of Biological Chemistry*, 281, 26, 18145–18155.

3

The Importance of ERα/ERβ Ratio in Breast Cancer: Mitochondrial Function and Oxidative Stress

Pilar Roca, Jordi Oliver, Jorge Sastre-Serra and Mercedes Nadal-Serrano
Universitat de les Illes Balears
Spain

1. Introduction

Breast cancer is the most commonly diagnosed malignancy within the female population of developed countries and is the first leading cause of cancer deaths in women. In the European Union (EU27) every year there are an estimated 319.000 new cases diagnosed, and approximately 131.000 deaths, which comprises 16.7% of all cancer caused deaths in women (Ferlay et al., 2007).

The causes of breast cancer are not fully understood, but the epidemiology of the disease clearly shows that hormonal factors play a key role. Estrogen production appears as one potential risk factor among women worldwide because it stimulates the proliferation of breast epithelial cells (Ekbom et al., 1997; Ferlay et al., 2007). Coincident with this proliferation, breast cancer risk increases in early menarche, late menopause and with obesity in postmenopausal women (situations where there is a direct association between estrogen and breast cancer risk). In general, breast cancer risk decreases around 5% with each year that menarche is delayed. Breast cancer incidence rates also increase more slowly after menopause; therefore a woman with a natural menopause at age 45 years has half the risk of developing this type of cancer that a woman with menopause at age 55 (Kelsey et al., 1993; Key et al., 2001).

Childbearing seems to have a dual effect on risk of breast cancer (Key et al., 2001). On one hand the immediate effect is to temporarily increase the risk after a birth, yet on the other, this risk diminishes in the long term and the overall effect of a pregnancy is to reduce the overall risk of developing this disease. It appears that the negative short term effect is due to the increase in estradiol levels in early pregnancy. However, has been seen that premenopausal parous women have lower global levels of circulating estradiol than in nulliparous premenopausal women. This effect is observed among postmenopausal women, suggesting that this diminution is stable (Ewertz et al., 1990). Women who have had at least one child have around a 25% reduction in breast cancer risk compared to nulliparous women (Layde et al., 1989; Ewertz et al., 1990).

Moreover, the use of menopausal hormonal therapy increases the risk of breast cancer; in fact, the use of these estrogen preparations over a period of 10 years, increases cancer risk by 35%(Key et al., 2001). Other risk factor associated with breast cancer is family history and genetic predisposition. Women with a first-degree relative have about a two-fold risk of

developing breast cancer. However the risk is lower when only second-degree relatives are affected (Pharoah et al., 1997). Several germline mutations that have a prediposition for the development of breast cancer have been identified: BRCA1, BRCA2, P53, PTEN, ATM, NBS1, RAD50, BRIP1, PALB2 and CHEK2 (Walsh and King, 2007). In addition, the International Agency for Research on Cancer (IARC) estimates that 25% of all cancers are associated with overweight and obesity. This increase in cancer risk is approximately linear with increasing body-mass index, yet is reduced in the more physically active, equivalent population (McTiernan, 2003). In the European Union, 13.000 cases of breast cancer could be avoided annually by maintaining a normal body weight (Devenish et al., 1979). The increased risk in obese postmenopausal women may be due to higher levels of circulating estrogens (Lahmann et al., 2004). For many years this risk has been linked to higher estrogenic synthesis by the aromatase process in the adipose tissue and recent studies showed that the hormones secreted for this tissue have the capacity to induce tumour cell proliferation and survival (Catalano et al., 2003; Lahmann et al., 2004; Garofalo and Surmacz, 2006).
The most common type of breast cancer is invasive ductal carcinoma (IDC), and about 80% of all breast cancers are of this histological type. The second most common type is invasive lobular carcinoma (ILC), represents approximately 10%. Tubular carcinoma of the breast is a rare subtype of invasive ductal carcinoma, and accounts for only 1-2% of all breast cancer cases (Novelli et al., 2008).

2. Estrogen receptors

2.1 History of estrogen

Estrogen is term derived from Greek *oistros*¸ a word which refers to oestrus, the phase in which females are sexually receptive. In women with active menstrual cycles, daily ovary estrogen production is between 70 and 500 micrograms, with 17β-estradiol (E_2) the most important one. Studies report that the production E_2 of increases under the influence of gonadotropins secreted by the pituitary gland and by the maturation of ovarian follicles. Follicular estrogens induce the growth and development of female sex organs and to maintain sexual characteristics, as well as influence female behaviour (Morani et al., 2008). Studies of action of E_2 on the uterus, directed by Jensen, led to the conclusion that the biological effects of estrogen occur through the activation of estrogen receptor (ER) (Jensen et al., 1972). In the classical scheme of reproductive organ development, estrogens were considered as "female hormones", while testosterone was thought to be the "male hormone". In the 1980's the studies began to analyse effects of estrogen in non-target organs for the action of this hormone, i.e. in organs that are not associated with reproduction. The importance of estrogens in the bone homeostasis was recognised because of the observed increased risk of osteoporosis in postmenopausal women. However, it was a publication in 1994 of a case report of male with an ER mutation who had abnormal bone density and impaired glucose tolerance that finally confirmed the importance of estrogens in both males and females (Smith et al., 1994).
It was only until 1985, 23 years after the discovery of ER by Jensen, that this receptor was identified as a member of nuclear receptor superfamily (Greene et al., 1980; Walter et al., 1985; Green et al., 1986). Ten years later, in 1995, Gustafsson's laboratory discovered a second ER. The "Jensen" receptor was than named ERα and the new receptor ERβ (Kuiper et al., 1996). ERα and ERβ have distinct tissue expression patterns (Kuiper et al., 1997). In

fact, many tissues previously thought to be "estrogen-insensitive tissue" were found to be ERβ positive and estrogen sensitive, with ERβ highly expressed and is almost the exclusive ER in ovarian granulose cells. ERα is the main ER subtype in the liver, breast and ovaries, while ERβ is predominantly in the prostate, colon and lung (Gustafsson, 1999; Pearce and Jordan, 2004). Thus, the proliferative actions of estrogens mediated via ERα can be opposed by ERβ (Pearce and Jordan, 2004; Chang et al., 2008; Jensen et al., 2010).

2.2 Estrogen receptors structure

ERα and ERβ have the typical structure of the nuclear receptor family (figure 1): a highly variable N-terminal region (A/B domain, involved in protein-protein interactions with transcriptional machinery and cofactors), a highly conserved DNA-binding domain (C), a hinge domain (D), a ligand-binding domain (E) and a C-terminal domain (F) (Giguere et al., 1986; Kumar et al., 1987).

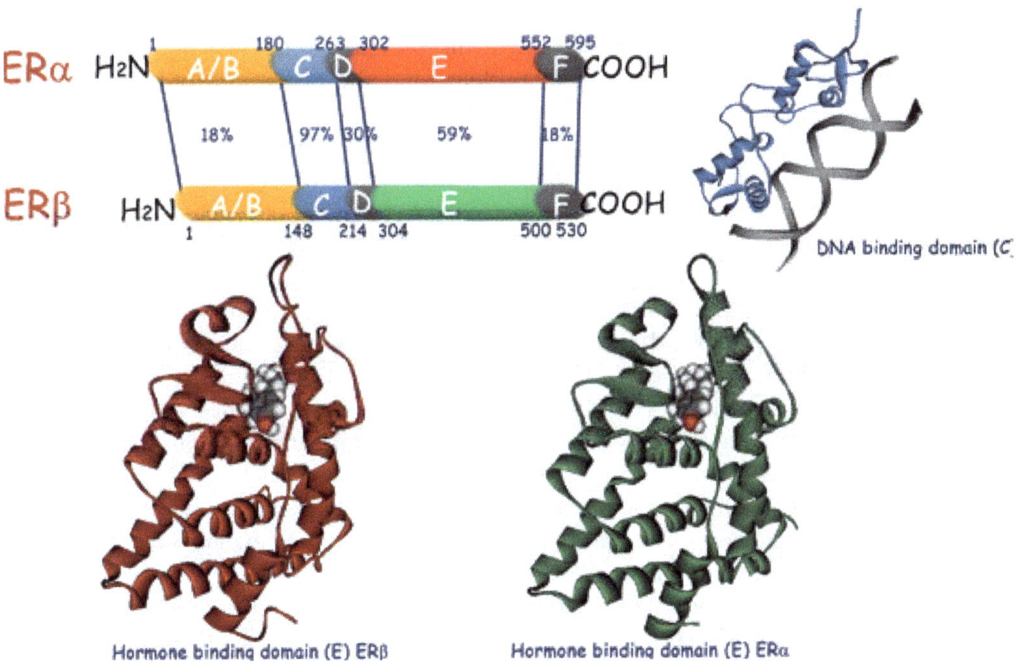

Fig. 1. ERα and ERβ structures. Schematic representation of the structure ERα and ERβ, structure DNA binding domain and structure of the hormone binding domain of both estrogen receptors.

ERα (595 aa) and ERβ (530 aa) receptors are codified by two different genes with less than 18% homology between them in A/B domain, although there is a 97% of homology between their respective DNA-binding domains (the most conserved). This domain (C) contains two zinc fingers and has a short motif, called a P-box, which is responsible for DNA specificity and is also involved in dimerization (Nilsson et al., 2001; Morani et al., 2008). Consequently both receptors ERα and ERβ bind to DNA in a similar manner, but the association with different cofactors enables them to modulate transcription genes (Giguere et al., 1986; Kumar et al., 1987). The D domain has nuclear localization signals and could provide malleability between the C and E domains. The E domain has the property for ligand binding, with its ligand-binding pocket formed by 12 alpha-helixes, and which is 60% conserved between the two estrogen receptors (Spithill et al., 1979; Morani et al., 2008). Moreover this domain is also involved in other functions such as receptor dimerization, nuclear localization and cofactor interaction. Finally, the F domain is extremely variable and contributes gene transactivation capacity (Morani et al., 2008).

2.3 Mechanisms of ER activation

Estrogens can act through different mechanisms and pathways to cause their biological effects (Gonzalez et al., 1993; Nilsson et al., 2001). There is a typical nuclear receptor superfamily mechanism to modulate the expression of several genes. Estrogen activates ER by ligand binding to the receptor, but this unity can occur in to forms. The first can occur when E_2-ER complex has formed in the cytoplasm and then is transported to the nucleus through cytoskeleton regulated mechanisms. The second form has the same final product, but occurs by a direct E_2 binding to the ER in the nucleus, with this union allowing for eventual ER dissociation of the chaperon proteins and the restoration of the ER to the inactive state. After this dissociation, ER can form either heterodimers or homodimers and bind directly to estrogen response element (ERE) through the DNA-binding domain as well as by association with different gene regulation co activators (Nilsson et al., 2001; Morani et al., 2008).

Another mechanism includes the involvement of the SP1 protein in the formation of the bridge between the activated estrogen receptor dimer and ERE (Kushner et al., 2000; Saville et al., 2000). This mechanism forms an indirect activation/inhibition of E_2 regulated genes and some authors have found differences dependant on the ERα and ERβ union to ERE (Sidhu and Tauro, 1979; Morani et al., 2008).

Another action of ERs, in a non-genomic process, involves the interaction of activated ERs with secondary messenger proteins (SM) with rapid, concomitant effects in many tissues, although this process is still not well understood (Heldring et al., 2007).

Furthermore, ERs have a ligand-independent activation mechanism, involving kinases that phosphorylate and activate ERs and this mechanism could explain the hormone-independent growth of some tumours.

Other factors have an important role in the activation mechanisms of ERs and serve as corregulators (or cofactors) recruited by the ERs to activate (coactivator) or to repress (corepressor) the transcriptional activity of ERs. These corregulators can modify the affinity of the ERs to EREs and can be in the form of acetylases/deacetylases, kinases/phosphatases and methylases/demethylases. It must be emphasized, however, that the pool of corregulators can differ according to the type of tissue, and it is the fact that has been proposed as an explanation for the differential tissue effects of estrogen and selective estrogen receptor modulator (SERMS).

Moreover, not only do corregulators differ according to tissue, the distribution of ERα and ERβ has also been reported to vary. In the tissues when both ERα and ERβ coexist, their effects seem to counteract each other. Thus, in the uterus, mammary glands and the immune systems, ERα promotes cell proliferation while ERβ has proapoptotic and cell differentiation functions (Morani et al., 2008).

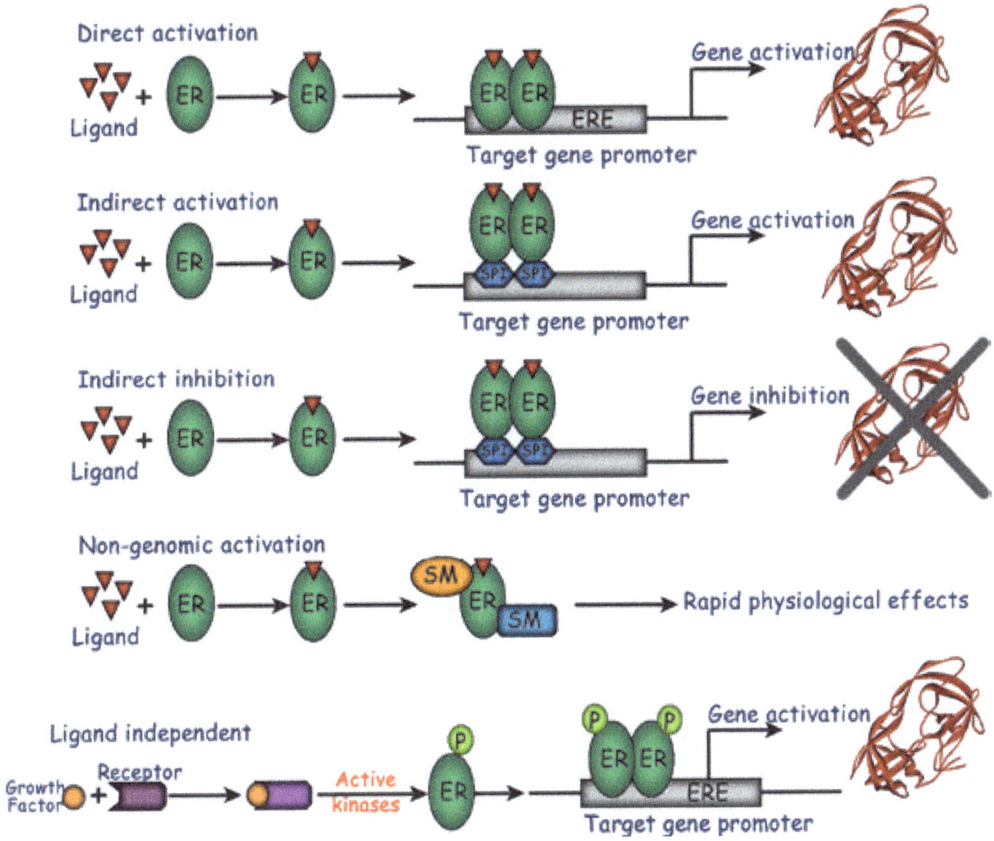

Fig. 2. Mechanisms ER activation.

3. Breast cancer and estrogens

3.1 Mammary gland and estrogens

Development and physiology of the mammary gland are under estrogen control and suffers important changes during a women's lifespan and estrogens have an active role in these changes. During puberty the glands undergoes an increased cellular division and in adult life there is a proliferation/involution cycle according to menstrual cycle (Russo et al., 1999). The role of estrogen in mammary epithelial proliferation has been unclear, because the proliferation markers in ductal epithelial cells never co localize with ERα (Saji et al., 2000).

For a long time, estrogens were believed to induce proliferation through indirect effects, such as growth factor secretion to the stroma. However, recent studies suggest that when ERα is activated by estrogen it is quickly lost in the beginning of the G1 phase of the cell cycle. This fact could be explain the non-colocalisation of ERα with proliferation markers, such as cyclin A or PCNA, tipycal from the S phase (Morani et al., 2008).

Ductal cells in the mammary gland appear to be one example of cells where ERα and ERβ counteract each other in estrogen-stimulated proliferation. The proliferative response to E_2 seems to be determined by the ratio of ERα / ERβ. The functions of ERβ in the breast are probably related to its antiproliferative as well as its prodifferentiative functions (Strom et al., 2004).

In studies with MCF7 cells, a breast cancer cell line expressing ERα but not ERβ, showed that E_2 increases proliferation, and when ERβ was artificially introduced into these cells, E_2-induced proliferation was inhibited (Schatz, 1979).

3.2 Breast cancer estrogen induction

Estrogens are a major risk factor for breast cancer initiation and progression, as they affect epithelial mammary cell growth and these cells are more susceptible to make DNA replication errors. Another point of view is that estrogens produce oxidant species for their metabolism (quinine metabolites) that can form adducts in DNA and generate reactive oxygen species (ROS) through a redox cycle (Russo et al., 2003; Yager and Davidson, 2006).

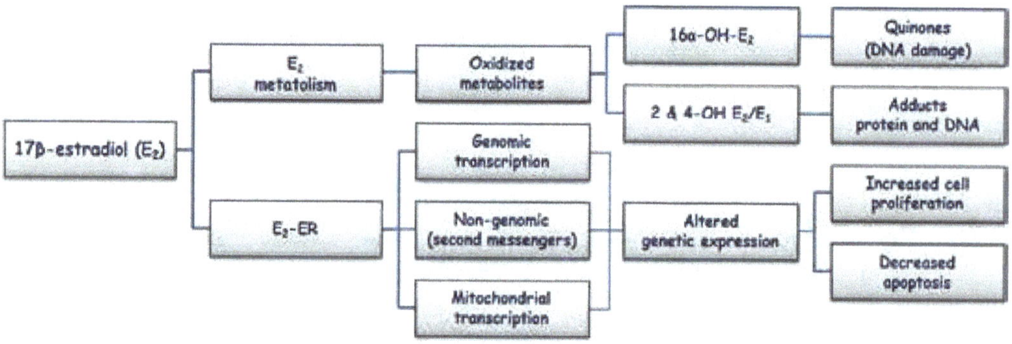

Fig. 3. Estrogen carcinogenesis mechanisms: E_2: 17β-estradiol. ER: estrogen receptor. 16α-OH-E_2: 16α-hydroxyE_2. 2-OH-E_2: 2-hydroxyE_2. 4-OH-E_2: 4-hydroxyE_2. 2-OH-E_1 2-hydroxyestrone. 4-OH-E_1 4-hydroxyestrone.

In recent years, EREs have been found in mitochondrial DNA, suggesting that the carcinogenic role of estrogen could be mediated by the action of these molecules in the mitochondria (Gonzalez et al., 1993; Sogl et al., 2000). Moreover, as mentioned earlier, the two subtypes of estrogen receptors have different actions in several tissues and therefore it is entirely possible that the effects will differ in mitochondria as well. Other papers have studied the localization of ERα and ERβ in the mitochondria and the regulation of mitochondrial genes (Gonzalez et al., 1993; Sogl et al., 2000; Chen et al., 2004; Pedram et al., 2006; Amutha et al., 2009; Usmanova et al., 2011). Furthermore, apoptotic pathways and the presence of estrogen receptor in the mitochondria could be important for carcinogenic processes (Gonzalez et al., 1993; Sogl et al., 2000).

The majority of ER-positive breast tumours contain both ERα and ERβ subtypes, although some tumours have only ERβ and may have distinct clinical behaviours and responses. In contrast to ERα, studies suggest that ERβ expression declines during breast tumourigenesis (Roger et al., 2001; Skliris et al., 2003; Bardin et al., 2004; Hartman et al., 2009). The mechanism by which ERβ is downregulated is not fully understood, but epigenetic changes could play an important role (Zhao et al., 2003). This downregulation of ERβ in breast cancers indicates a role for ERβ as a tumour suppressor (Novelli et al., 2008; Fox et al., 2008). Characterization of the role of ERβ in ERα negative tumors is basically unexplored, but available data suggest that the role of ERβ may differ depending if it is co-expressed with ERα or expressed alone (Fox et al., 2008; Skliris et al., 2008; Hartman et al., 2009). Classically, the ERα negative tumors are considered endocrine resistant since they lack a receptor to mediate the estrogenic response. However, it has been observed that approximately 50% of this subgroup expresses ERβ (Skliris et al., 2006). Several studies have been published different conclusions for correlations with ERβ, prognostic markers and clinical outcome. Reports have shown that tumours that co-expressed ERβ and ERα have a good prognosis and good clinical outcome with adjuvant therapy. Additional studies have considered the addition of ERβ to ERα as clinical tumor marker as beneficial (Murphy and Watson, 2006; Skliris et al., 2006; Gruvberger-Saal et al., 2007; Skliris et al., 2008; Hartman et al., 2009). Conversely, very few studies have focused on ERβ expression in ERα negative breast tumors; where ERβ has been described as a marker for poor prognosis and endocrine resistance (Leygue et al., 1998; Speirs et al., 1999; O'Neill et al., 2004; Skliris et al., 2006; Fox et al., 2008; Skliris et al., 2008; Hartman et al., 2009) (table 1).

ERα and ERβ status	Clinical outcome
ERα+/ ERβ+	Increased overall survival and disease-free survival correlated ERβ+
ERα+/ ERβ-	Worst prognosis
ERα-/ ERβ+	Less favorable prognosis, ERβ seems to correlate with the proliferation

Table 1. Clinical correlation between ERα/ ERβ expression and evaluation response to endocrine therapy in breast cancer.

An increased ERα/ERβ ratio respect to non tumoral breast tissue is an important factor for the development of the cancerous phenotype (Stossi et al., 2004; Strom et al., 2004; Adam et al., 2006; Garcia-Roves et al., 2007; Morani et al., 2008). On the contrary, a decrease in this ratio (due to ERβ increase) is indicative of a poor prognosis and problems with antiestrogen treatment (Power and Thompson, 2003). This evidence could also explain the different action of estrogens and phytoestrogens through varing ERα and ERβ levels (Sotoca et al., 2008).

Another difference between ERα and ERβ is estrogen activation, because estrogen stimulates both ERα and ERβ receptors, although it is 10 times more selective for ERα than ERβ (Kuiper et al., 1998; Quaedackers et al., 2001). Furthermore, several authors shave shown that estrogen regulation of ERα and ERβ expression, causing a decrease in ERα and an increase in ERβ in ERα-positive cell lines such as MCF-7 and T47D (Power and Thompson, 2003; Lee et al., 2005). In addition to this important fact, oxidative stress also regulates ERα and ERβ levels, and in the same manner, causes downregulation of ERα and upregulation of ERβ (Tamir et al., 2002).

4. Estrogens, mitochondria and oxidative stress

Classically, it has been suggested that estrogens induce growth in mammary gland epithelial cells. This high cell proliferation can increase susceptibility to the acquirement of error-induced mutations during DNA replication, which if not corrected can establish a malignant phenotype (Gonzalez et al., 1993). Another mechanism to explain this association is that estrogens can produce genotoxic metabolites during their metabolism (cathecol estrogens), that can make DNA adducts and create ROS through redox cycle (Russo et al., 2003; Yager and Davidson, 2006), but for these compounds to have a relevant impact, the estrogen concentration must be higher than physiological levels.

Recently, ERs have been found in the mitochondria, and in mitochondrial DNA there are EREs. Moreover, mitochondrial biogenesis and ROS production are under estrogen influence. For this reason, some authors give estrogens a new role in the carcinogenesis process, in the modulation of mitochondrial function (Addison and McCormick, 1978; Sogl et al., 2000). The changes in mitochondrial function cause an increase in ROS production, which alters the control that mitochondria exerts in cellular proliferation and apoptosis, and which could explain the action of estrogen in cancer development (Addison and McCormick, 1978; Gonzalez et al., 1993).

4.1 Mitochondria

Mitochondria are important organelles in eukaryotic cells. The structure of the mitochondrion is delimited by an outer and inner membrane. The former is wrinkled and completely surrounds the organelle. The later has infolding called cristae where the mitochondrial respiratory chain (MRC) resides. The inner compartment of mitochondria, the matrix, is a concentrated aqueous solution of many enzymes and chemical intermediates involved in energy-yielding metabolism. The outer membrane is a relatively simple phospholipid bilayer, containing protein structures called porins which render it permeable to molecules of about 10 kDA or less (the size of the smallest proteins). Ions, nutrient molecules, ATP, ADP, etc. can pass through the outer membrane with ease. The inner membrane is only freely permeable to oxygen, carbon dioxide, and water. Its structure is highly complex, including all of the complexes of the electron transport system, the ATP synthase complex and transport proteins.

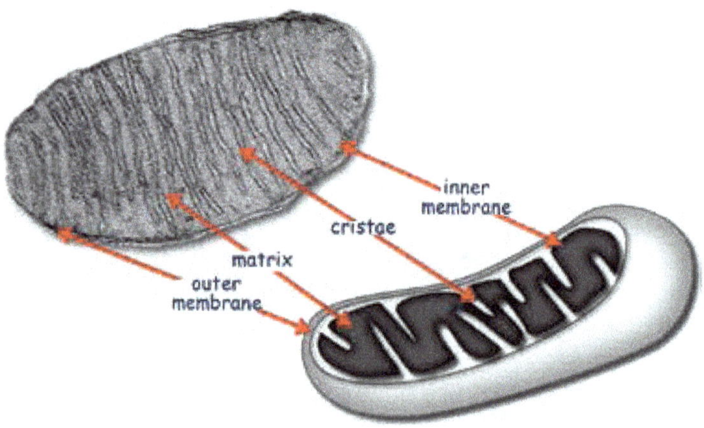

Fig. 4. Mitochondrial structure.

Mitochondria are the intracellular organelles responsible for the supply of ATP (generation of more than 90% of the cell's energy requirements) and are also the main intracellular source and target of reactive oxygen species (ROS). Mitochondria also participate in the regulation of intracellular calcium homeostasis by controlling various ion channels and transporters and participation in heme and steroid biosynthesis. In addition, mitochondria play a role in the regulation of cellular proliferation and apoptosis (Gonzalez et al., 1993).

The primary role of mitochondria is the generation of ATP through a complex process of controlled substrate degradation and oxygen consumption known as oxidative phosphorylation (OXPHOS) (Korb and Neupert, 1978). The inner membrane mitochondrial contains the large protein complexes that are necessary for energy transduction and ATP synthesis. Briefly, oxidation of reduced nutrient molecules, such as carbohydrates, lipids, and proteins, through cellular metabolism yields electrons in the form of the reduced hydrogen carriers $NADH^+$ and $FADH_2$. These reduced cofactors donate electrons to a series of protein complexes of the electron transport chain embedded in the inner mitochondrial membrane. These complexes (complex I, III and IV) use the energy released from electron transport for the active pumping of protons across the inner membrane, thereby generating an electrochemical gradient. The ultimate destiny of these electrons is the reduction of molecular oxygen at complex IV to yield a molecule of water, whereas the energy, conserved as a proton gradient, is used by the F_0F_1 ATP synthase (or complex V) to phosphorylate ADP through the return of protons into the mitochondrial matrix (Devenish et al., 1978).

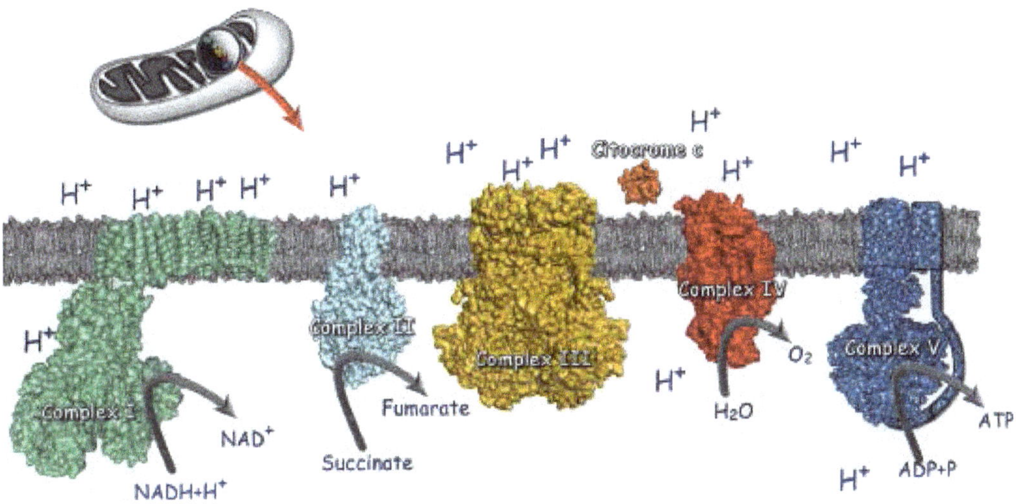

Fig. 5. The mitochondrial oxidative phosphorylation system.

Although mitochondria have their own genome, most of the proteins and enzymes that reside in the mitochondrial membranes are nuclear gene products. Each mammalian cell contains several hundred to more than a thousand mitochondria, and each organelle harbours 2–10 copies of mitochondrial DNA (mtDNA) (Amutha et al., 2008). The double-strand circular mtDNA consists of 16,500 base pairs (bp). This DNA encodes 13 protein coding genes (or polypeptides), 22 transfer RNA (or tRNA) and 2 ribosomal RNA (or rRNA) necessary for the translation. The 13 polypeptides including seven subunits of complex I-NADH dehydrogenase (ND1, ND2, ND3, ND4, ND4L, ND5, and ND6), three subunits of complex III-cytochrome c oxidase (COI, COII, and COIII), two subunits of complex V-F_0F_1ATPase (ATPase 6 and ATPase 8), and cytochrome b are encoded by mtDNA and synthesized in the organelle (Molina-Navarro et al., 2006). A single major noncoding region, referred to as the displacement loop (D-loop), contains the primary regulatory sequences for transcription and imitation of replication (Menassa et al., 1997). mtDNA is first transcribed to a larger mitochondrial transcript precursor, from which the 13 mRNAs, 22 tRNAs and 2 rRNAs are derived (Menassa et al., 1997).

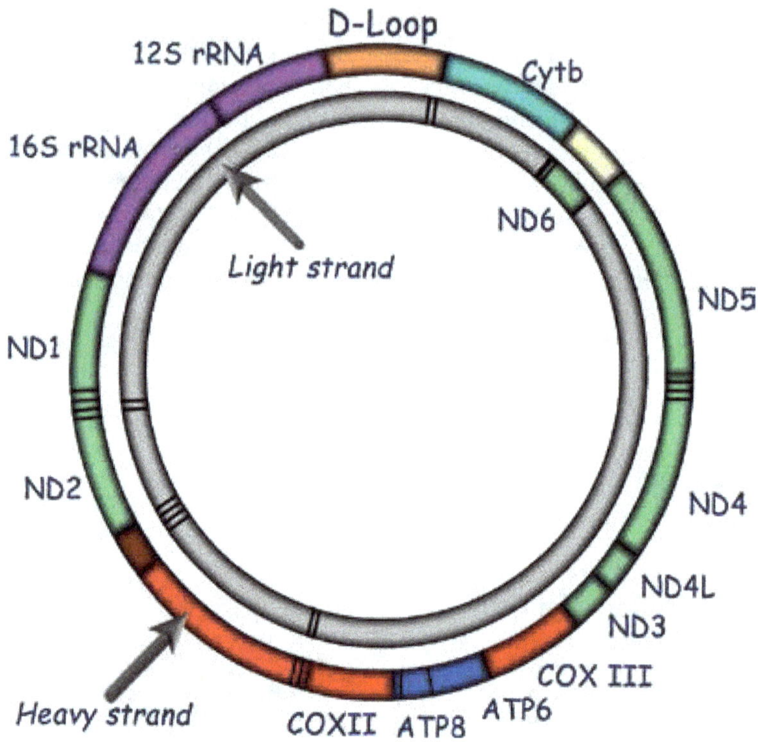

Fig. 6. The mitochondrial genome. The mammalian mitochondrial genome is a circular double stranded molecule, composed of one heavy and one light strand.

The assembly and functioning of the respiratory enzyme complexes in mammalian cells require coordinated expression and interaction between gene products of the mitochondrial and nuclear genomes (Menassa et al., 1997). Correct mitochondrial biogenesis relies on the spatiotemporally coordinated synthesis and import of ~1000 proteins encoded by the nuclear genome, of which some are assembled with proteins encoded by mitochondrial DNA within the newly synthesized phospholipid membranes of the inner and outer mitochondrial membranes. (Klingenspor et al., 1996).

	Complex I	Complex II	Complex III	Complex IV	Complex V
mtDNA	7	0	1	3	2
nDNA	39	4	9	10	10

Table 2. Nuclear and mitochondrial respiratory subunits.

Transcription and replication of mitochondrial DNA is driven by the nuclear-encoded mitochondrial transcription factor A (TFAM), which binds to a common upstream enhancer of the promoter sites of the two mitochondrial DNA strands. (Klingenspor et al., 1996) Additionally, two proteins that interact with the mammalian mitochondrial RNA polymerase and TFAM, TFB1M and TFB2M, can support promoter-specific mtDNA transcription (Addya et al., 1997). Nuclear respiratory factors 1 and 2 control (NRF1 and NRF2) play an important role in the regulation of mitochondrial respiratory function, as they on one hand control nuclear transcription of the subunits of the respiratory chain complexes (Schuster, 1994) as well as activate the expression of factors involved in the initiation of transcription of the mitochondrial genome, such as TFAM, and TFB2M TFB1M (Addya et al., 1997).

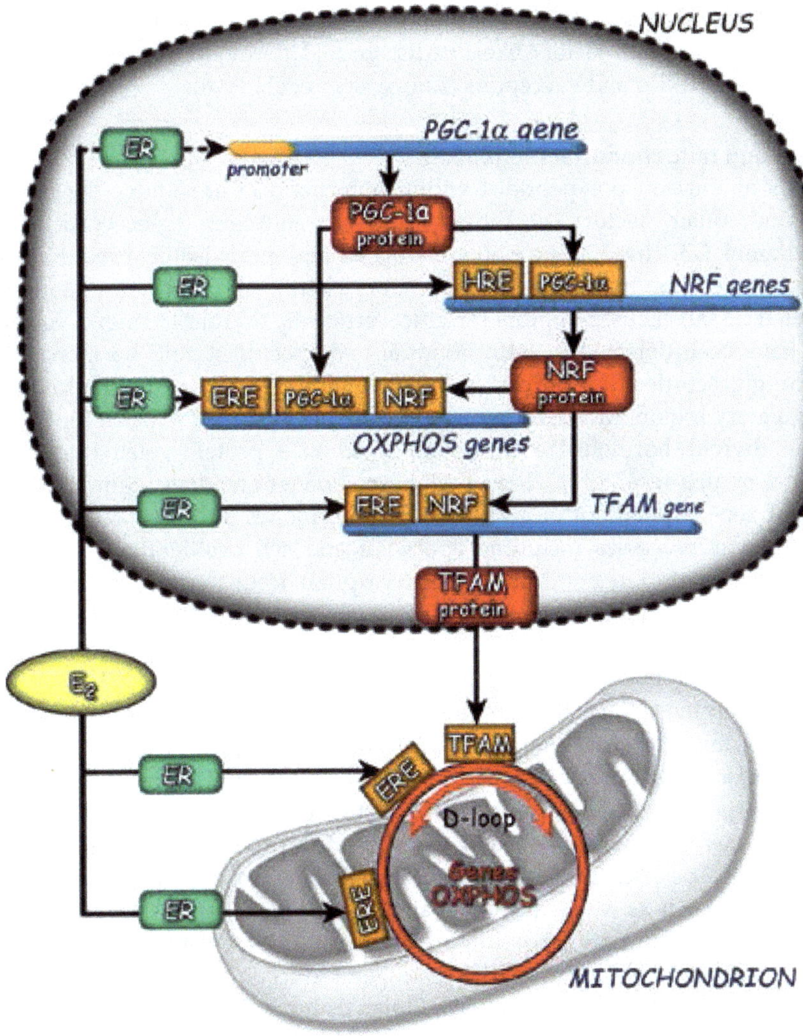

Fig. 7. Coordination of transcription of nuclear and mitochondrial genes encoding OXPHOS by steroid hormones.

The TFAM promoter contains recognition sites for NRF1 and/or NRF2, thus allowing coordination between mitochondrial and nuclear activation during mitochondrial biogenesis. However, there is a subset of genes that does not appear to be regulated by NRFs. For example, fatty acid transport proteins and oxidation enzyme genes are mainly regulated by the peroxisome proliferator-activated receptor alpha PPARα (Klingenspor et al., 1996).

Peroxisome proliferator-activated receptor gamma co-activator (PGC-1α) lacks DNA-binding activity but interacts with and co-activates numerous transcription factors including NRFs on the promoter of TFAM. Mitochondrial biogenesis and respiration are stimulated by PGC-1α through a powerful induction of NRF1 and NRF2 gene expression (Giege et al., 2008). Data are accumulating that show PGC-1α to be a master regulator of mitochondrial biogenesis in mammals (Klingenspor et al., 1996). In addition to NRFs, PGC-1α also interacts with and co-activates other transcription factors like PPARs, thyroid hormone, glucocorticoid, estrogen, and estrogen-related ERRα and γ receptors (Klingenspor et al., 1996).

4.2 Estrogen and mitochondrial biogenesis

The synthesis of thirteen polypeptides within mitochondria are under the regulation of hormones and other factors, including cortisol, androgen, glucocorticoids, 1,25α-dihydroxyvitamin D3, thyroid hormone, estrogens and peroxisome proliferators, which have profound effects on mitochondrial respiratory chain (MRC) activities (Gonzalez et al., 1993; Sogl et al., 2000). Thus, receptors for glucocorticoids, thyroid hormone, estrogens and androgens have been detected in mitochondrial and specific steroid hormone responsive elements for glucocorticoids, thyroid hormone and estrogen are found in the human mtDNA regulatory region. Moreover the ligand-activated glucocorticoid receptor, a variant form of the thyroid hormone receptor and a 45 kDa protein related to peroxisome proliferation-activated receptor γ2, have each been shown to mediate stimulatory effects on mitochondrial gene expression. In addition, these hormones and their receptors control a number of cellular processes including apoptosis and cell proliferation. It is likely that hormonal regulation of mitochondrial gene transcription occur through mechanisms similar to those that control nuclear gene transcription. These insights have extended our understanding of hormone action at the cellular level (Gonzalez et al., 1993).

In the last years, there has been increasing evidence pointing to the MRC as a novel and important target for the actions of E_2 and ERs in a number of cell types and tissues that have high demand for mitochondrial energy metabolism for their biological activities. This novel E2-mediated mitochondrial pathway involves the cooperation of the nuclear ERα and ERβ with mitochondrial localized ERs and their co-activators on the coordinate regulation of both-encoded genes and mtDNA-encoded genes for MRC proteins (Sogl et al., 2000).

ERα and ERβ have been detected in the mitochondria of several human cells, including breast cancer cells such as MCF7 (Chen et al., 2004; Pedram et al., 2006). Thus estrogens regulate the biogenesis and mitochondrial function through cross-talk between the nucleus and the mitochondria to control the estrogen-induced signaling involved in the proliferation, apoptosis and differentiation cellular (Felty and Roy, 2005). E_2 stimulates the expression of TFAM and possibly TFB1M and TFB2M via the activation of NRF-1 and NRF-2, and it is likely that E_2 and ERs stimulate the transcription via activation of the expression of these mitochondrial transcriptional factors (Sogl et al., 2000). Moreover, it has been found that E_2 significantly enhanced the amounts of mitochondrial ERα and ERβ in a time- and concentration-dependent manner and that these effects are accompanied by a significant increase in the transcript levels of mtDNA-encoded genes (Chen et al., 2004).

4.3 Estrogen and mitochondrial ROS production

Mitochondrial ROS production is under estrogen influence and the consequences of this production in the control that mitochondria exerts in cellular proliferation and apoptosis could be explain the action of estrogen in cancer development (Gonzalez et al., 1993; Sogl et al., 2000).

Mitochondria are the most important source of ROS production in mammalian cells, as under normal physiological conditions about 1% of electrons during transfer along the respiratory chain, escape and form a single electron reduction of molecular oxygen to form a superoxide anion ($O2^{\bullet-}$), which in turn is the precursor of other ROS (Fariss et al., 2005; Murphy, 2009). Aerobic respiration involves the complete reduction of oxygen to water, which is catalyzed by complex IV (or cytochrome c oxidase). Superoxide is rapidly converted to hydrogen peroxide (H_2O_2), either spontaneously or is enzymatically catalyzed by superoxide dismutase (SOD). H_2O_2, although not an oxygen free radical, can lead to the production, in the presence of ferrous iron via the Fenton reaction, of the highly reactive hydroxyl radical ($^{\bullet}OH$). ROS production can be significantly enhanced with a high mitochondrial potential membrane that can occur with abundant fuel supply (high NADH production) or with the functional impairment of complexes I or III of respiratory chain, while ROS production decreased with reduced energy demand (Lenaz, 2001; Chen et al., 2003; Fariss et al., 2005).

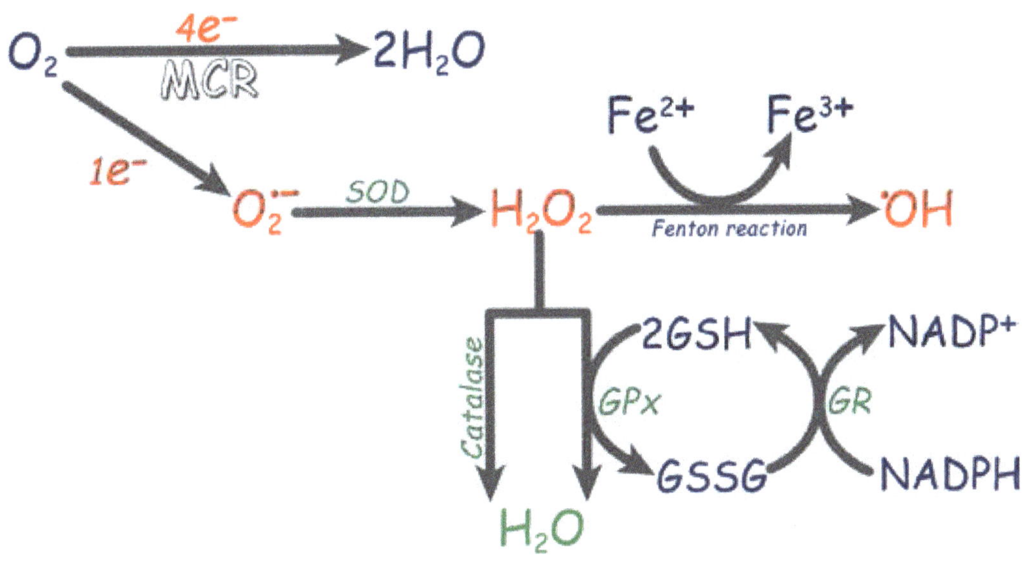

Fig. 8. ROS detoxification mechanisms.

ROS can be dissipated by the action of several enzymes, as SOD, glutation peroxidase (GPx) and glutation reductase (GR). SOD transforms $O2^{\bullet-}$ in H_2O_2, which is detoxified by the action of two enzymes, catalase and GPx yielding H_2O. Glutathione (GSH) is regenerated from glutathione disulfide (GSSG) by the action of GR, using NADPH as a reducing equivalent. Non-enzymatic antioxidants (as vitamins C and E) provide alternative targets to ROS reactivity, thus avoiding the deleterious effects on cell components (Fariss et al., 2005; Murphy, 2009).

Another mechanism to be included within the systems that can protect against oxidative damage are the uncoupling proteins or UCPs (Addison and McCormick, 1978; Echtay, 2007).

UCPs are a family of inner mitochondrial membrane proteins whose function is to allow the re-entry of protons into the mitochondrial matrix dissipate the proton gradient and, subsequently, decrease the membrane potential and ROS production (Addison and McCormick, 1978; Echtay, 2007).

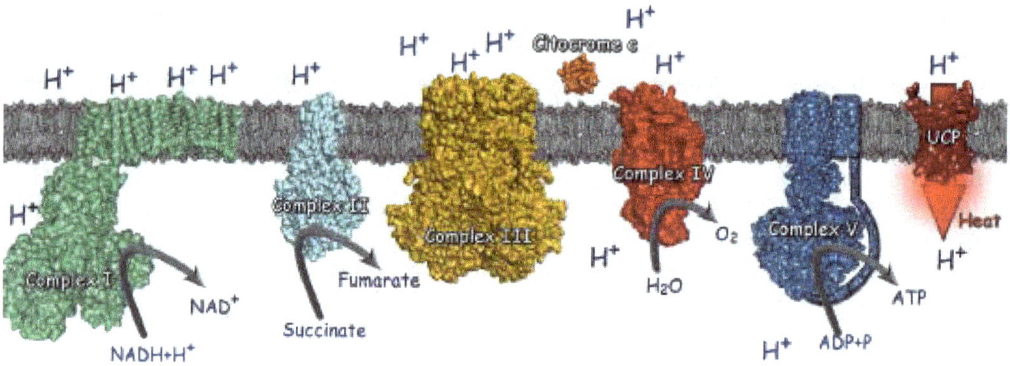

Fig. 9. Mitochondrial oxidative phosphorylation system and uncoupling protein.

When cellular production of ROS overwhelms the overall antioxidant defenses, free radicals may escape and exert their deleterious effects. This situation is oxidative stress, and is supposed to be responsible for the accrual of cellular damage during its lifetime, thereby playing a role in the etiogenesis and course of numerous pathologies and in the aging process (Addison and McCormick, 1978; Lenaz, 2001). Macromolecules within the mitochondria are more prone to ROS-induced damage due to their physical proximity to ROS sources. In addition, mitochondrial DNA, which lacks protective histone shields and also has limited DNA-repair systems, is especially vulnerable to such damage. It is worth noting that the damage exerted by ROS on mitochondrial DNA may lead to a higher degree of mitochondrial dysfunction and in turn, to a higher ROS production, leading to a vicious cycle of ROS amplification (Fariss et al., 2005).

Nevertheless, ROS should not be seen only in a negative light or as just damaging to molecules. It is worth noting that the rapidly-produced, short-lived, and highly diffusible ROS also perfectly fits the characteristics of a second messenger molecule. In fact, although ROS do cause damage, low levels of ROS are thought to participate in cell signaling processes such as cell proliferation, inflammation, apoptosis and phagocytosis (Obbink et al., 1977). Thus, it is well established by many studies that ROS may act as second messengers in cellular signaling transduction cascade pathways, including stress-activated protein kinases (SAPK) with both p38MAPK and c-Jun N-terminal kinase (JNK), p53 (universal sensor of genotoxic stress) through PI3K/PKB and NF-κB pathways (Harkness et al., 1994; Sauer et al., 2001; Martindale and Holbrook, 2002; Sanders et al., 2004; Murphy, 2009). In this complex context, low levels of ROS stimulate cellular proliferation, while high levels induce apoptosis. In summary, many cellular signal pathways are sensible to ROS levels and the final cellular response depends on the final cell interpretation, which is the result of equilibrium between apoptotic signals and proliferative and survival signals (Addison and McCormick, 1978).

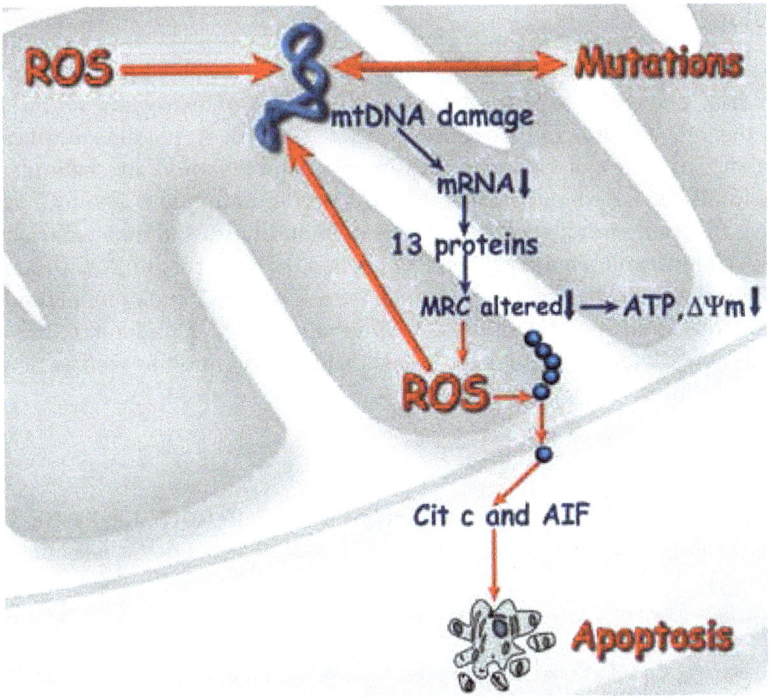

Fig. 10. Mitochondrial DNA and oxidative stress and apoptosis.

Estrogens can mediate in the complex process of ROS cellular level control. Thus, estrogens control mitochondrial biogenesis and maintenance, which are induced by signal pathways related to cellular proliferation, differentiation and apoptosis (Gonzalez et al., 1993). Moreover, mitochondrial ROS production can be regulated by estrogens through both nuclear and mitochondrial ER, with regulation by these via mitochondrial structure and function (Vic et al., 1982; Tam and Wong, 1991). Additionally estrogen controls the ROS dissipation, since expression of antioxidant enzymes and UCPs are induced by ERE (Chen et al., 2004). However, the literature is contradictory in this aspect, as the effect depends on tissue studied, estrogen concentration and *in vitro* or *in vivo* studies. For example, while oxidative stress induction in breast and prostate cancer cell lines has been described, in liver, brain, skeletal and cardiac muscle as well as adipose tissue, a protector role has been described to estrogen for the avoidance of oxidative stress (Valle et al., 2005; Colom et al., 2007a; Colom et al., 2007b; Valle et al., 2007a; Valle et al., 2007b; Guevara et al., 2008; Valle et al., 2008). This controversy could be attributed to the different ERα and ERβ ratios in different tissues. Thus in MCF7 breast cancer cell lines (with a high ratio of ERα/ERβ) estrogen induces oxidative stress either by or in combination with mitochondrial dysfunction, decrease in antioxidant enzymes and/or UCPs. On the contrary, in MDA-MB-231 breast cancer cell lines (with only ERα) no effects have been detected in the same conditions (Garcia-Roves et al., 2007). In addition it has been described , for prostrate cell lines which had the greatest levels of ERβ and the lowest ERα/ERβ ratio, that E_2 treatment caused the up-regulation of antioxidant enzymes and UCPs with a look-up decrease in ROS production. These effects were reversed when the cells were treated with E_2 in the presence of an ERβ antagonist (Houstek et al., 1990).

5. Conclusion

ERα and ERβ endowment can be of great importance in the establishment of oxidative stress in mitochondria, and may explain the opposite effects of estrogens found in different tissues. On the other hand, the presence of UCPs and their possible implication in the oxidative balance of breast cancer cell lines is notable and it should also be underscored that UCP expression is regulated, or sensible to, estrogen regulation and also to ERα/ERβ ratio. For the above mentioned evidence, a better understanding of the molecular action of ERα and ERβ, especially at mitochondrial level, is needed, as their role in ROS production could explain both the implication of estrogen in breast cancer development and its cancer protective role observed in other tissues. Additionally, a better understanding at this level could provide new dietary strategies for breast cancer prevention as well as new anticancer therapeutic procedures.

6. Acknowledgment

This work was supported by the Spanish Government (PS09/01637). J. Sastre-Serra and M. Nadal-Serrano were funded by grants of Comunidad Autónoma de las Islas Baleares.

7. References

Adam, A.C., Bornhovd, C., Prokisch, H., Neupert, W., & Hell, K. (2006). The Nfs1 interacting protein Isd11 has an essential role in Fe/S cluster biogenesis in mitochondria. *EMBO Journal,* Vol.25. No.1, (Jan 11). pp. 174-183, ISSN 0261-4189.

Addison, R., & McCormick, D.B. (1978). Biogenesis of flavoprotein and cytochrome components in hepatic mitochondria from riboflavin-deficient rats. *Biochemical and Biophysical Research Communications,* Vol.81. No.1, (Mar 15). pp. 133-138, ISSN 0006-291X.

Addya, S., Anandatheerthavarada, H.K., Biswas, G., Bhagwat, S.V., Mullick, J., & Avadhani, N.G. (1997). Targeting of NH2-terminal-processed microsomal protein to mitochondria: a novel pathway for the biogenesis of hepatic mitochondrial P450MT2. *Journal of Cell Biology,* Vol.139. No.3, (Nov 3). pp. 589-599, ISSN 0021-9525.

Amutha, B., Gordon, D.M., Dancis, A., & Pain, D. (2009). Chapter 14 Nucleotide-dependent iron-sulfur cluster biogenesis of endogenous and imported apoproteins in isolated intact mitochondria. *Methods in Enzymology,* Vol.456. pp. 247-266, ISSN 1557-7988.

Amutha, B., Gordon, D.M., Gu, Y., Lyver, E.R., Dancis, A., & Pain, D. (2008). GTP is required for iron-sulfur cluster biogenesis in mitochondria. *Journal of Biological Chemistry,* Vol.283. No.3, (Jan 18). pp. 1362-1371, ISSN 0021-9258.

Bardin, A., Boulle, N., Lazennec, G., Vignon, F., & Pujol, P. (2004). Loss of ERbeta expression as a common step in estrogen-dependent tumor progression. *Endocrine-Related Cancer,* Vol.11. No.3, (Sep). pp. 537-551, ISSN 1351-0088.

Catalano, S., Marsico, S., Giordano, C., Mauro, L., Rizza, P., Panno, M.L., & Ando, S. (2003). Leptin enhances, via AP-1, expression of aromatase in the MCF-7 cell line. *Journal of Biological Chemistry,* Vol.278. No.31, (Aug 1). pp. 28668-28676, ISSN 0021-9258.

Colom, B., Alcolea, M.P., Valle, A., Oliver, J., Roca, P., & Garcia-Palmer, F.J. (2007). Skeletal muscle of female rats exhibit higher mitochondrial mass and oxidativephosphorylative capacities compared to males. *Cellular Physiology and Biochemistry,* Vol.19. No.1-4, pp. 205-212, ISSN 1015-8987.

Colom, B., Oliver, J., Roca, P., & Garcia-Palmer, F.J. (2007). Caloric restriction and gender modulate cardiac muscle mitochondrial H2O2 production and oxidative damage. *Cardiovascular Research,* Vol.74. No.3, (Jun 1). pp. 456-465, ISSN 0008-6363.

Chang, E.C., Charn, T.H., Park, S.H., Helferich, W.G., Komm, B., Katzenellenbogen, J.A., & Katzenellenbogen, B.S. (2008). Estrogen Receptors alpha and beta as determinants of gene expression: influence of ligand, dose, and chromatin binding. *Molecular Endocrinology,* Vol.22. No.5, (May). pp. 1032-1043, ISSN 0888-8809.

Chen, J.Q., Delannoy, M., Cooke, C., & Yager, J.D. (2004). Mitochondrial localization of ERalpha and ERbeta in human MCF7 cells. *American Journal of Physiology Endocrinology and Metabolism,* Vol.286. No.6, (Jun). pp. E1011-1022, ISSN 0193-1849.

Chen, Q., Vazquez, E.J., Moghaddas, S., Hoppel, C.L., & Lesnefsky, E.J. (2003). Production of reactive oxygen species by mitochondria: central role of complex III. *Journal of Biological Chemistry,* Vol.278. No.38, (Sep 19). pp. 36027-36031, ISSN 0021-9258.

Devenish, R.J., Englisn, K.J., Hall, R.M., Linnase, A.W., & Lukins, H.B. (1978). Biogenesis of mitochondria 49 identification and mapping of a new mitochondrial locus (tsr1) which maps within polar region of yeast mitochondrial genome. *Molecular and General Genetics,* Vol.161. No.3, (May 31). pp. 251-259, ISSN 0026-8925.

Devenish, R.J., Hall, R.M., Linnane, A.W., & Lukins, H.B. (1979). Biogenesis of mitochondria. 52. Deletions in petite strains occurring in the mitochondrial gene for the 21 S ribosomal RNA, that affect the properties of mitochondrial recombination. *Molecular and General Genetics,* Vol.174. No.3, (Jul 24). pp. 297-305, ISSN 0026-8925.

Echtay, K.S. (2007). Mitochondrial uncoupling proteins--what is their physiological role? *Free Radical Biology and Medicine,* Vol.43. No.10, (Nov 15). pp. 1351-1371, ISSN 0891-5849.

Ekbom, A., Hsieh, C.C., Lipworth, L., Adami, H.Q., & Trichopoulos, D. (1997). Intrauterine environment and breast cancer risk in women: a population-based study. *Journal of the National Cancer Institute,* Vol.89. No.1, (Jan 1). pp. 71-76, ISSN 0027-8874.

Ewertz, M., Duffy, S.W., Adami, H.O., Kvale, G., Lund, E., Meirik, O., Mellemgaard, A., Soini, I., & Tulinius, H. (1990). Age at first birth, parity and risk of breast cancer: a meta-analysis of 8 studies from the Nordic countries. *International Journal of Cancer,* Vol.46. No.4, (Oct 15). pp. 597-603, ISSN 0020-7136.

Fariss, M.W., Chan, C.B., Patel, M., Van Houten, B., & Orrenius, S. (2005). Role of mitochondria in toxic oxidative stress. *Molecular Interventions,* Vol.5. No.2, (Apr). pp. 94-111, ISSN 1534-0384.

Felty, Q., & Roy, D. (2005). Estrogen, mitochondria, and growth of cancer and non-cancer cells. *Journal of Carcinogenesis,* Vol.4. No.1, (Jan 15). pp. 1, ISSN 1477-316.

Ferlay, J., Autier, P., Boniol, M., Heanue, M., Colombet, M., & Boyle, P. (2007). Estimates of the cancer incidence and mortality in Europe in 2006. *Annals of Oncology,* Vol.18. No.3, (Mar). pp. 581-592, ISSN 0923-7534.

Fox, E.M., Davis, R.J., & Shupnik, M.A. (2008). ERbeta in breast cancer--onlooker, passive player, or active protector? *Steroids,* Vol.73. No.11, (Oct). pp. 1039-1051, ISSN 0039-128X.

Garcia-Roves, P., Huss, J.M., Han, D.H., Hancock, C.R., Iglesias-Gutierrez, E., Chen, M., & Holloszy, J.O. (2007). Raising plasma fatty acid concentration induces increased biogenesis of mitochondria in skeletal muscle. *Proceedings of the National Academy of Sciences of the United States of America,* Vol.104. No.25, (Jun 19). pp. 10709-10713, ISSN 0027-8424.

Garofalo, C., & Surmacz, E. (2006). Leptin and cancer. *Journal of Cellular Physiology,* Vol.207. No.1, (Apr). pp. 12-22, ISSN 0021-9541.

Giege, P., Grienenberger, J.M., & Bonnard, G. (2008). Cytochrome c biogenesis in mitochondria. *Mitochondrion,* Vol.8. No.1, (Jan). pp. 61-73, ISSN 1567-7249.

Giguere, V., Hollenberg, S.M., Rosenfeld, M.G., & Evans, R.M. (1986). Functional domains of the human glucocorticoid receptor. *Cell,* Vol.46. No.5, (Aug 29). pp. 645-652, ISSN 0092-8674.

Gonzalez, D.H., Bonnard, G., & Grienenberger, J.M. (1993). A gene involved in the biogenesis of c-type cytochromes is co-transcribed with a ribosomal protein gene in wheat mitochondria [corrected]. *Current Genetics,* Vol.24. No.3, (Sep). pp. 248-255, ISSN 0172-8083.

Green, S., Walter, P., Greene, G., Krust, A., Goffin, C., Jensen, E., Scrace, G., Waterfield, M., & Chambon, P. (1986). Cloning of the human oestrogen receptor cDNA. *Journal of Steroid Biochemistry and Molecular Biology,* Vol.24. No.1, (Jan). pp. 77-83, ISSN 0022-4731.

Greene, G.L., Nolan, C., Engler, J.P., & Jensen, E.V. (1980). Monoclonal antibodies to human estrogen receptor. *Proceedings of the National Academy of Sciences of the United States of America,* Vol.77. No.9, (Sep). pp. 5115-5119, ISSN 0027-8424.

Gruvberger-Saal, S.K., Bendahl, P.O., Saal, L.H., Laakso, M., Hegardt, C., Eden, P., Peterson, C., Malmstrom, P., Isola, J., Borg, A., & Ferno, M. (2007). Estrogen receptor beta expression is associated with tamoxifen response in ERalpha-negative breast carcinoma. *Clinical Cancer Research,* Vol.13. No.7, (Apr 1). pp. 1987-1994, ISSN 1078-0432.

Guevara, R., Santandreu, F.M., Valle, A., Gianotti, M., Oliver, J., & Roca, P. (2008). Sex-dependent differences in aged rat brain mitochondrial function and oxidative stress. *Free Radical Biology and Medicine.* (Oct 17). ISSN 0891-5849.

Gustafsson, J.A. (1999). Estrogen receptor beta--a new dimension in estrogen mechanism of action. *Journal of Endocrinology,* Vol.163. No.3, (Dec). pp. 379-383, ISSN 0022-0795.

Harkness, T.A., Nargang, F.E., van der Klei, I., Neupert, W., & Lill, R. (1994). A crucial role of the mitochondrial protein import receptor MOM19 for the biogenesis of mitochondria. *Journal of Cell Biology,* Vol.124. No.5, (Mar). pp. 637-648, ISSN 0021-9525.

Hartman, J., Strom, A., & Gustafsson, J.A. (2009). Estrogen receptor beta in breast cancer--diagnostic and therapeutic implications. *Steroids,* Vol.74. No.8, (Aug). pp. 635-641, ISSN 1878-5867.

Heldring, N., Pike, A., Andersson, S., Matthews, J., Cheng, G., Hartman, J., Tujague, M., Strom, A., Treuter, E., Warner, M., & Gustafsson, J.A. (2007). Estrogen receptors: how do they signal and what are their targets. *Physiological Reviews,* Vol.87. No.3, (Jul). pp. 905-931, ISSN 0031-9333.

Houstek, J., Kopecky, J., Baudysova, M., Janikova, D., Pavelka, S., & Klement, P. (1990). Differentiation of brown adipose tissue and biogenesis of thermogenic mitochondria in situ and in cell culture. *Biochimica et Biophysica Acta,* Vol.1018. No.2-3, (Jul 25). pp. 243-247, ISSN 0006-3002.

Jensen, E.V., Jacobson, H.I., Smith, S., Jungblut, P.W., & De Sombre, E.R. (1972). The use of estrogen antagonists in hormone receptor studies. *Gynecologic Investigation,* Vol.3. No.1, pp. 108-123, ISSN 0017-5986.

Jensen, E.V., Jacobson, H.I., Walf, A.A., & Frye, C.A. (2010). Estrogen action: a historic perspective on the implications of considering alternative approaches. *Physiology & Behavior,* Vol.99. No.2, (Feb 9). pp. 151-162, ISSN 1873-507X.

Kelsey, J.L., Gammon, M.D., & John, E.M. (1993). Reproductive factors and breast cancer. *Epidemiologic Reviews,* Vol.15. No.1, pp. 36-47, ISSN 0193-936X.

Key, T.J., Verkasalo, P.K., & Banks, E. (2001). Epidemiology of breast cancer. *The Lancet Oncology,* Vol.2. No.3, (Mar). pp. 133-140, ISSN 1470-2045.

Klingenspor, M., Ivemeyer, M., Wiesinger, H., Haas, K., Heldmaier, G., & Wiesner, R.J. (1996). Biogenesis of thermogenic mitochondria in brown adipose tissue of Djungarian hamsters during cold adaptation. *Biochemical Journal,* Vol.316 (Pt 2). (Jun 1). pp. 607-613, ISSN 0264-6021.

Korb, H., & Neupert, W. (1978). Biogenesis of cytochrome c in Neurospora crassa. Synthesis of apocytochrome c, transfer to mitochondria and conversion to Holocytochrome c. *European Journal of Biochemistry,* Vol.91. No.2, (Nov 15). pp. 609-620, ISSN 0014-2956.

Kuiper, G.G., Carlsson, B., Grandien, K., Enmark, E., Haggblad, J., Nilsson, S., & Gustafsson, J.A. (1997). Comparison of the ligand binding specificity and transcript tissue distribution of estrogen receptors alpha and beta. *Endocrinology,* Vol.138. No.3, (Mar). pp. 863-870, ISSN 0013-7227.

Kuiper, G.G., Enmark, E., Pelto-Huikko, M., Nilsson, S., & Gustafsson, J.A. (1996). Cloning of a novel receptor expressed in rat prostate and ovary. *Proceedings of the National Academy of Sciences of the United States of America,* Vol.93. No.12, (Jun 11). pp. 5925-5930, ISSN 0027-8424.

Kuiper, G.G., Lemmen, J.G., Carlsson, B., Corton, J.C., Safe, S.H., van der Saag, P.T., van der Burg, B., & Gustafsson, J.A. (1998). Interaction of estrogenic chemicals and phytoestrogens with estrogen receptor beta. *Endocrinology,* Vol.139. No.10, (Oct). pp. 4252-4263, ISSN 0013-7227.

Kumar, V., Green, S., Stack, G., Berry, M., Jin, J.R., & Chambon, P. (1987). Functional domains of the human estrogen receptor. *Cell,* Vol.51. No.6, (Dec 24). pp. 941-951, ISSN 0092-8674.

Kushner, P.J., Agard, D.A., Greene, G.L., Scanlan, T.S., Shiau, A.K., Uht, R.M., & Webb, P. (2000). Estrogen receptor pathways to AP-1. *Journal of Steroid Biochemistry and Molecular Biology,* Vol.74. No.5, (Nov 30). pp. 311-317, ISSN 0960-0760.

Lahmann, P.H., Hoffmann, K., Allen, N., van Gils, C.H., Khaw, K.T., Tehard, B., Berrino, F., Tjonneland, A., Bigaard, J., Olsen, A., Overvad, K., Clavel-Chapelon, F., Nagel, G., Boeing, H., Trichopoulos, D., Economou, G., Bellos, G., Palli, D., Tumino, R., Panico, S., Sacerdote, C., Krogh, V., Peeters, P.H., Bueno-de-Mesquita, H.B., Lund, E., Ardanaz, E., Amiano, P., Pera, G., Quiros, J.R., Martinez, C., Tormo, M.J., Wirfalt, E., Berglund, G., Hallmans, G., Key, T.J., Reeves, G., Bingham, S., Norat, T., Biessy, C., Kaaks, R., & Riboli, E. (2004). Body size and breast cancer risk: findings from the European Prospective Investigation into Cancer And Nutrition (EPIC). *International Journal of Cancer,* Vol.111. No.5, (Sep 20). pp. 762-771, ISSN 0020-7136.

Layde, P.M., Webster, L.A., Baughman, A.L., Wingo, P.A., Rubin, G.L., & Ory, H.W. (1989). The independent associations of parity, age at first full term pregnancy, and duration of breastfeeding with the risk of breast cancer. Cancer and Steroid Hormone Study Group. *Journal of Clinical Epidemiology,* Vol.42. No.10, pp. 963-973, ISSN 0895-4356.

Lee, Y.R., Park, J., Yu, H.N., Kim, J.S., Youn, H.J., & Jung, S.H. (2005). Up-regulation of PI3K/Akt signaling by 17beta-estradiol through activation of estrogen receptor-alpha, but not estrogen receptor-beta, and stimulates cell growth in breast cancer cells. *Biochemical and Biophysical Research Communications,* Vol.336. No.4, (Nov 4). pp. 1221-1226, ISSN 0006-291X.

Lenaz, G. (2001). The mitochondrial production of reactive oxygen species: mechanisms and implications in human pathology. *IUBMB Life,* Vol.52. No.3-5, (Sep-Nov). pp. 159-164, ISSN 1521-6543.

Leygue, E., Dotzlaw, H., Watson, P.H., & Murphy, L.C. (1998). Altered estrogen receptor alpha and beta messenger RNA expression during human breast tumorigenesis. *Cancer Research,* Vol.58. No.15, (Aug 1). pp. 3197-3201, ISSN 0008-5472.

Martindale, J.L., & Holbrook, N.J. (2002). Cellular response to oxidative stress: signaling for suicide and survival. *Journal of Cellular Physiology,* Vol.192. No.1, (Jul). pp. 1-15, ISSN 0021-9541.

McTiernan, A. (2003). Behavioral risk factors in breast cancer: can risk be modified? *Oncologist,* Vol.8. No.4, pp. 326-334, ISSN 1083-7159.

Menassa, R., El-Rouby, N., & Brown, G.G. (1997). An open reading frame for a protein involved in cytochrome c biogenesis is split into two parts in Brassica mitochondria. *Current Genetics,* Vol.31. No.1, (Jan). pp. 70-79, ISSN 0172-8083.

Molina-Navarro, M.M., Casas, C., Piedrafita, L., Belli, G., & Herrero, E. (2006). Prokaryotic and eukaryotic monothiol glutaredoxins are able to perform the functions of Grx5 in the biogenesis of Fe/S clusters in yeast mitochondria. *FEBS Letters,* Vol.580. No.9, (Apr 17). pp. 2273-2280, ISSN 0014-5793.

Morani, A., Warner, M., & Gustafsson, J.A. (2008). Biological functions and clinical implications of oestrogen receptors alfa and beta in epithelial tissues. *Journal of Internal Medicine,* Vol.264. No.2, (Aug). pp. 128-142, ISSN 1365-2796.

Murphy, L.C., & Watson, P.H. (2006). Is oestrogen receptor-beta a predictor of endocrine therapy responsiveness in human breast cancer? *Endocrine-Related Cancer,* Vol.13. No.2, (Jun). pp. 327-334, ISSN 1351-0088.

Murphy, M.P. (2009). How mitochondria produce reactive oxygen species. *Biochemical Journal,* Vol.417. No.1, (Jan 1). pp. 1-13, ISSN 1470-8728.

Nilsson, S., Makela, S., Treuter, E., Tujague, M., Thomsen, J., Andersson, G., Enmark, E., Pettersson, K., Warner, M., & Gustafsson, J.A. (2001). Mechanisms of estrogen action. *Physiological Reviews,* Vol.81. No.4, (Oct). pp. 1535-1565, ISSN 0031-9333.

Novelli, F., Milella, M., Melucci, E., Di Benedetto, A., Sperduti, I., Perrone-Donnorso, R., Perracchio, L., Venturo, I., Nistico, C., Fabi, A., Buglioni, S., Natali, P.G., & Mottolese, M. (2008). A divergent role for estrogen receptor-beta in node-positive and node-negative breast cancer classified according to molecular subtypes: an observational prospective study. *Breast Cancer Research,* Vol.10. No.5, pp. R74, ISSN 1465-5411.

O'Neill, P.A., Davies, M.P., Shaaban, A.M., Innes, H., Torevell, A., Sibson, D.R., & Foster, C.S. (2004). Wild-type oestrogen receptor beta (ERbeta1) mRNA and protein expression in Tamoxifen-treated post-menopausal breast cancers. *British Journal of Cancer,* Vol.91. No.9, (Nov 1). pp. 1694-1702, ISSN 0007-0920.

Obbink, D.J., Spithill, T.W., Maxwell, R.J., & Linnane, A.W. (1977). Biogenesis of mitochondria 48: mikamycin resistance in Saccharomyces cerevisiae--a mitochondrial mutation conferring resistance to an antimycin A-like contaminant in mikamycin. *Molecular and General Genetics,* Vol.151. No.2, (Mar 7). pp. 127-136, ISSN 0026-8925.

Pearce, S.T., & Jordan, V.C. (2004). The biological role of estrogen receptors alpha and beta in cancer. *Critical Reviews in Oncology/Hematology,* Vol.50. No.1, (Apr). pp. 3-22, ISSN 1040-8428.

Pedram, A., Razandi, M., Wallace, D.C., & Levin, E.R. (2006). Functional estrogen receptors in the mitochondria of breast cancer cells. *Molecular Biology of the Cell,* Vol.17. No.5, (May). pp. 2125-2137, ISSN 1059-1524.

Pharoah, P.D., Day, N.E., Duffy, S., Easton, D.F., & Ponder, B.A. (1997). Family history and the risk of breast cancer: a systematic review and meta-analysis. *International Journal of Cancer,* Vol.71. No.5, (May 29). pp. 800-809, ISSN 0020-7136.

Power, K.A., & Thompson, L.U. (2003). Ligand-induced regulation of ERalpha and ERbeta is indicative of human breast cancer cell proliferation. *Breast Cancer Research and Treatment,* Vol.81. No.3, (Oct). pp. 209-221, ISSN 0167-6806.

Quaedackers, M.E., Van Den Brink, C.E., Wissink, S., Schreurs, R.H., Gustafsson, J.A., Van Der Saag, P.T., & Van Der Burg, B.B. (2001). 4-hydroxytamoxifen trans-represses nuclear factor-kappa B activity in human osteoblastic U2-OS cells through estrogen receptor (ER)alpha, and not through ER beta. *Endocrinology,* Vol.142. No.3, (Mar). pp. 1156-1166, ISSN 0013-7227.

Roger, P., Sahla, M.E., Makela, S., Gustafsson, J.A., Baldet, P., & Rochefort, H. (2001). Decreased expression of estrogen receptor beta protein in proliferative preinvasive mammary tumors. *Cancer Research,* Vol.61. No.6, (Mar 15). pp. 2537-2541, ISSN 0008-5472.

Russo, J., Ao, X., Grill, C., & Russo, I.H. (1999). Pattern of distribution of cells positive for estrogen receptor alpha and progesterone receptor in relation to proliferating cells in the mammary gland. *Breast Cancer Research and Treatment,* Vol.53. No.3, (Feb). pp. 217-227, ISSN 0167-6806.

Russo, J., Hasan Lareef, M., Balogh, G., Guo, S., & Russo, I.H. (2003). Estrogen and its metabolites are carcinogenic agents in human breast epithelial cells. *Journal of Steroid Biochemistry and Molecular Biology,* Vol.87. No.1, (Oct). pp. 1-25, ISSN 0960-0760.

Saji, S., Jensen, E.V., Nilsson, S., Rylander, T., Warner, M., & Gustafsson, J.A. (2000). Estrogen receptors alpha and beta in the rodent mammary gland. *Proceedings of the National Academy of Sciences of the United States of America,* Vol.97. No.1, (Jan 4). pp. 337-342, ISSN 0027-8424.

Sanders, L.M., Henderson, C.E., Hong, M.Y., Barhoumi, R., Burghardt, R.C., Wang, N., Spinka, C.M., Carroll, R.J., Turner, N.D., Chapkin, R.S., & Lupton, J.R. (2004). An increase in reactive oxygen species by dietary fish oil coupled with the attenuation of antioxidant defenses by dietary pectin enhances rat colonocyte apoptosis. *The Journal of Nutrition,* Vol.134. No.12, (Dec). pp. 3233-3238, ISSN 0022-3166.

Sauer, H., Wartenberg, M., & Hescheler, J. (2001). Reactive oxygen species as intracellular messengers during cell growth and differentiation. *Cellular Physiology and Biochemistry,* Vol.11. No.4, pp. 173-186, ISSN 1015-8987.

Saville, B., Wormke, M., Wang, F., Nguyen, T., Enmark, E., Kuiper, G., Gustafsson, J.A., & Safe, S. (2000). Ligand-, cell-, and estrogen receptor subtype (alpha/beta)-dependent activation at GC-rich (Sp1) promoter elements. *Journal of Biological Chemistry,* Vol.275. No.8, (Feb 25). pp. 5379-5387, ISSN 0021-9258.

Schatz, G. (1979). Biogenesis of yeast mitochondria: synthesis of cytochrome c oxidase and cytochrome c. *Methods in Enzymology,* Vol.56. pp. 40-50, ISSN 0076-6879.

Schuster, W. (1994). The highly edited orf206 in Oenothera mitochondria may encode a component of a heme transporter involved in cytochrome c biogenesis. *Plant Molecular Biology,* Vol.25. No.1, (Apr). pp. 33-42, ISSN 0167-4412.

Sidhu, R.S., & Tauro, P. (1979). Biogenesis of mitochondria in yeast Saccharomyces cerevisiae: Part I--Nuclear control of mitochondria biogenesis. *Indian Journal of Experimental Biology,* Vol.17. No.1, (Jan). pp. 19-23, ISSN 0019-5189.

Skliris, G.P., Leygue, E., Curtis-Snell, L., Watson, P.H., & Murphy, L.C. (2006). Expression of oestrogen receptor-beta in oestrogen receptor-alpha negative human breast tumours. *British Journal of Cancer,* Vol.95. No.5, (Sep 4). pp. 616-626, ISSN 0007-0920.

Skliris, G.P., Leygue, E., Watson, P.H., & Murphy, L.C. (2008). Estrogen receptor alpha negative breast cancer patients: estrogen receptor beta as a therapeutic target. *Journal of Steroid Biochemistry and Molecular Biology,* Vol.109. No.1-2, (Mar). pp. 1-10, ISSN 0960-0760.

Skliris, G.P., Munot, K., Bell, S.M., Carder, P.J., Lane, S., Horgan, K., Lansdown, M.R., Parkes, A.T., Hanby, A.M., Markham, A.F., & Speirs, V. (2003). Reduced expression of oestrogen receptor beta in invasive breast cancer and its re-expression using DNA methyl transferase inhibitors in a cell line model. *The Journal of Pathology,* Vol.201. No.2, (Oct). pp. 213-220, ISSN 0022-3417.

Smith, E.P., Boyd, J., Frank, G.R., Takahashi, H., Cohen, R.M., Specker, B., Williams, T.C., Lubahn, D.B., & Korach, K.S. (1994). Estrogen resistance caused by a mutation in the estrogen-receptor gene in a man. *New England Journal of Medicine,* Vol.331. No.16, (Oct 20). pp. 1056-1061, ISSN 0028-4793.

Sogl, B., Gellissen, G., & Wiesner, R.J. (2000). Biogenesis of giant mitochondria during insect flight muscle development in the locust, Locusta migratoria (L.). Transcription, translation and copy number of mitochondrial DNA. *European Journal of Biochemistry,* Vol.267. No.1, (Jan). pp. 11-17, ISSN 0014-2956.

Sotoca, A.M., Ratman, D., van der Saag, P., Strom, A., Gustafsson, J.A., Vervoort, J., Rietjens, I.M., & Murk, A.J. (2008). Phytoestrogen-mediated inhibition of proliferation of the human T47D breast cancer cells depends on the ERalpha/ERbeta ratio. *Journal of Steroid Biochemistry and Molecular Biology,* Vol.112. No.4-5, (Dec). pp. 171-178, ISSN 0960-0760.

Speirs, V., Malone, C., Walton, D.S., Kerin, M.J., & Atkin, S.L. (1999). Increased expression of estrogen receptor beta mRNA in tamoxifen-resistant breast cancer patients. *Cancer Research,* Vol.59. No.21, (Nov 1). pp. 5421-5424, ISSN 0008-5472.

Spithill, T.W., Nagley, P., & Linnane, A.W. (1979). Biogenesis of mitochondria 51: biochemical characterization of a mitochondrial mutation in Saccharomyces cerevisiae affecting the mitochondrial ribosome by conferring resistance to aminoglycoside antibiotics. *Molecular and General Genetics,* Vol.173. No.2, (Jun 7). pp. 159-170, ISSN 0026-8925.

Stossi, F., Barnett, D.H., Frasor, J., Komm, B., Lyttle, C.R., & Katzenellenbogen, B.S. (2004). Transcriptional profiling of estrogen-regulated gene expression via estrogen receptor (ER) alpha or ERbeta in human osteosarcoma cells: distinct and common target genes for these receptors. *Endocrinology,* Vol.145. No.7, (Jul). pp. 3473-3486, ISSN 0013-7227.

Strom, A., Hartman, J., Foster, J.S., Kietz, S., Wimalasena, J., & Gustafsson, J.A. (2004). Estrogen receptor beta inhibits 17beta-estradiol-stimulated proliferation of the breast cancer cell line T47D. *Proceedings of the National Academy of Sciences of the United States of America,* Vol.101. No.6, (Feb 10). pp. 1566-1571, ISSN 0027-8424.

Tam, C.C., & Wong, Y.C. (1991). Ultrastructural study of the effects of 17 beta-oestradiol on the lateral prostate and seminal vesicle of the castrated guinea pig. *Acta Anatomica (Basel),* Vol.141. No.1, pp. 51-62, ISSN 0001-5180.

Tamir, S., Izrael, S., & Vaya, J. (2002). The effect of oxidative stress on ERalpha and ERbeta expression. *Journal of Steroid Biochemistry and Molecular Biology,* Vol.81. No.4-5, (Aug). pp. 327-332, ISSN 0960-0760.

Usmanova, N., Tomilin, N., Zhivotovsky, B., & Kropotov, A. (2011). Transcription factor GABP/NRF-2 controlling biogenesis of mitochondria regulates basal expression of peroxiredoxin V but the mitochondrial function of peroxiredoxin V is dispensable in the dog. *Biochimie,* Vol.93. No.2, (Feb). pp. 306-313, ISSN 1638-6183.

Valle, A., Catala-Niell, A., Colom, B., Garcia-Palmer, F.J., Oliver, J., & Roca, P. (2005). Sex-related differences in energy balance in response to caloric restriction. *American Journal of Physiology Endocrinology and Metabolism,* Vol.289. No.1, (Jul). pp. E15-22, ISSN 0193-1849.

Valle, A., Garcia-Palmer, F.J., Oliver, J., & Roca, P. (2007). Sex differences in brown adipose tissue thermogenic features during caloric restriction. *Cellular Physiology and Biochemistry,* Vol.19. No.1-4, pp. 195-204, ISSN 1015-8987.

Valle, A., Guevara, R., Garcia-Palmer, F.J., Roca, P., & Oliver, J. (2007). Sexual dimorphism in liver mitochondrial oxidative capacity is conserved under caloric restriction conditions. *American Journal of Physiology. Cell Physiology,* Vol.293. No.4, (Oct). pp. C1302-1308, ISSN 0363-6143.

Valle, A., Guevara, R., Garcia-Palmer, F.J., Roca, P., & Oliver, J. (2008). Caloric restriction retards the age-related decline in mitochondrial function of brown adipose tissue. *Rejuvenation Research,* Vol.11. No.3, (Jun). pp. 597-604, ISSN 1549-1684.

Vic, P., Vignon, F., Derocq, D., & Rochefort, H. (1982). Effect of estradiol on the ultrastructure of the MCF7 human breast cancer cells in culture. *Cancer Research,* Vol.42. No.2, (Feb). pp. 667-673, ISSN 0008-5472.

Walsh, T., & King, M.C. (2007). Ten genes for inherited breast cancer. *Cancer Cell,* Vol.11. No.2, (Feb). pp. 103-105, ISSN 1535-6108.

Walter, P., Green, S., Greene, G., Krust, A., Bornert, J.M., Jeltsch, J.M., Staub, A., Jensen, E., Scrace, G., Waterfield, M., & et al. (1985). Cloning of the human estrogen receptor cDNA. *Proceedings of the National Academy of Sciences of the United States of America,* Vol.82. No.23, (Dec). pp. 7889-7893, ISSN 0027-8424.

Yager, J.D., & Davidson, N.E. (2006). Estrogen carcinogenesis in breast cancer. *New England Journal of Medicine,* Vol.354. No.3, (Jan 19). pp. 270-282, ISSN 1533-4406.

Zhao, C., Lam, E.W., Sunters, A., Enmark, E., De Bella, M.T., Coombes, R.C., Gustafsson, J.A., & Dahlman-Wright, K. (2003). Expression of estrogen receptor beta isoforms in normal breast epithelial cells and breast cancer: regulation by methylation. *Oncogene,* Vol.22. No.48, (Oct 23). pp. 7600-7606, ISSN 0950-9232.

4

Role of ING Family Tumor Suppressors in Breast Cancer

Mehmet Gunduz[1], Esra Gunduz[2], Mikdat Bozer[3] and Ramazan Yigitoglu[4]

[2]Department of Medical Genetics,
[3]Department of General Surgery-Surgical Oncology Section,
[4]Department of Medical Biochemistry,
School of Medicine, Fatih University, Ankara,
Turkey

1. Introduction

Today cancer is one of the leading diseases, which treat human life and enormous efforts are being done for its eradication. Currently many cancer types including breast cancer are treated by extensive surgery as well as chemo-radiotherapy. These treatment modalities usually present extensive damage to the patient both anatomically, physiologically and psychologically. In addition, chemo-radiotherapy shows extreme side effects of the other system in the body and their efficiencies are quite limited especially in disseminated metastatic cases. Recent developments and progress in human genome technology provided us to develop novel therapeutic methods. This progress also provided novel biomarkers, which early diagnose the cancer and predict the sensitivity of the current chemo-radiation therapies.

Tight control by various regulatory mechanisms is applied on cell proliferation and growth in normal cells. However, certain genetic and epigenetic alterations permit the normal cells to avoid these mechanisms allowing indefinite cellular activities. Cancer is basically a genetic disease. The collection of genetic and epigenetic alterations of multiple genes and chromosomes lead to the development of cancer. In this regard, two major groups of tumor-associated genes, oncogenes and tumor suppressor genes (TSGs), have been implicated in the carcinogenic process **(Figure 1).**

TSGs have been defined as genetic elements whose loss or mutational inactivation allows cell to display one or more phenotypes of neoplastic growth [1]. TSG protein products are known to be involved in negative regulation of the cell cycle and proliferation and induction of apoptosis by different mechanisms. Thus inactivation of TSGs is one of the crucial steps during carcinogenetic process. In this process according to Knudson two-hit hypothesis for inactivation of TSGs [2], the deletion of targeted chromosomal regions (location of TSGs) eliminates one allele, while inactivating events (mutation, deletion, or epigenetic events such as promoter hypermethylation) affect the other allele of a concerning TSG [2]. The detection of frequent loss of heterozygosity (LOH) in a chromosomal locus is considered to be critical evidence for the localization of a TSG.

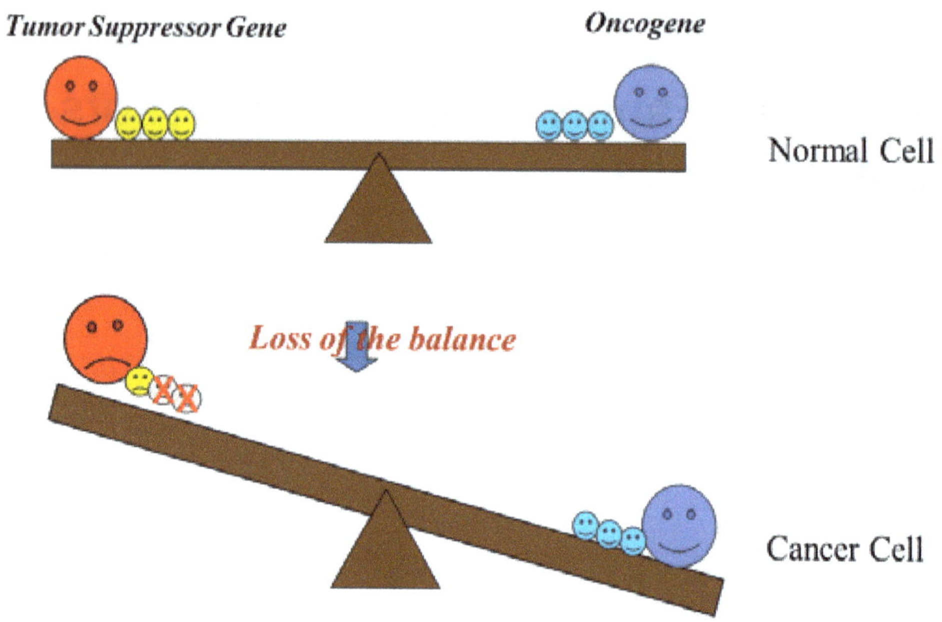

Fig. 1. Role of Oncogene and Tumor Suppressor Gene in Cancer.
Two group of genes (oncogene and tumor suppressor gene) influence on physiological cell proliferation and growth. In cancer development, balance between these two groups of genes is broken. Either oncogene activation or tumor suppressor gene inactivation promotes cancer development.

In fact many TSGs including well-known p53, RB1, p16, p21, and FHIT etc have been recently identified by using LOH analysis and then positional cloning. Inactivation of these classical TSGs usually occurs through deletion of one of its allele and mutation in the rest allele (Class I TSG, Knudson hypothesis). However, a novel class of TSGs with haploid insufficiency, in which one allele is lost and the remaining allele is haplo-insufficient, has been described recently, and the patients with these hemizygous TSGs in their genome are accepted as carriers for deficient allele of a TSG and they show a tumor-prone phenotype especially when challenged with carcinogens such as smoking, alcohol, x-ray, chemicals etc (Class II TSG) [3-7] **(Figure 2)**.
The novel TSG family, inhibitor of growth (ING), belongs to the group of genes that encodes proteins containing structural motifs involved in chromatin remodeling and transcription regulation. The ING family is classified as type II tumor suppressor since its inactivation has been implicated in neoplastic growth of various tumors [8-10]. Five human ING genes (ING1-5) have been identified and among them, ING1 is the founding member and the most widely studied. ING1 was first isolated using subtractive hybridization between short segments of cDNAs from normal and a number of breast cancer cell lines [11]. These randomly fragmented cDNAs interfered with the activity of tumor suppressors by either blocking protein production through anti-sense sequences or abrogating function in a dominant-negative fashion through truncated sense fragments [11]. Acute expression of transfected constructs encoding this gene inhibited cell growth while chronic expression of

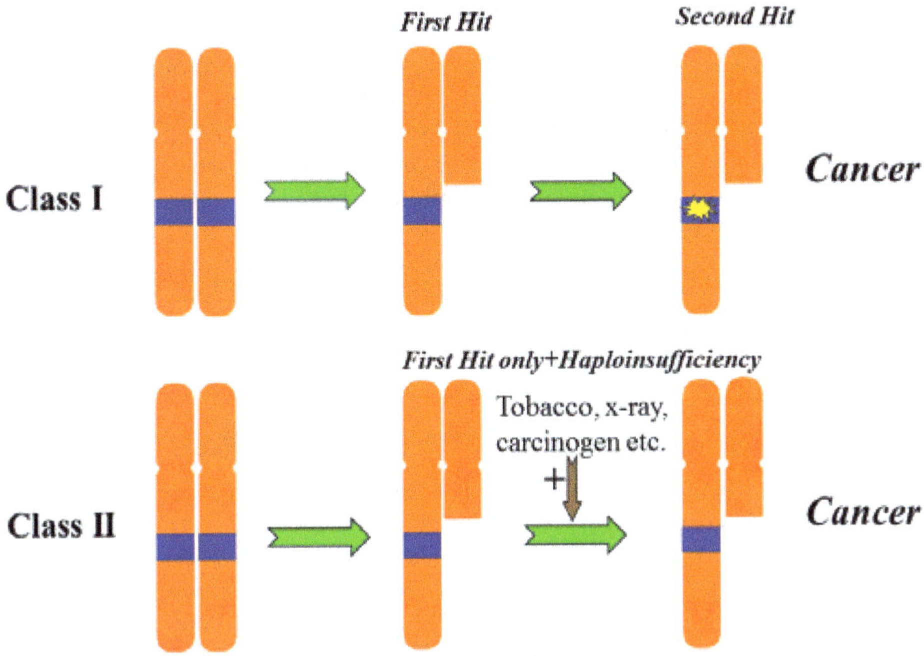

Fig. 2. Cancer Development through Inactivation of Tumor Suppressor Genes.
Knudson two-hit hypothesis for inactivation of TSGs, the deletion of targeted chromosomal regions (location of TSGs) eliminates one allele, while inactivating events (mutation, deletion, or epigenetic events such as promoter hypermethylation) affect the other allele of a concerning TSG (Class I). TSG with haploid insufficiency, in which one allele is lost and the remaining hemizygous allele is not enough to provide full suppression on cellular proliferation. These patients are carrier for deficient allele of a TSG and they show a tumor-prone phenotype especially when challenged with carcinogens such as smoking, alcohol, x-ray, chemicals etc (Class II).

antisense ING1 constructs promoted transformation of mouse breast epithelial cells and increased the frequency of focus formation with NIH3T3 cells and protected cells from apoptosis [11, 12]. Using radiation hybrid analysis, ING1 gene was mapped on human chromosome 13q33-34 [13]. The other four members have been disclosed through sequence homologies with ING1, followed by functional in-vitro and then in-vivo cancer patient tissue analysis [9, 10, 14-16]. However, recent researches demonstrated opposite findings for some of ING family members such as ING2 as a possible oncogene in specific conditions. In fact, ING2 expression was found to be increased in colorectal cancer and knock-down of ING2 suppressed cell growth and induced cell cycle arrest or apoptosis [17].

2. Structure and function of ING family genes

All members of ING family have distinct N-termini, which dictate the specific role of the ING members and, in certain instances, their antagonistic regulatory function [9,10,14-16]. Also all ING family members exhibit a highly conserved C-terminal plant homeodomain (PHD) that is commonly found in various chromatin remodeling proteins [9,10,14-22]

(**Figure 3**). The PHD motif consists of about 60 amino acids and shows a C4HC3 ring structure that typically binds two Zn2+ ions [16]. Approximately 150 distinct PHD domain-bearing proteins have been predicted to occur in humans [16]. PHD domains have been implicated in chromatin remodeling due to presence of their proteins as known components of larger chromatin remodeling complexes, and may function by strengthening a separate chromatin-binding activity of either the same protein or an associated protein [16]. Mutations within the PHD fingers of numerous proteins have been reported to be linked to tumorigenesis, immuno-deficiency syndromes, autoimmune syndromes, and several other genetic disorders [15, 23-26]. These mutations mainly occur at zinc-coordinating residues, suggesting that zinc ligation and hence integrity of the PHD finger fold are critical for the function of PHD finger-containing proteins [15].

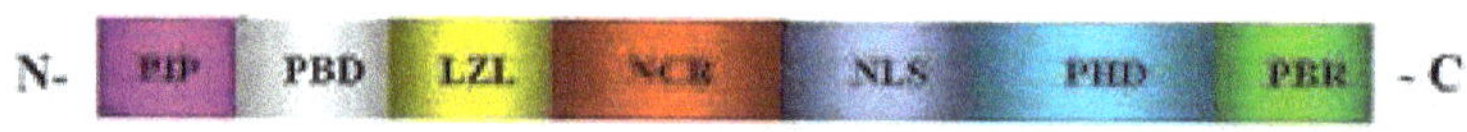

Fig. 3. Structure and Interacting Domains of ING Family Proteins.
All ING family proteins have a highly conserved plant homeodomain (PHD) finger motif, Novel Conserved Region (NCR) and Nuclear Localization Sequence (NLS). NLS directs ING to the nucleus through binding of the karyopherin/importins. NCR serves as an interacting site for lamin A as well as HAT/HDACs. The PHD finger binds to histone H3 and has a role in chromatin regulation. PCNA-interacting motif (PIP) and Partial Bromodomain (PBD) are specific to ING1. The PIP motif binds to PCNA and promotes ING1-mediated apoptosis. PBD domain binds SAP30 of mSin3A-HDAC1 and has a role in transcription regulation. All ING proteins except ING1 include LZL domain, which has roles in apoptosis and nucleotide excision repair of DNA. Both ING1 and ING2 include a short polybasic region called as PBR, to which PtdIns3P and PtdIns4P bind.

All ING proteins contain nuclear conserved region (NCR) domain, which was identified by sequence analyses and is the second most highly conserved domain in the ING family proteins [15]. This N-terminal region of ING1 has been reported to interact directly with lamin A, suggesting that the association with nuclear lamina is a common feature of this family [27].
All ING proteins contain a nuclear localization signal (NLS) at the carboxy terminal, and some of ING proteins have multiple NLS. Deletion of the NLS of ING1 resulted in cytoplasmic accumulation of the protein [28,29]. Translocation of ING proteins into the nucleus has been thought to be critical for their function because these molecules are nuclear proteins, and also it is clearly considered to be so by the observation of loss of nuclear ING1 staining in a number of cancers [16, 30]. Deletion of the entire NLS of ING4 resulted in a protein that could no longer bind p53 in co-transfection experiments [31]. Moreover, two copies of a putative nucleolar translocation signal (NTS) were found within the NLS of ING1, and translocation of ING1 into the nucleolus following exposure to UV light was suggested to be required for ING1-associated apoptosis [16,28].
All ING proteins, except ING1, contain leucine zipper-like (LZL) domain at the N-terminus. LZL domain forms a hydrophobic patch consisting of four to five conserved leucine or isoleucine residues spanning every seven amino acids. Similar leucine distribution has also been reported for ING3 to ING5 [15,32,33]. There is few information about the function of LZL and it been has reported that the LZL domain of ING2 is required for the induction of apoptosis and NER [34]. ING2 deletion mutants lacking the LZL domain do not show

increased apoptosis following UV exposure, suggesting that this domain is necessary for ING2-mediated apoptosis [34]. RNAi-mediated knockdown of ING2 has also been reported to abrogate the nucleotide excision repair (NER) capacity of melanoma cells [35].

Within ING family members, only ING1 includes PCNA binding domain called as PIP box in a DNA damage-inducible manner at N-terminus. This domain indicates the role of ING1 in DNA repair since PCNA has roles for DNA replication and repair. The interaction of this domain is specifically induced upon UV damage and has been thought to change PCNA activity away from DNA replication towards DNA repair [36]. Another unique domain present only in ING1b is called as PBD (partial bromodomain because of its sequence homology to bromodomains), which binds SAP30 of mSin3A-HDAC1, suggesting its role in transcriptional regulation of some genes [37].

Both ING1 and ING2 include a short polybasic region called as PBR at C-terminus. Though exact functions of this domain remain unknown, it has been reported that PtdIns3P and PtdIns4P can bind to the PBR [10,38], while PtdIns5P binds to the PHD motif of ING2 [10,39].

3. Genomic location, structure and expression of ING family genes

Most ING family genes are ubiquitously expressed in human tissues. We characterized genomic structure of human ING1 gene, and demonstrated that the human ING1 gene contains three exons (1a, 1b and 2) and two introns [8]. The gene has been mapped to chromosome 13 (13q33-34), and it has been found to encode 4 different mRNA variants. ING1 is ubiquitously expressed in various tissues [8]. The second member of the ING family, ING2 gene, has been mapped on chromosome 4 (4q35.1) and has been known to have 2 variants; ING2a and ING2b [40]. ING2 has 3 exons including ex1a, ex1b and 2 [41]. Our group identified the ING3 gene on chromosome 7 (7q31). The ING3 also encodes 2 different variants [9,10,41,42]. ING3 has 12 exons at its genomic location. The ING4 gene has been mapped on chromosome 12 (12q13.3) and encodes 8 variants with 8 exons [9,10,43,44]. The ING5 gene has been mapped on chromosome 2 (2q37.3) and encodes at least 5 different splicing variants with 8 exons [9,10,45].

4. Biological functions of ING family genes

ING proteins are involved in regulation of various cellular processes and signaling pathways such as angiogenesis, growth regulation, senescence, apoptosis, chemosensitivity, cell cycle, cell migration and DNA repair through p53-dependent and -independent pathways. ING proteins form complexes with HAT/HDAC [9,10,46]. After discovery of ING family genes prototype ING1, most of the functional studies have been conducted using ING1 variants, but fewer recently increasing studies, involving other ING family members, have also identified similar roles for these ING proteins. In addition, inhibition of ING proteins has been shown to increase cell spreading as well as migration, and relieve contact inhibition.

p33ING1b physically associates with the p53 tumor suppressor protein and seems to be a critical cofactor in p53-mediated regulation of cell growth and apoptosis [9,10,46,47]. However in a separate study, p37Ing1, mouse variant of human p33ING1b, blocked cell proliferation regardless of p53 and did not affect p53-mediated cell growth arrest following DNA damage [48]. p37Ing1 in mice regulated Bax levels in a negative way and worked as a prosurvival molecule following DNA damage independent of p53 status, complicating the function of ING1 in mouse and human and in various other circumstances. Moreover, recent experiments have also suggested that there are p53-independent functions for the ING proteins, including regulation of the NF-kB and hypoxia inducible factor (HIF) pathways [49-52].

ING2 shows a high rate of homology with ING1 about 70% [9,10,30,34,53]. Similar to other members of the ING family, ING2 is reported to have function in cooperation with p53, which is important for modulation of p53-mediated chromatin remodeling [54]. p33ING2 induces G1 phase cell cycle arrest or apoptosis in a p53-dependent manner following DNA damage [53]. ING2 has important roles in senescence, cellular response to DNA damage and DNA repair [34, 54]. Recently ING2 was also shown to interact with members of the transforming growth factor (TGF)-β signaling pathways enhancing transcription of target genes and cell cycle arrest [55]. However, overexpression of ING2 in colorectal cancer, burkitt lymphoma and cervical cancer and decreased expression in others such as head and neck carcinoma suggested that ING2 might have different function in various cancers [9,10,19,41,56,57]. Moreover, ING2 has 2 splicing variants and knockout experiments suggested oncogenic function of this gene [40,41]. In a recent study, a new function of ING2 was identified for the control of DNA replication and the maintenance of genome stability [58].

We identified ING3 for the first time by a homology search in human genome and showed ING3 as a candidate tumor suppressor in head and neck cancer [42]. Overexpression of p47ING3 protein resulted in a decreased population of cells in S phase, a diminished colony-forming efficiency, and induced apoptosis in RKO cells with wild type p53, but not in RKO-E6 cells with inactivated p53, suggesting necessity of p53 protein for at least some of its functions [59]. Histone acetyl transferase (HAT) complexes are important regulators of gene expression and among these, the NuA4 complex, first characterized in yeast, stands out as it controls multiple key nuclear functions in eukaryotic cells such as regulation of transcription, cell-cycle progression as well as the process of DNA repair [60]. p47ING3 activates p53-transactivated promoters, including promoters of p21/waf1 [61] and ING3 has been a stable component of Tip60/NuA4 HAT complex that cooperates with p53 and blocked cell cycle by activating the p21/waf1 gene [9,10,62,63]. Tip60 is an important transcriptional cofactor for p53-, NF-kB- and Myc-dependent transcription activation, suggesting that ING3 might have functions for many processes such as apoptosis and metastasis suppression at the transcription level through its association with the Tip60/NuA4 complex [63]. ING3 expression significantly promoted apoptosis by activating the Fas/caspase-8 pathway, suggesting that ING3 may also be involved in the death-receptor pathways [9,10,15,64]. Recently ING3 has been reported to be degraded by the ubiquitin-proteasome pathway through the SCF (Skp2) complex and interruption of ING3 degradation enhanced the tumor-suppressive function of ING3 [65].

p29ING4 was identified by Shiseki et al [66]. Overexpression of ING4 protein resulted in a diminished colony-forming efficiency, a decreased cell population in S phase, and the induction of apoptosis in a p53-dependent manner. p29ING4 also activated the p21/waf1 promoter, and induce p21/WAF1 expression [66].

ING4 has been proposed to regulate cell cycling and apoptosis. ING4 has been reported to inhibit angiogenesis by various studies besides its role for cellular processes common for all ING family members [67-69]. It has been demonstrated that ING4 physically interacts with p65 (RelA), a subunit of nuclear factor NF-kB, and that ING4 regulates angiogenesis through transcriptional repression of NF-kB-responsive genes in brain tumors [70]. ING4 functional studies suggest that this gene in addition to the common functions of the ING proteins could play a completely different role in tumorigenesis. Actually, ING4 is likely to be involved in inhibition of the cell's spreading and migration as well as tumor angiogenesis. Indeed, its loss results in loss of contact inhibition, activation of NF-kB transcriptional activity and enhanced cell migration. Thus ING4 deficiency may be a crucial step in malignant progression, especially for glioblastoma [9,10,15,16,66,71-75].

ING4 also associates with HBO1 (HAT binding to ORC1)/HAT complex [63,76]. It was shown that interaction between ING4 and H3K4me3 augments HBO1 acetylation activity on H3 tails and drives H3 acetylation at ING4 target promoters, which facilitates apoptosis in response to genotoxic stress and inhibits anchorage-independent cell growth, and these functions depend on ING4 interaction with H3K4me3 [77]. ING4 was recently reported to interact with tumor suppressor p53 through interaction with NLS domain and negatively regulate the cell growth with significant G2/M arrest of cell cycle in HepG2 cells through up-regulation of p53-inducible gene p21 [31,78].

Similar to ING4, ING5 was also identified by Shiseki et al [66]. Overexpression of ING5 protein also resulted in a diminished colony-forming efficiency, a decreased cell population in S phase, and the induction of apoptosis in a p53-dependent manner. p28ING5 protein activated the p21/waf1 promoter, and induced p21/WAF1 expression [66]. Relatively little information is available in the literature for ING5. Doyon et al. recently identified MOZ (monocytic leukemia zinc finger protein)/MORF (MOZ related factor) and HBO1 to be catalytic native subunits of ING5 complexes, which are necessary for their activity [63]. The MOZ, and the related factor MORF also form tetrameric complexes with Esa1-associated factor 6 ortholog (EAF6), and the bromodomain- and PHD finger protein (BRPF)-1, -2, or -3. BRPF proteins are rich in domains found in chromatin-associated factors, like PHD fingers and bromodomain. Ullah and his group found that BRPF proteins bridge the association of MOZ and MORF with ING5 and a homolog of yeast Esa-1 associated factor 6 (EAF6) [9,10,79]. ING5 as an adapter molecule links the MOZ/MORF and HBO1/HAT complexes. PHD fingers of ING proteins recognize histone H3 methylated at lysine 4 at the chromatin, suggesting the functional role of ING5 in the chromatin remodeling process [79, 80].

5. Disorders of ING family genes in human tumors

Rearrangement of ING1 gene locus was demonstrated in one neuroblastoma cell line and reduced expression in primary cancers and cell lines in early clinical studies at the time of ING1 cloning [8-11]. Following ING1 cDNA cloning, we identified the genomic structure of the human ING1 gene and showed its tumor suppressor character for the first time by finding its chromosomal deletion at the 13q34 locus and tumor-specific mutations in a number of head and neck squamous cell carcinoma (HNSCC) samples [8].

Few studies have analyzed the mRNA expression status of ING family genes in various human cancers. Toyama et al. found decrease of ING1 mRNA expression in about half of breast cancer samples and all of the breast cancer cell lines they examined [47]. Another study also revealed reduced expression of breast cancer samples [81]. Down-regulation of ING1 mRNA has also been demonstrated in various other cancer types, including lymphoid malignancies, gastric tumors, brain tumors, lung cancer, ovarian cancer and esophagogastric carcinomas, though no comprehensive clinical correlation was performed [9,10,15,16,82-90]. Uncommon missense mutations and reduced protein expression of ING1 have also been detected in esophageal carcinomas [91], and colon cancer cell lines [83] while no mutation was detected in leukemia [84,92], oral cancers [93] and lymphoid malignancies [82].

For loss of ING gene and their protein functions, loss of heterozygosity (LOH), promoter CpG hypermetylation and nucleo-cytoplasmic protein mislocalization have been proposed [9,10,15,16]. Using methylation-specific PCR, the p33ING1b promoter was methylated and silenced in almost a quarter of all cases in primary ovarian tumors [89]. No differences or increased expression of ING1 were observed in recent studies of myeloid leukemia or melanoma [92,94].

Recently reduced expression of ING2 mRNA as well as protein was observed in hepatocellular carcinoma (HCC) [95]. Decreased ING2 expression (but not ING2 mutation) has been observed in lung cancer [96]. Decrease of nuclear ING2 protein was observed in melanoma [57]. On the other hand increased expression of ING2 mRNA was shown in colon cancer [97]. We recently demonstrated that frequent deletion of ING2 locus at 4q35.1 associated with advanced tumor stage in HNSCC [98]. Moreover, ING2 may play a role in melanoma initiation, since reduction of nuclear ING2 has been reported in radial as well as vertical growth phases, and metastatic melanoma as compared to dysplastic nevi [57]. On the other hand, reduced ING2 expression was associated with tumor progression and shortened survival time in HCC [95]. These epidemiological studies suggest that ING2 loss or reduction may be important for tumor initiation and/or progression [9,10,15,16].

We showed frequent allelic loss of ING3 in HNSCC [42]. But ING3 mutation was very rare in our study (a sole missense mutation of ING3 at codon 20). In another recent study using a large study population, we revealed that down-regulation of ING3 was more evident in late-stage tumors as compared with early stage patients, and patients with low ING3 mRNA expression demonstrated worse survival rates as compared to the patients with normal-high ING3 expression [99]. As shown for ING2, decreased nuclear ING3 protein expression was associated with a poor survival rate. The survival rate was 93% for the patients with strong nuclear ING3 staining, whereas it declined to 44% for the patients with negative-to-moderate nuclear staining [100]. In a recent study, we also demonstrated frequent deletion of chromosomal locus of each of ING family member including ING3 in ameloblastomas [101].

ING4 mRNA was decreased in glioblastoma and associated with tumor progression [70]. Decreased ING4 has been associated with increased expression of IL-8 and osteopontin (OPN) in myeloma [9,102]. In both reports, decreased ING4 expression was associated with higher tumor grade and increased tumor angiogenesis. In myeloma, it was also associated with increased expression of interleukin-8 and osteopontin [9,102]. Expression of ING4 was decreased in malignant melanoma as compared to dysplastic nevi, and was found to be an independent poor prognostic factor for the patients [73]. ING4 was found to suppress the loss of contact inhibition and growth. Moreover some mutation and deletion were detected in cell lines derived from human cancers such as breast and lung [103].

We reported reduced expression level of ING4 and frequent LOH of the ING4 locus in HNSCC [43]. No mutation of the ING4 gene was found in head and neck cancers. Significant reduced expression of ING4 was detected in gliomas as compared with normal human brain tissue, and the extent of reduction correlated with the progression from lower to higher grades of tumours [70]. Klironomos et al. investigated immunohistochemically the expression pattern of ING-4, NF-kappaB and the NF-kappaB downstream targets MMP-2, MMP-9 and u-PA in human astrocytomas from 101 patients. They found that ING-4 expression was significantly reduced in astrocytomas, and it was associated with tumor grade progression. Expression of a NF-kappaB subunit p65 was significantly higher in grade

IV than in grade III and grade I/II tumors, and a statistical significant negative correlation between expression of ING-4 and expression of nuclear p65 was noticed [104].

Recently Nagahama et al. reported up-regulation of ING4 in a human gastric carcinoma cell line (MKN-1) by promoting mitochondria-mediated apoptosis via the activation of p53 [105]. Both mRNA and protein of ING4 expression were down regulated in hepatocellular carcinoma tissues. ING4 expression level correlated with prognosis and metastatic potential of hepatocellular carcinoma [106]. In another recent study, ING4 mRNA and protein expression were examined in gastric adenocarcinoma tissues and human gastric adenocarcinoma cell lines by RT-PCR, real-time RT-PCR, tissue microarray immunohistochemistry, and western blot analysis [107]. Their data showed that ING4 mRNA and protein were dramatically reduced in stomach adenocarcinoma cell lines and tissues, and significantly less in female than in male patients. Decrease of ING4 mRNA expression was found to correlate with the stage of the tumour [107]. Wang et al. examined ING4 protein expression in 246 lung cancer samples and overall reduced ING4 expression and higher ING4 expression in cytoplasm than in nucleus of tumour cells were detected, suggesting its involvement in the initiation and progression of lung cancers [108].

In a recent study, nuclear expression of ING4 was found to gradually decrease from non-cancerous epithelium and dysplasia to HNSCC and was negatively correlated with a poorly-differentiated status, T staging, and TNM staging in HNSCC. On the other hand, cytoplasmic expression of ING4 was significantly enhanced in HNSCC and was significantly associated with lymph node metastasis and 14-3-3η expression. Moreover, nuclear expression of ING4 was positively correlated with p21 and p300 expression and with the apoptotic index. Their results suggested that the decreases in nuclear ING4 and cytoplasmic translocation of ING4 protein play important roles in tumorigenesis, progression and tumor differentiation in HNSCC [109].

Examination of ING4 protein expression levels in colorectal cancer samples from 97 patients showed that ING4 protein was down regulated in adenoma relative to normal mucosa and further reduced in colorectal cancer tissues. Decrease of ING4 protein expression was also related to the more advanced Dukes' stages and ING4 expression levels in patients with lymphatic metastasis were lower than those without metastasis, suggesting that ING4 play a role in colorectal carcinoma progression [110].

Our group reported the first study linking ING5 chromosome locus to a human cancer. We demonstrated a high ratio of LOH in oral cancer using 16 microsatellite markers on the long arm of chromosome 2q21-37.3 [111]. ING5 appeared to be a strong candidate tumor suppressor in this study though several other candidate TSGs including ILKAP, HDAC4, PPP1R7, DTYMK, STK25, BOK are also localized at the area, where frequent deletion has been detected [9,10,111]. Moreover, our recent study revealed decreased expression of ING5 mRNA and mutations in oral cancer samples as compared to their corresponding normal controls, suggesting its tumor suppressive role in cancer [45]. Examination of 172 cases of HNSCC for ING5 protein by immunohistochemistry using tissue microarray, and in 3 oral SCC cell lines by immunohistochemistry and Western blot showed that a decrease in nuclear ING5 localization and cytoplasmic translocation were detected, supporting the previous studies and strong involvement of ING5 in tumorigenesis and tumor differentiation in HNSCC [112].

Xing et al. analyzed ING5 expression in gastric carcinoma tissues and cell lines (MKN28, MKN45, AGS, GT-3 TKB, and KATO-III) by Western blot and reverse transcriptase-polymerase chain reaction. An increased expression of ING5 messenger RNA was found in gastric carcinoma in comparison with paired mucosa and lower expression of nuclear ING5 protein and cytoplasmic translocation was detected in gastric dysplasia and carcinoma than that in nonneoplastic mucosa [113]. Nuclear ING5 expression was negatively correlated with tumor size, depth of invasion, lymph node metastasis, and clinicopathologic staging, whereas cytoplasmic ING5 was positively associated with depth of invasion, venous invasion, lymph node metastasis, and clinicopathologic staging [113].

6. Abnormalities of ING family genes in breast cancer

Abnormalities of ING family members are linked to etiopathogenesis of various cancers including breast cancer. In fact, ING1, the founding member, was first isolated using a method that combined PCR-mediated subtractive hybridization of cDNAs from normal and breast cancerous cells [11]. Later same group examined ING1 mutation and mRNA expression in breast cancer cell lines and in a large number of primary breast cancers [47]. Within 377 breast cancer patients analyzed for mutation of ING1, one germ-line missense and three germ-line silent alterations were detected. Then mRNA analysis was randomly examined in 48 breast cancer samples. Their results showed that ING1 mRNA expression was decreased (2-10-fold) in 44% (21 out of 48 cases) of breast cancer tissues compared to adjacent normal tissues, while 33% (16/48) of the tumors demonstrated levels similar to control sample and 23% (11/48) showed increases in ING1 mRNA. All of the 10 breast cancer lines displayed decreased ING1 mRNA expression. Using in situ hybridization, decrease of mRNA in breast cancer cells was also confirmed as compared to adjacent normal cells. Using a monoclonal antibody against ING1, similar levels of the protein was also demonstrated in randomly selected 10 breast cancer samples [47]. When the relationship between ING1 mRNA expression levels and clinicopathological factors of breast cancer samples was examined, probability of metastasis to regional lymph nodes was significantly increased in ING1-decreased samples. Only one of 11 tumors (%9) with increased ING1 mRNA expression metastasized to lymph nodes, whereas 11 of 19 cases (58%) with decreased expression of ING1 showed metastasis to lymph nodes [47].

Tokunaga et al. examined the expression of ING1 mRNA in breast cancer cell lines and clinical breast cancer tissues, using quantitative RT-PCR and real-time TaqMan™ technology [81]. Decreased expression of ING1 mRNA was found in 71% of the breast cancer samples as compared to adjacent normal tissues. The authors has also examined p53 mutation status by immunohistochemistry and decreased ING1 expression was detected in 9 of 15 tumors that were negative for p53 immunostaining (i.e, wild type). Decrease of ING1 mRNA was speculated to be responsible for malfunction of p53 in these cases [9,10,81].

In an immunohistochemical study performed by Nouman et al, 69 (80%) out of 86 breast cancer cases showed reduced expression of p33ING1b protein. On the other hand, strong nuclear expression of ING1 protein was detected in normal breast lobules and adjacent stroma. Correlation of each of estrogen and progesterone receptor status demonstrated a positive response with nuclear expression of p33ING1b protein. Nuclear loss of ING1 protein was associated with a concomitant enhancement of cytoplasmic p33ING1b expression in a proportion of the cases, suggesting as a cause for loss of normal function of the ING1 protein [114]. Similar reduced nuclear expression of p33ING1b protein was also shown in acute lymphoblastic leukemia [115], melanoma [116].

Toyama et al. reported that p33ING1b increased ERα transcriptional activity stimulated by estrogen through AF2 domain [10, 117]. In another research, p40, a protein highly homologous to breast carcinoma metastasis suppressor 1 (BRMS1), was found to be unit of the mammalian Sin3A co-repressor complex including RBP1 and p33ING1b and overexpression of p40 in human cells inhibited cell growth by recruiting the HDAC1 deacetylase complex. When tethered to the promoter by Gal-DNA binding domain, p40 can repress transcription of the luciferase reporter gene [118].

Kim et al. tried to identify genes that can suppress oncogenic properties such as loss of contact inhibition elicited by overexpression of MYCN. Their screen data revealed ING4 as a suppressor of loss of contact inhibition. Then they hypothesized that a deficiency of ING4 may play a role in tumorigenesis. For this aim, they examined ING4 transcripts in human cancer cell lines. They found a common deletion in various cancer cell lines including a breast cancer cell, T47D. Deletion of the four highly charged amino acid residues (KGKK) would result in mislocalization of the ING4 protein, thereby impairing its function [103]. Later this deletion was reported to be a source of alternative splicing variants of ING4 and was linked to abnormalities of subcellular localization of ING4 [71]. Besides Kim et al. also performed southern blot analysis for ING4 locus deletion in 55 breast cancer cell lines using 2 BAC probe within ING4 locus at 12p13.31. These probes, BAC RP11-272L6 and BAC RP11-59H1, were shown to be deleted in 24% and 11% of the cells including T47D breast cancer cell line, respectively [103].

In a recent study, ING4 was found to suppress an initial hyperplastic response to the oncogene MYC in a mouse model of breast cancer. In addition, they showed that a C-terminal truncation mutant of ING4 found in a human neuroblastoma cell line induced mammary hyperplasia and exacerbated MYC-initiated mammary tumorigenesis, suggesting that ING4 can function as a tumor suppressor gene in breast tissue [119].

In another recent report, therapeutic effect of adenovirus-mediated ING4 (Ad-ING4) gene therapy was investigated in human breast cancers in vitro and in vivo in an athymic nude mouse model, using two human breast carcinoma cell lines MDA-MB-231 (mutant p53) and MCF-7 (wild-type p53). The results displayed that Ad-ING4 treatment could induce in vitro significant growth suppression in both mutant p53 MDA-MB-231 and wild-type p53 MCF-7 breast carcinoma cells despite p53 status. Moreover the study further revealed that Ad-ING4 gene transfer resulted in G2/M phase arrest and apoptosis, upregulation of p21, p27, and Bax, downregulation of Bcl-2, IL-8, and Ang-1, promoted cytochrome c release from mitochondria into cytosol, and activated caspase-9, caspase-3, and PARP in mutant p53 MDA-MB-231 breast carcinoma cells. Furthermore, intratumoral injections of Ad-ING4 in nude mice bearing mutant p53 MDA-MB-231 breast tumors clearly inhibited the human breast xenografted tumor growth and decreased CD34 expression of tumor vessels and microvessel density. All these results suggest that Ad-ING4 is a potential candidate for breast cancer gene therapy [120].

ING4 was detected to be deleted in 170 (16.5%) of 1033 breast cancer samples using two color FISH with a probe of BAC RP11-433J6 including ING4 locus. Comparison of clinicopathological variables with ING4 deletion status in these breast cancer samples showed significant difference for Her2 expression status. Thirty- nine (23.8%) of 164 of tumors with ING4 deletion were HER2 positive, as compared with 115 (14.1%) of 814 of tumors without deletion. In another way, 25.3% (39/ 154) of HER2-positive tumors harbored ING4 deletion as compared to 15.1% (125/824) of HER2-negative tumors, indicating that ING4 deletion is more common in HER2- positive tumors [121]. In breast cancer, there is no report yet regarding with other members of ING family, ING2, 3 and 5. A summary of alterations of ING family genes in breast cancer is shown in table 1.

ING Gene	Alteration	Reference
ING1	Mutation,↓ mRNA expression, ↓protein expression	47
ING1	↓ mRNA expression	81
ING1	↓ Nuclear protein,↑ Cytoplasmic protein	114
ING1	Induction of ERα activity	117
ING4	Deletion at chromosomal locus	103
ING4	Suppression of MYC-induced carcinogenesis	119
ING4	Ad-ING4-treated suppression of cancer cells and tumor growth	120
ING4	Deletion at chromosomal locus	121

Table 1. Alterations of ING Family Genes in Breast Cancer.

7. Future prospects

Nearly 15 years of research after discovery of the first member of ING family gene, ING1, there are more accumulating data which show importance of these gene family in multiple cellular functions such as transcription, chromatin regulation, cell cycling, angiogenesis, cell transformation, apoptosis, growth regulation, senescence, DNA repair and tumorigenesis etc. Recent knowledge on this family displays that the family members have common and separate functions in human cancer. Though at the beginning, all members were considered to be tumor suppressor, recent evidences show a complex situation with oncogenic functions for at least some of the members and in some specific conditions. Thus both diagnostic and therapeutic approach should be revisited according to their functional roles in various conditions and tumor types. Though much work is necessary for clarifying the exact functions of these genes to provide therapy for various human cancers, promising results are noticed at the moment for usability of these genes as a therapeutic and diagnostic target. Thus progress on the knowledge of functions of ING family genes as well as the relationship with p53 and other unknown molecules will clarify their roles in cancer, which will result in their uses in cancer diagnostics as well as therapy soon.

8. References

Hinds PW and Weinberg RA. Tumor suppressor genes. Curr Opin Genet Dev 4: 135-141, 1994

Knudson AG Jr. Mutation and cancer: statistical study of retinoblastoma. Proc Natl Acad Sci USA 68: 820-823, 1971

Tang B, Bottinger EP, Jakowlew SB, Bagnall KM, Mariano J, Anver MR, Letterio JJ and Wakefield LM. Transforming growth factor-b1 is a new form of tumor suppressor with true haploid insufficiency. Nat Med 4: 802-807, 1998

Bai F, Pei XH, Godfrey VL and Xiong Y. Haploinsufficiency of p18 (INK4c) sensitizes mice to carcinogen-induced tumorigenesis. Mol Cell Biol 23: 1269-1277, 2003

Mduff FK, Hook CE, Tooze RM, Huntly BJ, Pandolfi PP, Turner SD. Determining the contribution of NPM1 heterozygosity to NPM-ALK-induced lymphomagenesis. Lab Invest. 2011 Jun 27. doi: 10.1038/labinvest.2011.96. [Epub ahead of print]

Huang H, Wei X, Su X, Qiao F, Xu Z, Gu D, Fan H, Chen J. Clinical significance of expression of Hint1 and potential epigenetic mechanism in gastric cancer. Int J Oncol 38:1557-64, 2011

Zhou XZ, Huang P, Shi R, Lee TH, Lu G, Zhang Z, Bronson R, Lu KP. The telomerase inhibitor PinX1 is a major haploinsufficient tumor suppressor essential for chromosome stability in mice. J Clin Invest 121(4):1266-82, 2011

Gunduz M, Ouchida M, Fukushima K, Hanafusa H, Etani T, Nishioka S, Nishizaki K and Shimizu K. Genomic structure of the human ING1 gene and tumor-specific mutations detected in head and neck squamous cell carcinomas. Cancer Res 60: 3143-3146, 2000

Gunduz M, Gunduz E, Rivera RS, Nagatsuka H. The inhibitor of growth (ING) gene family: potential role in cancer therapy. Curr Cancer Drug Targets 8:275-84, 2008

Gunduz M, Demircan K, Gunduz E, Katase N, Tamamura R, Nagatsuka H. Potential usage of ING family members in cancer diagnostics and molecular therapy. Curr Drug Targets. 10(5):465-76, 2009

Garkavtsev I, Kazarov A, Gudkov A and Riabowol K. Suppression of the novel growth inhibitor p33ING1 promotes neoplastic transformation. Nat Genet 14: 415-420, 1996

Helbing CC, Veilette C, Riabowol K, Johnston RN and Garkavtsev I. A novel candidate tumor suppressor gene, ING1, is involved in the regulation of apoptosis. Cancer Res 57: 1255-1258, 1997

Zeremski M, Horrigan SK, Grigorian IA, Westbrook CA and Gudkov AV. Localization of the candidate tumor suppressor gene ING1 to human chromosome 13q34. Somatic Cell Mol Genet 23: 233-236, 1997

Feng X, Hara Y and Riabowol K. Different HATS of the ING1 gene family. Trends Cell Biol 12: 532-538, 2002

Aguissa-Touré AH, Wong RP, Li G. Cell Mol Life Sci. The ING family tumor suppressors: from structure to function. 68:45-54, 2011

Coles AH, Jones SN. The ING gene family in the regulation of cell growth and tumorigenesis. J Cell Physiol 218:45-57, 2009

Unoki M, Kumamoto K, Harris CC. ING proteins as potential anticancer drug targets. Curr Drug Targets 10:442-54, 2009

Aasland R, Gibson TJ, Stewart AF. The PHD finger: implications for chromatin-mediated transcriptional regulation. Trends Biochem Sci 20:56-59, 1995

Shimada Y, Saito A, Suzuki M, Takahashi E, Horie M. Cloning of a novel gene (ING1L) homologous to ING1, a candidate tumor suppressor. Cytogenet Cell Genet 83:232- 235, 1998

Ha S, Park S, Yun CH, Choi Y. Characterization of nuclear localization signal in mouse ING1 homolog protein. Biochem Biophys Res Commun 293:163-166, 2002

Scott M, Boisvert FM, Vieyra D, Johnston RN, Bazett-Jones DP, Riabowol K. UV induces nucleolar translocation of ING1 through two distinct nucleolar targeting sequences. Nucleic Acids Re 29:2052-2058, 2001

Zeremski M, Hill JE, Kwek SS, Grigorian IA, Gurova KV, Garkavtsev IV, Diatchenko L, Koonin EV, Gudkov AV. Structure and regulation of the mouse ing1 gene. Three alternative transcripts encode two phd finger proteins that have opposite effects on p53 function. J Biol Chem 274:32172-32181, 1999

Pascual J, Martinez-Yamout M, Dyson HJ, Wright PE. Structure of the PHD zinc finger from human Williams-Beuren syndrome transcription factor. J Mol Biol 304:723-9, 2000

Gibbons RJ, Bachoo S, Picketts DJ, Aftimos S, Asenbauer B, Bergoffen J, Berry SA, Dahl N, Fryer A, Keppler K, Kurosawa K, Levin ML, Masuno M, Neri G, Pierpont ME, Slaney SF, Higgs DR. Mutations in transcriptional regulator ATRX establish the functional significance of a PHD-like domain. Nat Genet 17:146-8, 1997

Saugier-Veber P, Drouot N, Wolf LM, Kuhn JM, Frébourg T, Lefebvre H. Identification of a novel mutation in the autoimmune regulator (AIRE-1) gene in a French family with autoimmune polyendocrinopathy-candidiasis-ectodermal dystrophy. Eur J Endocrinol 144:347-51, 2001

Elkin SK, Ivanov D, Ewalt M, Ferguson CG, Hyberts SG, Sun ZY, Prestwich GD, Yuan J, Wagner G, Oettinger MA, Gozani OP. A PHD finger motif in the C terminus of RAG2 modulates recombination activity. J Biol Chem 280:28701-10, 2005

Han X, Feng X, Rattner JB, Smith H, Bose P, Suzuki K, Soliman MA, Scott MS, Burke BE, Riabowol K. Tethering by lamin A stabilizes and targets the ING1 tumour suppressor. Nat Cell Biol 10:1333–1340, 2008

Scott M, Boisvert FM, Vieyra D, Johnston RN, Bazett-Jones DP, Riabowol K. UV induces nucleolar translocation of ING1 through two distinct nucleolar targeting sequences. Nucleic Acids Res 29:2052–2058, 2001

Ha S, Park S, Yun CH, Choi Y. Characterization of nuclear localization signal in mouse ING1 homolog protein. Biochem Biophys Res Commun 293:163–166, 2002

Gong W, Suzuki K, Russell M, Riabowol K. Function of the ING family of PHD proteins in cancer. Int J Biochem Cell Biol 37:1054–1065, 2005

Zhang X, Wang KS, Wang ZQ, Xu LS, Wang QW, Chen F, Wei DZ, Han ZG. Nuclear localization signal of ING4 plays a key role in its binding to p53. Biochem Biophys Res Commun 331:1032–1038, 2005

Soliman MA, Riabowol K. After a decade of study-ING, a PHD for a versatile family of proteins. Trends Biochem Sci 32:509–519, 2007

He GH, Helbing CC, Wagner MJ, Sensen CW, Riabowol K. Phylogenetic analysis of the ING family of PHD finger proteins. Mol Biol Evol 22:104–116, 2005

Wang Y, Wang J, Li G. Leucine zipper-like domain is required for tumor suppressor ING2-mediated nucleotide excision repair and apoptosis. FEBS Lett 580:3787–3793, 2006

Wang J, Chin MY, Li G. The novel tumor suppressor p33ING2 enhances nucleotide excision repair via inducement of histone H4 acetylation and chromatin relaxation. Cancer Res 66:1906–1911, 2006

Scott M, Bonnefin P, Vieyra D, Boisvert FM, Young D, Bazett- Jones DP, Riabowol K. UV-induced binding of ING1 to PCNA regulates the induction of apoptosis. J Cell Sci 114:3455–3462, 2001

Kuzmichev A, Zhang Y, Erdjument-Bromage H, Tempst P, Reinberg D. Role of the

Sin3-histone deacetylase com- plex in growth regulation by the candidate tumor suppressor p33(ING1). Mol Cell Biol 22:835–848, 2002

Kaadige MR, Ayer DE. The polybasic region that follows the plant homeodomain zinc finger 1 of Pf1 is necessary and sufficient for specific phosphoinositide binding. J Biol Chem 281:28831–28836, 2006

Huang W, Zhang H, Davrazou F, Kutateladze TG, Shi X, Gozani O, Prestwich GD. Stabilized phosphatidylinositol- 5-phosphate analogues as ligands for the nuclear protein ING2: chemistry, biology, and molecular modeling. J Am Chem Soc 129:6498–6506, 2007

Unoki M, Kumamoto K, Robles AI, Shen JC, Zheng ZM, Harris CC. A novel ING2 isoform, ING2b, synergizes with ING2a to prevent cell cycle arrest and apoptosis. FEBS Lett 582:3868-74, 2008

Unoki M, Kumamoto K, Takenoshita S, Harris CC. Reviewing the current classification of inhibitor of growth family proteins. Cancer Sci 100:1173-9, 2009

Gunduz M, Ouchida M, Fukushima K, Ito S, Jitsumori Y, Nakashima T, Nagai N, Nishizaki K, Shimizu K. Allelic loss and reduced expression of the ING3, a candidate tumor suppressor gene at 7q31, in human head and neck cancers. Oncogene 21:4462-70, 2002

Gunduz M, Nagatsuka H, Demircan K, Gunduz E, Cengiz B, Ouchida M, Tsujigiwa H, Yamachika E, Fukushima K, Beder L, Hirohata S, Ninomiya Y, Nishizaki K, Shimizu K, Nagai N. Frequent deletion and down-regulation of ING4, a candidate tumor suppressor gene at 12p13, in head and neck squamous cell carcinomas. Gene 15;356:109-117, 2005

Ythier D, Larrieu D, Brambilla C, Brambilla E, Pedeux R. The new tumor suppressor genes ING: genomic structure and status in cancer. Int J Cancer 123:1483-90, 2008

Cengiz B, Gunduz E, Gunduz M, Beder LB, Tamamura R, Bagci C, Yamanaka N, Shimizu K, Nagatsuka H. Tumor-specific mutation and downregulation of ING5 detected in oral squamous cell carcinoma. Int J Cancer 127:2088-94, 2010

Campos EI, Chin MY, Kuo WH, Li G. Biological functions of the ING family tumor suppressors. Cell Mol Life Sci 61(19-20):2597-613, 2004

Toyama T, Iwase H, Watson P, Muzik H, Saettler E, Magliocco A, DiFrancesco L, Forsyth P, Garkavtsev I, Kobayashi S, Riabowol K. Suppression of ING1 expression in sporadic breast cancer. Oncogene 18:5187-93, 1999

Coles AH, Liang H, Zhu Z, Marfella CG, Kang J, Imbalzano AN, Jones SN. Deletion of p37Ing1 in mice reveals a p53-independent role for Ing1 in the suppression of cell proliferation, apoptosis, and tumorigenesis. Cancer Res 67:2054-61, 2007

Ozer A, Bruick RK. Regulation of HIF by prolyl hydroxylases: recruitment of the candidate tumor suppressor protein ING4. Cell Cycle 4:1153-6, 2005

Ozer A, Wu LC, Bruick RK. The candidate tumor suppressor ING4 represses activation of the hypoxia inducible factor (HIF). Proc Natl Acad Sci U S A 102:7481-6, 2005

Coles AH, Gannon H, Cerny A, Kurt-Jones E, Jones SN. Inhibitor of growth-4 promotes IkappaB promoter activation to suppress NF-kappaB signaling and innate immunity. Proc Natl Acad Sci U S A 107:11423-8, 2010

Nozell S, Laver T, Moseley D, Nowoslawski L, De Vos M, Atkinson GP, Harrison K, Nabors LB, Benveniste EN. The ING4 tumor suppressor attenuates NF-kappaB activity at the promoters of target genes. Mol Cell Biol 28:6632-45, 2008

Nagashima M, Shiseki M, Miura K, Hagiwara K, Linke SP, Pedeux R, Wang XW,

Yokota J, Riabowol K, Harris CC. DNA damage-inducible gene p33ING2 negatively regulates cell proliferation through acetylation of p53. Proc Natl Acad Sci U S A 98:9671-6, 2001

Pedeux R, Sengupta S, Shen JC, Demidov ON, Saito S, Onogi H, Kumamoto K, Wincovitch S, Garfield SH, McMenamin M, Nagashima M, Grossman SR, Appella E, Harris CC. ING2 regulates the onset of replicative senescence by induction of p300-dependent p53 acetylation. Mol Cell Biol 25:6639-48, 2005

Sarker KP, Kataoka H, Chan A, Netherton SJ, Pot I, Huynh MA, Feng X, Bonni A, Riabowol K, Bonni S. ING2 as a novel mediator of transforming growth factor-beta- dependent responses in epithelial cells. J Biol Chem 283:13269-79, 2008

Borkosky SS, Gunduz M, Nagatsuka H, Beder LB, Gunduz E, Ali MA, Rodriguez AP, Cilek MZ, Tominaga S, Yamanaka N, Shimizu K, Nagai N. Frequent deletion of ING2 locus at 4q35.1 associates with advanced tumor stage in head and neck squamous cell carcinoma. J Cancer Res Clin Oncol 135:703-13, 2009

Lu F, Dai DL, Martinka M, Ho V, Li G. Nuclear ING2 expression is reduced in human cutaneous melanomas. Br J Cancer 95:80-6, 2006

Larrieu D, Ythier D, Binet R, Brambilla C, Brambilla E, Sengupta S, Pedeux R. ING2 controls the progression of DNA replication forks to maintain genome stability. EMBO Rep 10:1168-74, 2009

Nagashima M, Shiseki M, Pedeux RM, Okamura S, Kitahama-Shiseki M, Miura K, Yokota J, Harris CC. A novel PHD-finger motif protein, p47ING3, modulates p53- mediated transcription, cell cycle control, and apoptosis. Oncogene 22:343-50, 2003

Doyon Y, Côté J.The highly conserved and multifunctional NuA4 HAT complex. Curr Opin Genet Dev 14:147-5, 2004

Kataoka H, Bonnefin P, Vieyra D, Feng X, Hara Y, Miura Y, Joh T, Nakabayashi H, Vaziri H, Harris CC, Riabowol K. ING1 represses transcription by direct DNA binding and through effects on p53. Cancer Res 63:5785-92, 2003

Doyon Y, Selleck W, Lane WS, Tan S, Côté J. Structural and functional conservation of the NuA4 histone acetyltransferase complex from yeast to humans. Mol Cell Biol 24:1884-9, 2004

Doyon Y, Cayrou C, Ullah M, Landry AJ, Côté V, Selleck W, Lane WS, Tan S, Yang XJ, Côté J. ING tumor suppressor proteins are critical regulators of chromatin acetylation required for genome expression and perpetuation. Mol Cell 21:51-64, 2006

Wang Y, Li G. J. ING3 promotes UV-induced apoptosis via Fas/caspase-8 pathway in melanoma cells. Biol Chem 281:11887-93, 2006

Chen G, Wang Y, Garate M, Zhou J, Li G. The tumor suppressor ING3 is degraded by SCF (Skp2)-mediated ubiquitin-proteasome system. Oncogene 29:1498-508, 2010

Shiseki M, Nagashima M, Pedeux RM, Kitahama-Shiseki M, Miura K, Okamura S, Onogi H, Higashimoto Y, Appella E, Yokota J, Harris CC. p29ING4 and p28ING5 bind to p53 and p300, and enhance p53 activity. Cancer Res 63:2373-8, 2003

Li J, Li G. Cell cycle regulator ING4 is a suppressor of melanoma angiogenesis that is regulated by the metastasis suppressor BRMS1. Cancer Res 70:10445-53, 2010

Xie YF, Sheng W, Xiang J, Zhang H, Ye Z, Yang J. Adenovirus-mediated ING4 expression suppresses pancreatic carcinoma cell growth via induction of cell-cycle alteration, apoptosis, and inhibition of tumor angiogenesis. Cancer Biother Radiopharm 24:261-9, 2009

Zhu Y, Lv H, Xie Y, Sheng W, Xiang J, Yang J. Enhanced tumor suppression by an ING4/IL-24 bicistronic adenovirus-mediated gene cotransfer in human non-small cell lung cancer cells. Cancer Gene Ther. 2011 Jun 10. doi: 10.1038/cgt.2011.31. [Epub ahead of print]

Garkavtsev I, Kozin SV, Chernova O, Xu L, Winkler F, Brown E, Barnett GH, Jain RK. The candidate tumour suppressor protein ING4 regulates brain tumour growth and angiogenesis. Nature 428:328-32, 2004

Unoki M, Shen JC, Zheng ZM, Harris CC. Novel splice variants of ING4 and their possible roles in the regulation of cell growth and motility. J Biol Chem 281:34677- 86, 2006

Shen JC, Unoki M, Ythier D, Duperray A, Varticovski L, Kumamoto K, Pedeux R, Harris CC. Inhibitor of growth 4 suppresses cell spreading and cell migration by interacting with a novel binding partner, liprin alpha1. Cancer Res 67:2552-8, 2007

Li J, Martinka M, Li G. Role of ING4 in human melanoma cell migration, invasion and patient survival. Carcinogenesis 29:1373-9, 2008

Cai L, Li X, Zheng S, Wang Y, Wang Y, Li H, Yang J, Sun J. Inhibitor of growth 4 is involved in melanomagenesis and induces growth suppression and apoptosis in melanoma cell line M14. Melanoma Res 19:1-7, 2009

Li X, Cai L, Chen H, Zhang Q, Zhang S, Wang Y, Dong Y, Cheng H, Qi J. Inhibitor of growth 4 induces growth suppression and apoptosis in glioma U87MG. Pathobiology 76:181-92, 2009

Saksouk N, Avvakumov N, Champagne KS, Hung T, Doyon Y, Cayrou C, Paquet E, Ullah M, Landry AJ, Côté V, Yang XJ, Gozani O, Kutateladze TG, Côté J. HBO1 HAT complexes target chromatin throughout gene coding regions via multiple PHD finger interactions with histone H3 tail. Mol Cell 33:257-65, 2009

Hung T, Binda O, Champagne KS, Kuo AJ, Johnson K, Chang HY, Simon MD, Kutateladze TG, Gozani O. ING4 mediates crosstalk between histone H3 K4 trimethylation and H3 acetylation to attenuate cellular transformation. Mol Cell 33:248-56, 2009

Zhang X, Xu LS, Wang ZQ, Wang KS, Li N, Cheng ZH, Huang SZ, Wei DZ, Han ZG. ING4 induces G2/M cell cycle arrest and enhances the chemosensitivity to DNA- damage agents in HepG2 cells. FEBS Lett 570:7-12, 2004

Ullah M, Pelletier N, Xiao L, Zhao SP, Wang K, Degerny C, Tahmasebi S, Cayrou C, Doyon Y, Goh SL, Champagne N, Côté J, Yang XJ. Molecular architecture of quartet MOZ/MORF histone acetyltransferase complexes. Mol Cell Biol 28:6828-43, 2008 Erratum in: Mol Cell Biol. 2009 Feb;29:942

Champagne KS, Saksouk N, Peña PV, Johnson K, Ullah M, Yang XJ, Côté J, Kutateladze TG. The crystal structure of the ING5 PHD finger in complex with an H3K4me3 histone peptide. Proteins 72:1371-6, 2008

Tokunaga E, Maehara Y, Oki E, Kitamura K, Kakeji Y, Ohno S, Sugimachi K. Diminished expression of ING1 mRNA and the correlation with p53 expression in breast cancers. Cancer Lett 152:15-22, 2000

Ohmori M, Nagai M, Tasaka T, Koeffler HP, Toyama T, Riabowol K, Takahara J. Decreased expression of p33ING1 mRNA in lymphoid malignancies. Am J Hematol 62:118-9, 1999 Erratum in: Am J Hematol 2000 May;64(1):82.

Oki E, Maehara Y, Tokunaga E, Kakeji Y, Sugimachi K. Reduced expression of p33 (ING1) and the relationship with p53 expression in human gastric cancer. Cancer Lett 147:157-62, 1999

Ito K, Kinjo K, Nakazato T, Ikeda Y, Kizaki M. Expression and sequence analyses of p33(ING1) gene in myeloid leukemia. Am J Hematol 69:141-3, 2002

Hara Y, Zheng Z, Evans SC, Malatjalian D, Riddell DC, Guernsey DL, Wang LD, Riabowol K, Casson AG. ING1 and p53 tumor suppressor gene alterations in adenocarcinomas of the esophagogastric junction. Cancer Lett 192:109-16, 2003

Tallen G, Riabowol K, Wolff JE. Expression of p33ING1 mRNA and chemosensitivity in brain tumor cells. Anticancer Res 23(2B):1631-5, 2003

Tallen G, Kaiser I, Krabbe S, Lass U, Hartmann C, Henze G, Riabowol K, von Deimling A No ING1 mutations in human brain tumours but reduced expression in high malignancy grades of astrocytoma. Int J Cancer 109:476-9, 2004

Takahashi M, Ozaki T, Todo S, Nakagawara A. Decreased expression of the candidate tumor suppressor gene ING1 is associated with poor prognosis in advanced neuroblastomas. Oncol Rep 12:811-6, 2004

Shen DH, Chan KY, Khoo US, Ngan HY, Xue WC, Chiu PM, Ip P, Cheung AN. Epigenetic and genetic alterations of p33ING1b in ovarian cancer. Carcinogenesis 26:855-63, 2005

Kameyama K, Huang CL, Liu D, Masuya D, Nakashima T, Sumitomo S, Takami Y, Kinoshita M, Yokomise H. Reduced ING1b gene expression plays an important role in carcinogenesis of non-small cell lung cancer patients. Clin Cancer Res 9:4926-34, 2003

Chen L, Matsubara N, Yoshino T, Nagasaka T, Hoshizima N, Shirakawa Y, Naomoto Y, Isozaki H, Riabowol K, Tanaka N. Genetic alterations of candidate tumor suppressor ING1 in human esophageal squamous cell cancer. Cancer Res 61:4345-9, 2001

Bromidge T, Lynas C. Relative levels of alternative transcripts of the ING1 gene and lack of mutations of p33/ING1 in haematological malignancies. Leuk Res 26:631-5, 2002

Krishnamurthy J, Kannan K, Feng J, Mohanprasad BK, Tsuchida N, Shanmugam G. Mutational analysis of the candidate tumor suppressor gene ING1 in Indian oral squamous cell carcinoma. Oral Oncol 37:222-4, 2001

Stark M, Puig-Butille JA, Walker G, Badenas C, Malvehy J, Hayward N, Puig S. Mutation of the tumour suppressor p33ING1b is rare in melanoma. Br J Dermatol 155:94-9, 2006

Zhang HK, Pan K, Wang H, Weng DS, Song HF, Zhou J, Huang W, Li JJ, Chen MS, Xia JC. Decreased expression of ING2 gene and its clinicopathological significance in hepatocellular carcinoma. Cancer Lett 261:183-92, 2008

Okano T, Gemma A, Hosoya Y, Hosomi Y, Nara M, Kokubo Y, Yoshimura A, Shibuya M, Nagashima M, Harris CC, Kudoh S. Alterations in novel candidate tumor suppressor genes, ING1 and ING2 in human lung cancer. Oncol Rep 15:545-9, 2006

Kumamoto K, Fujita K, Kurotani R, Saito M, Unoki M, Hagiwara N, Shiga H, Bowman ED, Yanaihara N, Okamura S, Nagashima M, Miyamoto K, Takenoshita S, Yokota J, Harris CC. ING2 is upregulated in colon cancer and increases invasion by enhanced MMP13 expression. Int J Cancer 125:1306-15, 2009

Borkosky SS, Gunduz M, Nagatsuka H, Beder LB, Gunduz E, Ali MA, Rodriguez AP,

Cilek MZ, Tominaga S, Yamanaka N, Shimizu K, Nagai N. Frequent deletion of ING2 locus at 4q35.1 associates with advanced tumor stage in head and neck squamous cell carcinoma. J Cancer Res Clin Oncol 135:703-13, 2009

Gunduz M, Beder LB, Gunduz E, Nagatsuka H, Fukushima K, Pehlivan D, Cetin E, Yamanaka N, Nishizaki K, Shimizu K, Nagai N. Downregulation of ING3 mRNA expression predicts poor prognosis in head and neck cancer. Cancer Sci 99:531-8, 2008

Wang Y, Dai DL, Martinka M, Li G. Prognostic significance of nuclear ING3 expression in human cutaneous melanoma. Clin Cancer Res 13:4111-6, 2007

Borkosky SS, Gunduz M, Beder L, Tsujigiwa H, Tamamura R, Gunduz E, Katase N, Rodriguez AP, Sasaki A, Nagai N, Nagatsuka H. Allelic loss of the ING gene family loci is a frequent event in ameloblastoma. Oncol Res 18:509-18, 2010

Colla S, Tagliaferri S, Morandi F, Lunghi P, Donofrio G, Martorana D, Mancini C, Lazzaretti M, Mazzera L, Ravanetti L, Bonomini S, Ferrari L, Miranda C, Ladetto M, Neri TM, Neri A, Greco A, Mangoni M, Bonati A, Rizzoli V, Giuliani N. The new tumor-suppressor gene inhibitor of growth family member 4 (ING4) regulates the production of proangiogenic molecules by myeloma cells and suppresses hypoxia- inducible factor-1 alpha (HIF-1alpha) activity: involvement in myeloma-induced angiogenesis. Blood 110:4464-75, 2007. Epub 2007 Sep 11. Erratum in Blood. 2008 Sep 1;112:2170.

Kim S, Chin K, Gray JW, Bishop JM. A screen for genes that suppress loss of contact inhibition: identification of ING4 as a candidate tumor suppressor gene in human cancer. Proc Natl Acad Sci U S A 101:16251-6, 2004

Klironomos G, Bravou V, Papachristou DJ, Gatzounis G, Varakis J, Parassi E, Repanti M, Papadaki H. Loss of inhibitor of growth (ING-4) is implicated in the pathogenesis and progression of human astrocytomas. Brain Pathol 20:490-7, 2010

Nagahama Y, Ishimaru M, Osaki M, Inoue T, Maeda A, Nakada C, Moriyama M, Sato K, Oshimura M, Ito H. Apoptotic pathway induced by transduction of RUNX3 in the human gastric carcinoma cell line MKN-1. Cancer Sci 99:23-30, 2008

Fang F, Luo LB, Tao YM, Wu F, Yang LY. Decreased expression of inhibitor of growth 4 correlated with poor prognosis of hepatocellular carcinoma. Cancer Epidemiol Biomarkers Prev 18:409-16, 2009

Li M, Jin Y, Sun WJ, Yu Y, Bai J, Tong DD, Qi JP, Du JR, Geng JS, Huang Q, Huang XY, Huang Y, Han FF, Meng XN, Rosales JL, Lee KY, Fu SB. Reduced expression and novel splice variants of ING4 in human gastric adenocarcinoma. J Pathol 219:87-95, 2009

Wang QS, Li M, Zhang LY, Jin Y, Tong DD, Yu Y, Bai J, Huang Q, Liu FL, Liu A, Lee KY, Fu SB. Down-regulation of ING4 is associated with initiation and progression of lung cancer. Histopathology 57:271-81, 2010

Li XH, Kikuchi K, Zheng Y, Noguchi A, Takahashi H, Nishida T, Masuda S, Yang XH, Takano Y. Downregulation and translocation of nuclear ING4 is correlated with tumorigenesis and progression of head and neck squamous cell carcinoma. Oral Oncol 47:217-23, 2011

You Q, Wang XS, Fu SB, Jin XM. Downregulated Expression of Inhibitor of Growth 4 (ING4) in Advanced Colorectal Cancers: A Non-Randomized Experimental Study. Pathol Oncol Res. 2011 May 31. [Epub ahead of print]

Cengiz B, Gunduz M, Nagatsuka H, Beder L, Gunduz E, Tamamura R, Mahmut N, Fukushima K, Ali MA, Naomoto Y, Shimizu K, Nagai N. Fine deletion mapping of chromosome 2q21-37 shows three preferentially deleted regions in oral cancer. Oral Oncol 43:241-7, 2007

Li X, Nishida T, Noguchi A, Zheng Y, Takahashi H, Yang X, Masuda S, Takano Y. Decreased nuclear expression and increased cytoplasmic expression of ING5 may be linked to tumorigenesis and progression in human head and neck squamous cell carcinoma. J Cancer Res Clin Oncol 136:1573-83, 2010

Xing YN, Yang X, Xu XY, Zheng Y, Xu HM, Takano Y, Zheng HC. The altered expression of ING5 protein is involved in gastric carcinogenesis and subsequent progression. Hum Pathol 42:25-35, 2011

Zheng HC, Xia P, Xu XY, Takahashi H, Takano Y. The nuclear to cytoplasmic shift of ING5 protein during colorectal carcinogenesis with their distinct links to pathologic behaviors of carcinomas. Hum Pathol 42:424-33, 2011

Nouman GS, Anderson JJ, Crosier S, Shrimankar J, Lunec J, Angus B. Downregulation of nuclear expression of the p33(ING1b) inhibitor of growth protein in invasive carcinoma of the breast. J Clin Pathol 56:507-11, 2003

Nouman GS, Anderson JJ, Wood KM, Lunec J, Hall AG, Reid MM, Angus B. Loss of nuclear expression of the p33(ING1b) inhibitor of growth protein in childhood acute lymphoblastic leukaemia. J Clin Pathol 55:596-601, 2002

Nouman GS, Anderson JJ, Mathers ME, Leonard N, Crosier S, Lunec J, Angus B. Nuclear to cytoplasmic compartment shift of the p33ING1b tumour suppressor protein is associated with malignancy in melanocytic lesions. Histopathology 40:360-6, 2002

Toyama T, Iwase H, Yamashita H, Hara Y, Sugiura H, Zhang Z, Fukai I, Miura Y, Riabowol K, Fujii Y. p33(ING1b) stimulates the transcriptional activity of the estrogen receptor alpha via its activation function (AF) 2 domain. J Steroid Biochem Mol Biol 87:57-63, 2003

Nikolaev AY, Papanikolaou NA, Li M, Qin J, Gu W. Identification of a novel BRMS1-homologue protein p40 as a component of the mSin3A/p33(ING1b)/HDAC1 deacetylase complex. Biochem Biophys Res Commun 323:1216-22, 2004

Kim S, Welm AL, Bishop JM. A dominant mutant allele of the ING4 tumor suppressor found in human cancer cells exacerbates MYC-initiated mouse mammary tumorigenesis. Cancer Res 70:5155-62, 2010

Li Z, Xie Y, Sheng W, Miao J, Xiang J, Yang J. Tumor-suppressive effect of adenovirus-mediated inhibitor of growth 4 gene transfer in breast carcinoma cells in vitro and in vivo. Cancer Biother Radiopharm 25:427-37, 2010

Tapia C, Zlobec I, Schneider S, Kilic E, Güth U, Bubendorf L, Kim S. Deletion of the inhibitor of growth 4 (ING4) tumor suppressor gene is prevalent in human epidermal growth factor 2 (HER2)-positive breast cancer. Hum Pathol 42:983-90, 2011

5

Steroid Receptor Coactivators and their Expression, Regulation and Functional Role in Endocrine Responsive and Resistant Breast Cancer

Line L. Haugan Moi[1,3], Marianne Hauglid Flågeng[1], Ingvild S. Fenne[1], Jennifer Gjerde[1], Ernst A. Lien[1,2] and Gunnar Mellgren[1,2]
[1]*Institute of Medicine, University of Bergen*
[2]*The Hormone Laboratory, Haukeland University Hospital*
[3]*Department of Clinical Pathology, University Hospital of North Norway*
Norway

1. Introduction

Breast cancer is the most frequent malignancy and one of the leading causes to cancer related deaths in women. Most human breast cancers express the estrogen receptor (ER) which belongs to the family of nuclear receptors and is a ligand-regulated transcription factor. It is well established that the natural ligand of ER, estrogen, has pro-carcinogenic and growth promoting effects in the mammary epithelium by stimulating proliferation and leaving the cells prone to mutations during cell cycle progression (Foster et al., 2001). Endocrine treatment of hormone sensitive breast cancer targets the estrogen activity in breast cancer cells by blocking the ER with a selective ER modulator (SERM) such as tamoxifen or inhibiting estrogen synthesis using aromatase inhibitors such as anastrozole or letrozole. Endocrine treatment decreases mortality, prolongs disease-free survival and can even reduce the incidence of breast cancer in women at increased risk (Cuzick et al., 2003). Approximately 70 % of women with ER positive tumors respond to endocrine therapy, but resistance do occur, either *de novo* or develop over time. The molecular mechanism involved in endocrine resistance is one of the central areas of breast cancer research.

The trancriptional activity of the ER is not only regulated by its ligands, but also by the level and activity of coregulator proteins. Nuclear receptor coactivators serve as adapters between the receptor and the trancriptional machinery. They possess diverse enzymatic acitivities such as histone acetyltransferase, histone methyltransferase, chromatin remodeling and ubiquitin-conjugation activity and are involved in every step of ER regulated transcription, from chromatin remodeling to transcriptional termination. The members of the p160 family of coactivators are some of the best studied coactivators. These steroid receptor coactivators (SRCs) are small proteins of 160 kDa with similar structural and functional properties, and include SRC-1, SRC-2/transcription intermediary factor-2 (TIF-2) and SRC-3/amplified in breast cancer 1 (AIB1). The SRCs are not only crucial to ER mediated effects in normal tissue. They have also been shown to be involved in the carcinogenic process and are overexpressed in breast cancer. In addition, the SRCs are of relevance to the tissue-specific effects of tamoxifen and data suggest that they may be important to the cellular sensitivity to endocrine treatment. The SRCs and their expression, regulation and functional role during endocrine treatment in breast cancer *in vitro* and *in vivo* are the focus of this chapter.

2. Expression and functional role of SRCs in breast tissue

The SRCs are genetically distinct, but have structural similarities with 40 - 55 % sequence homology (Xu & Li, 2003). Although the SRCs have similar functional properties, experimental evidence indicates different physiological functions for the SRCs, which in part can be explained by tissue-specific expression levels, different affinities for the various nuclear receptors and variations in post-translational modifications (Chauchereau et al., 2003; Fenne et al., 2008; Hoang et al., 2004; Wu et al., 2004; Xu et al., 2009). In the classical activation of ER-mediated gene transcription, the ligand estradiol (E2) binds to the ER and promotes binding of the ER-E2 complex to the estrogen receptor element (ERE) of the target gene promoter. Here they recruit coregulatory proteins to a multi-subunit complex for gene transcription (Mangelsdorf et al., 1995; Pearce & Jordan, 2004). The ER has an activation function-1 (AF-1) domain in the N-terminus whereas the centrally located DNA-binding domain (DBD) is responsible for specific binding of the ER to EREs on target genes. The dimerization domain contains the ligand binding domain (LBD) and the AF-2. The AF-1 contributes to the constitutive estrogen-independent activation by the receptor and is separated by a hinge region from the AF-2. The SRCs have a basic helix-loop-helix (bHLH) domain, a Per-Arnt-Sim (PAS) domain and a nuclear hormone interaction domain (NID) including three LXXLL-sequences where L is leucine and X any amino acid (Fig. 1).

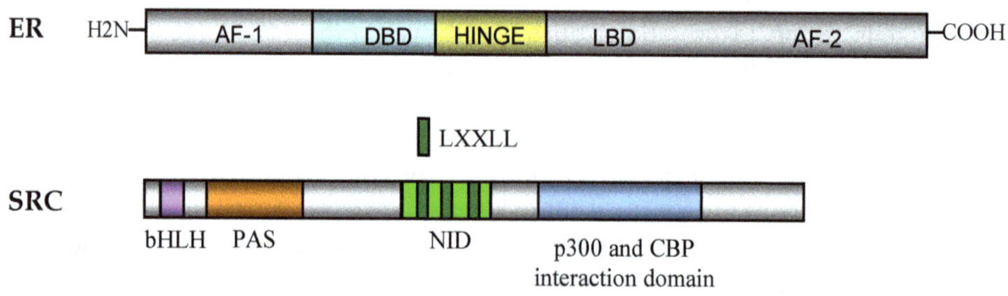

Fig. 1. Schematic presentation of the functional domains of the ER and the SRCs.

Upon ligand binding, the helix 12 of the ER is positioned across the LBD, and together with helices 3-5 form a hydrophobic groove where the LXXLL motifs of coactivators can bind (Heery et al., 1997). The coactivators in the multi-subunit protein complex alter the chromatin structure and facilitate recruitment of the RNA polymerase II and the basal transcriptional machinery in a programmed cyclic manner to initiate transcription of the target gene (Metivier et al., 2003).

The SRC family members are widely expressed and are detected in tissues such as placenta, testis, pancreas, lung, kidney, liver and brain (Xu & O'Malley, 2002; Xu & Li, 2003). The expression levels of the three SRC proteins in normal human breast epithelial cells are variable, but usually very low (Xu et al., 2009). SRCs are known to be overexpressed in several types of human cancers, including breast cancer, where their overexpression is due to enhanced cellular amplification of their genes, and/or by a decrease in the intracellular degradation process of the coactivators (Xu et al., 2009). The SRCs are known to contribute to proliferation and development of breast cancers by mechanisms such as stimulation of the G1 to S phase transition during cell cycle by regulation of expression of mitogenic genes such as *c-MYC* and *cyclin D1* (Dubik & Shiu, 1992; Sabbah et al., 1999).

2.1 SRC-1

SRC-1 was the first nuclear receptor coactivator to be cloned and identified (Onate et al., 1995). The gene is located on the short arm of chromosome 2 at position 2p23 (Carapeti et al., 1998). SRC-1$^{-/-}$ mice show partial steroid hormone resistance and hepatic insufficiency (Xu et al., 1998; Louet et al., 2010). Noteworthy, ovariectomized female SRC-1$^{-/-}$ mice have decreased uterine growth and reduced mammary gland ductal side branching and alveolar formation in response to estrogen compared with wild-type mice, indicating a role of SRC-1 in estrogen-regulated breast development (Xu et al., 1998; Xu & Li, 2003). We found higher SRC-1 mRNA levels by real-time RT-PCR in human breast cancer samples compared to normal breast tissue (Haugan Moi et al., 2010), and the same has been observed at the protein level (Hudelist et al., 2003; Fleming et al., 2004b; Myers et al., 2004). SRC-1 protein expression in breast cancer has been reported to associate positively with human epidermal growth factor receptor 2/neu (HER-2/neu) and negatively with ERβ (Fleming et al., 2004b). *In vitro* studies indicate that SRC-1 plays an important role in ER-mediated growth of breast cancer cells. Overexpression of SRC-1 potentiates E2-stimulated growth of MCF-7 breast cancer cells in accordance with an increase in the expression of estrogen-responsive genes (Tai et al., 2000). SRC-1 has also been reported to specifically promote breast cancer metastasis, possibly by promoting migration and invasion by enhancing PEA3 mediated transcriptional activation of Twist, a master regulator of metastasis (Qin et al., 2009). Furthermore, SRC-1 may promote metastasis in mammary tumors by facilitating Ets-2 mediated HER-2/neu expression and activating colony stimulating factor-1 expression to recruit macrophages to mammary tumors in mice (Wang et al., 2009).

2.2 SRC-2/TIF-2

The human SRC-2/TIF-2 gene is located on the long arm of chromosome 8 at position 8q21 (Kalkhoven et al., 1998). Knock-out experiments indicate that SRC-2/TIF-2 are of special relevance to fertility and fat metabolism where SRC-2/TIF-2$^{-/-}$ mice have defective spermatogenesis, testicular degeneration, placenta hypoplasia, male and female hypofertility, higher lipolysis in white fat, higher energy expenditure in brown fat and resistance to obesity (Gehin et al., 2002; Picard et al., 2002). Increased levels of SRC-2/TIF-2 mRNA have been observed in intraductal and invasive carcinoma compared to normal breast tissue (Kurebayashi et al., 2000; Haugan Moi et al., 2010). Knockdown of SRC-2/TIF-2 has been shown to inhibit growth of MCF-7 breast cancer cells due to decreased cell proliferation, increased apoptosis and reduced ER mediated transcriptional activity (Cavarretta et al., 2002; Karmakar et al., 2009). However, overall SRC-2/TIF-2 is the least studied of the coactivators in breast cancer.

2.3 SRC-3/AIB1

The third member of the SRC family, SRC-3/AIB1, is located on the long arm of chromosome 20 at position 20q12 in humans and was first identified as a gene amplified and overexpressed in several human breast cancer cell lines (Anzick et al., 1997). The *SRC-3/AIB1* gene is found to be amplified in 5-10% of breast cancer cases, and SRC-3/AIB1 are overexpressed at mRNA and protein level in 20-60 % of breast cancer patients (Anzick et al., 1997; Takeshita et al., 1997; Bautista et al., 1998; Murphy et al., 2000; Bouras et al., 2001; List et al., 2001; Hudelist et al., 2003; Zhao et al., 2003). Female SRC-3/AIB1$^{-/-}$ mice have significantly lower levels of estrogen and delayed mammary gland development, indicating a proliferative role of this coactivator in breast tissue (Xu et al., 2000). In transgenic mice, overexpression of SRC-3/AIB1 leads to development of tumors in several organs including breast, in addition to increased expression of the insulin-like growth factor-1 (IGF-1) and activation of intracellular pathways suggesting that SRC-3/AIB1 is acting as an oncogene (Torres-Arzayus et al., 2004). The oncogenic potential of SRC-3/AIB1 has been ascribed to mechanisms such as enhanced interaction between ER and the *cyclin D1* promoter, hence leading to increased levels of cyclin D1 and stimulation of cell cycle progression (Planas-Silva et al., 2001). Conversely, cyclin D1 expression has been shown to be reduced in SRC-3/AIB1 knock-out cells (Karmakar et al., 2009), and mice with reduced SRC-3/AIB1 expression have a decrease in epithelial proliferation associated with a reduction in cyclin expression (Fereshteh et al., 2008). Overexpression of SRC-3/AIB1 also stimulates the Akt signaling pathway which promotes cell growth (Torres-Arzayus et al., 2004; Zhou et al., 2003). Matrix metalloproteinases (MMPs) are zink-dependent enzymes involved in the degradation of extracellular matrix and are essential to the metastatic process. Experimental evidence suggests that SRC-3/AIB1 promotes breast cancer metastasis by stimulating the transcription factor PEA3 to enhance expression of MMP2 and MMP9 (Qin et al., 2008).

2.4 Regulation of SRCs expression during endocrine treatment

Most studies seem to indicate higher levels of the SRCs in malignant breast tumors compared to normal breast tissue. However, the expression levels of the SRCs have been shown to change during endocrine treatment in breast cancer. In a clinical study of preoperative tamoxifen treatment for 4 weeks using tamoxifen doses from 1 to 20 mg/daily, we found the mRNA levels of all three SRCs to be significantly upregulated in tamoxifen treated normal and malignant breast tissue compared to samples from untreated patients. The increase in coactivator mRNA expression was especially evident for SRC-3/AIB1 (Haugan Moi et al., 2010). In a clinical study on neoadjuvant treatment with aromatase inhibitors in locally advanced breast cancer, we also found the mRNA levels of coactivators in tumors to increase during treatment, especially for SRC-1 (Flågeng et al., 2009). This is in line with *in vitro* studies. E2 has been shown to repress SRC-3/AIB1 mRNA and protein expression in MCF-7 human breast cancer cells primarily by suppressing SRC-3/AIB1 gene transcription (Lauritsen et al., 2002). Conversely, total SRC-3/AIB1 mRNA levels were increased when MCF-7 breast cancer cells were treated with the antiestrogen 4-hydroxytamoxifen. 4-hydroxtamoxifen has also been shown to increase the stability and hence steady-state levels of SRC-1 and SRC-3/AIB1 proteins in a MCF-7 breast cancer-derived cell line (Lonard et al., 2004). We also found an increase in the mRNA levels of HER-2/neu and a positive correlation between SRC-1 and HER-2/neu in human breast tissue treated with aromatase inhibitors. This finding is interesting in light of *in vitro* assays suggesting that ER and HER-2/neu compete for the coactivator SRC-1. Under antiestrogenic conditions, SRC-1 will be released from the ER and may instead bind to the HER-2/neu enhancer and facilitate transcription of HER-2/neu, leading to increased expression of HER-2/neu under estrogen deprived conditions (Newman et al., 2000).

3. SRCs and endocrine treatment in breast cancer: Molecular mechanisms

The regulation of SRCs during endocrine treatment is especially interesting since the coactivators are directly involved in the molecular mechanisms underlying the antiestrogenic effects. The natural ligand of ER, estrogen, is converted from androgens by the enzyme aromatase. Endocrine treatment of ER positive breast cancer includes aromatase inhibitors or the SERM tamoxifen. Aromatase inhibitors block the synthesis of estrogens by binding to and suppressing the aromatase enzyme that converts androgens to estrogens. Tamoxifen binds to the ER and functions as an antagonist in breast tissue and prevents estrogen from binding to the ER. The net effect of both therapeutic regiments is to block ER-dependent transcriptional regulation of genes and prevent proliferation (Fig. 2).

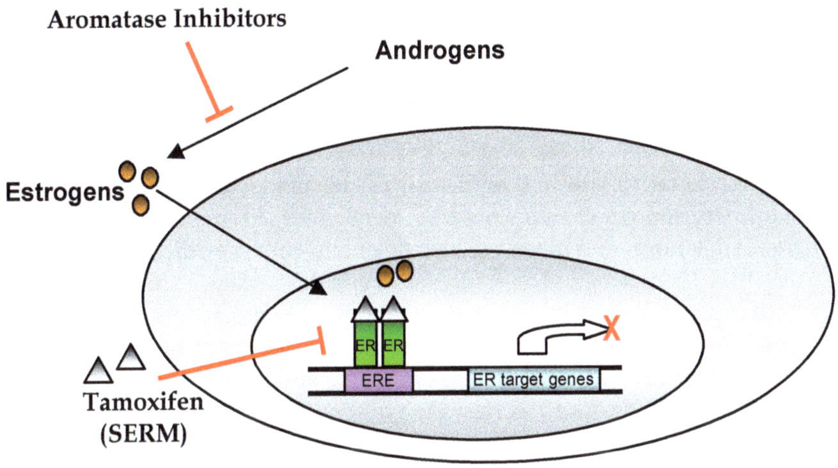

Fig. 2. Schematic presentation of the mechanisms of action of endocrine treatment in breast cancer using tamoxifen or aromatase inhibitors.

3.1 The SERM tamoxifen

Tamoxifen is a synthetic estrogen antagonist which has been in clinical use for over 30 years. While the success of tamoxifen in breast cancer therapy is based on its ER antagonistic effects in malignant breast tissue, tamoxifen demonstrates ER agonistic effects in other organ systems such as bone and liver. ER appears to bind to corepressors in the presence of SERMs in breast tissue, while coactivator recruitment is favored when E2 is bound to ER. Upon binding to ER, SERMs inhibit ER transcriptional activity by competing with E2 for the binding site and by blocking the AF-2 activity of ER (Shiau et al., 1998; Brzozowski et al., 1997). The potent ER antagonistic metabolite 4-hydroxytamoxifen induces a displacement and rotation of the receptor's helix 12. The helix 12 then binds to the hydrophobic pocket via a sequence resembling the NR box of the coactivators, and thereby inhibits coactivator recruitment (Brzozowski et al., 1997; Shiau et al., 1998). The binding of 4-hydroxytamoxifen instead favors recruitment of the two corepressors silencing mediator for retinoid and thyroid hormone receptor (SMRT) and nuclear receptor corepressor (NCoR). These corepressors are associated with histone deacetylase activity and inhibit ER regulated gene transcription (Webb et al., 2003; Fleming et al., 2004a).

However, tamoxifen may exert ER agonistic effects depending on the coactivator context. For example, it has been shown that overexpression of SRC-3/AIB1 and the growth factor HER-2/neu increases the ER agonistic properties of tamoxifen (Shou et al., 2004) and that tamoxifen resistance develops when SRC-3/AIB1 is high and the transcriptional repressor paired box 2 (PAX2) is low in breast cancer cells (Hurtado et al., 2008). Elevated expression of SRC-1 in the uterine derived Ishikawa cell line increases the agonist behavior of 4-hydroxytamoxifen, whereas lower expression of SRC-1 in MCF-7 cells contributed to an ER-antagonistic behavior of tamoxifen (Shang & Brown., 2002). Studies have shown that the estrogenic effects of tamoxifen can be mediated by the constitutive active AF-1 domain of ER which can be stimulated by several mechanisms, including high levels of coactivators (Webb et al., 1998). Hence, the levels of SRCs may determine the response to tamoxifen treatment, at least *in vitro*.

3.2 Aromatase inhibitors

Aromatase inhibitors work by blocking the estrogen synthesis and depriving the breast cancer cells of this important growth factor. In premenopausal women, estrogens are primarily synthesized by the granulose cells in the ovaries, but aromatase activity and conversion of androgens to estrogens also take place in tissues such as subcutaneous fat, breast tissue and bone which are the primary sources of estrogens after menopause. Aromatase is a cytochrome P450 enzyme where the haem protein binds the androgen and catalyzes the formation of the phenolic A-ring which is characteristic for estrogens. Type 1 aromatase inhibitors such as formestane and exemestane, also known as steroidal inhibitors, are analogues to androstenedione and work by competitive binding to the active site of aromatase. Type 2 aromatase inhibitors include the first generation compound aminoglutethimide, the second generation drug fadrozole and the third generation compounds anastrozole and letrozole, which are widely used clinically. These non-steroidal aromatase inhibitors work by binding to an iron atom in the haem group of aromatase and have proved very effective in inhibiting aromatase activity. In the absence of agonist, the ER will be locacted in the cytoplasm associated with heat shock protein (hsp), and dimerization, conformational changes and coactivator recruitment will be inhibited, hence leading to reduced transcription of ER-regulated genes. However, resistance to aromatase inhibitors does occur. In the frequently used cellular model system for resistance to aromatase inhibitors, breast cancer cells are grown in estrogen-deprived conditions for 1-6 months. These long-term estrogen deprived cells (LTED) develop enhanced sensitivity to E2 (Masamura et al., 1995; Santen et al., 2005). This hypersensitivity is associated with upregulation of ERα and the mitogen activated protein kinases (MAPKs) (Jeng et al., 1998; Jeng et al., 2000). The MAPKs are found downstream of several growth factor receptors including HER-2/neu and could phosphorylate and influence the activity of the SRCs, but also the ER. Accumulated evidence points to an important crosstalk between ER and growth factor pathways where posttranslational modifications of the SRCs are involved. These modifications could influence not only SRC activity, but also the effect of endocrine treatment in breast cancer over time.

4. SRCs and growth factor signaling

4.1 Posttranslational modifications of SRCs with functional aspects

The SRCs are components and targets of multiple cell signaling pathways that modulate their activity. Extracellular stimuli such as hormones, growth factors and cytokines induce a variety of posttranslational modifications of SRCs, including acetylation, methylation, phosphorylation, ubiquitination and sumoylation. These modifications influence the SRCs transcriptional activity and/or the SRC protein levels and stability (Baek & Rosenfeld, 2004; Li & Shang, 2007; Xu et al., 2009).

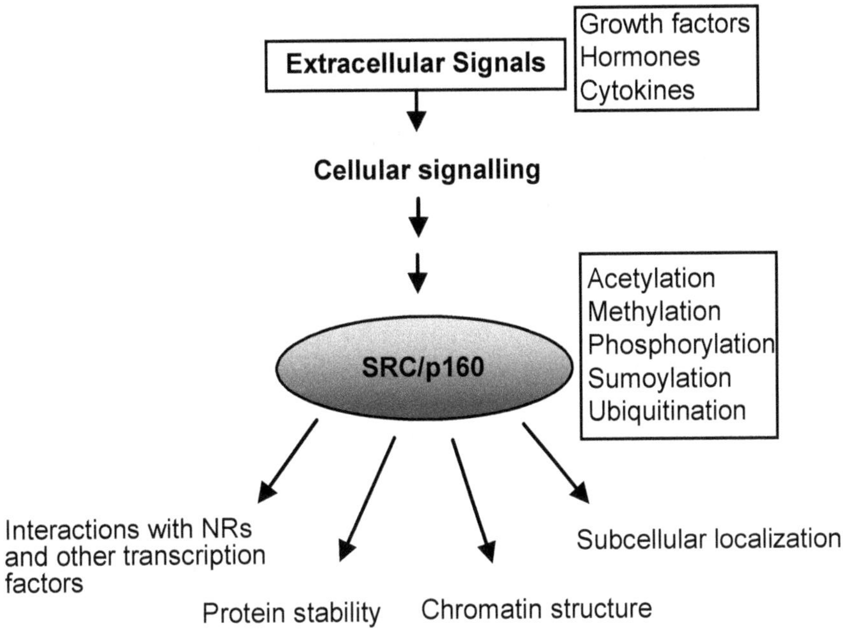

Fig. 3. Functional aspects of posttranslational modifications of the SRCs.

Phosphorylation of coactivators modulates ER-dependent gene transcription by regulating coactivator function in various ways. Three SRC-1 phosphorylation sites with corresponding kinases have been identified (S395, T1179 and S1185), one SRC-2/TIF-2 (S736) and sixteen SRC-3/AIB1 phosphorylation sites (T24, S505, S543, S601, S857, S860, S867, S1033, S1042, S1048, T1059, S1062, T1064, T1067, T1114 and Y1357) (Bulynko & O'Malley, 2011). Comparison of these sites reveals little conservation of sequences among the SRCs, indicating that phosphorylation is a significant determinant of the specificity of the SRCs (Wu et al., 2005).

Phosphorylation may influence the function and acitivity of the SRCs. It is shown *in vitro* using COS-1 cells that positions S395 and T1179/S1185 of SRC-1 are phosphorylated by the MAPK family members ERK1 and ERK2 (Rowan et al., 2000b) where MAPK-mediated phosphorylation on T1179 and S1185 has been shown to increase the affinity of SRC-1 for androgen receptor (AR) in prostate cancer cells (Ueda et al., 2002; Gregory et al., 2004). ERK2 may also phosphorylate SRC-3/AIB1 *in vitro* which stimulates the recruitment of p300 and associated histone acetyltransferase activity (Font de Mora & Brown, 2000). cAMP regulated phosphorylation of SRC-1 occurs through an indirect pathway in which protein kinase A (PKA) induces the activity of ERK1 and ERK2 (Rowan et al., 2000a). SRC-3/AIB1 phosphorylation-defective mutants exhibit reduced ability to interact with ER compared to wild type SRC-3/AIB1, both in the absence and presence of E2 (Wu et al., 2004). Epidermal growth factor (EGF)-induced activation of ER-, progesterone receptor (PR)- and AR-dependent transcription is shown to be regulated through phosphorylation of SRC-2/TIF-2 at S736 by the EGF-activated ERK MAPK and p38MAPK which stimulate SRC-2/TIF-2 coactivator function (Lopez et al., 2001; Gregory et al., 2004; Frigo et al., 2006).

Phosphorylation and dephosphorylation of proteins also regulate the nuclear import and export by modifying the nuclear localization signals (NLS) and nuclear export signals (NES) of the proteins (Whitmarsh & Davis, 2000). The sequence of the bHLH domain of the SRCs has been shown to be important for their nuclear localization. SRC-1 and SRC-3/AIB1 contain a conserved bipartite NLS in their bHLH-PAS domain (Amazit et al., 2003; Li et al., 2007). Furthermore, specific residues in the NLS of SRC-3/AIB1 are identified to signal proteasome-dependent turnover of SRC-3/AIB1 in the nucleus (Li et al., 2007). SRC-1 also contains a non-conserved sequence localized in its C-terminal region that is suggested to serve as a NES. The return of SRC-1 to the cytoplasm is proposed to be involved in termination of hormone action (Amazit et al., 2003).

Phosphorylation does not only influence the activation and subcellular localization of the SRCs, but also regulate the ubiquitination and degradation of the coactivators. Phosphorylated SRCs are suggested to be targets for enzymes in the ubiquitin-proteasome pathway. The ubiquitin-proteasome degradation pathway is regarded as an important mechanism to control the steady state levels of SRCs, thereby modulating growth responses to various growth-promoting factors (Lonard & O'Malley, 2005). Retinoic acid-induced phosphorylation of SRC-3/AIB1 by p38MAPK at S860, and phosphorylation at S505 by Akt/protein kinase B (PKB)-activated glycogen synthase kinase-3 (GSK3) have been shown to mediate SRC-3/AIB1 degradation (Gianni et al., 2006; Wu et al., 2007). On the other hand, atypical PKC-induced phosphorylation of the C-terminal region of SRC-3/AIB1 was reported to increase its stabilization by protecting it from proteasome-mediated degradation leading to an increased estrogen-induced breast cancer cell growth (Yi et al., 2008).

Growth factor pathways regulate SRC function not only through phosphorylation. We found activation of the cAMP/PKA pathway to stimulate association of SRC-2/TIF-2 with an ER-transcription complex prior to its degradation by the ubiquitin-proteasome system (Fenne et al., 2008). MCF-7 breast cancer cells were transfected with an expression plasmid encoding HA-GRIP1, the rodent homologue to SRC-2/TIF-2, along with the luciferase reporter construct ERE-TATA-luc. Cells were treated with cAMP analog and cAMP-elevating agents for different time-lengths and after 48 hours the cells where lysed and subjected to luciferase assay. A time-dependent regulation of cAMP/PKA on SRC-2/TIF-2 coactivator function was observed (Fig. 4A). PKA is activated when hormones bind to a G-protein coupled receptor (GPCR). The activated receptor interacts with adenylyl cyclase (AC) which catalyses the conversion of ATP to cAMP, further activating the cAMP dependent PKA (Fig. 4b). PKA can regulate SRC-2/TIF-2 coactivator function in a time-dependent matter. Short-term treatment stimulated SRC-2/TIF-2 coactivator function, whereas long-term treatments inhibited SRC-2/TIF-2 function due to ubiquitin-proteasome-mediated degradation (Hoang et al., 2004; Fenne et al., 2008).

All three SRCs can also be modified by site-specific sumoylation of lysine residues in their respective NIDs (Kotaja et al., 2002; Chauchereau et al., 2003). Sumoylation of SRC-2/TIF-2 has been shown to increase its coactivation of AR by enhancing their interaction (Kotaja et al., 2002). Conversely, sumoylation of SRC-1 increases its interaction with the PR and leads to prolonged retention of SRC-1 in the nucleus (Chauchereau et al., 2003). In contrast to SRC-1 and SRC-2/TIF-2, sumoylation of SRC-3/AIB1 seems to attenuate its coactivation function (Wu et al., 2006).

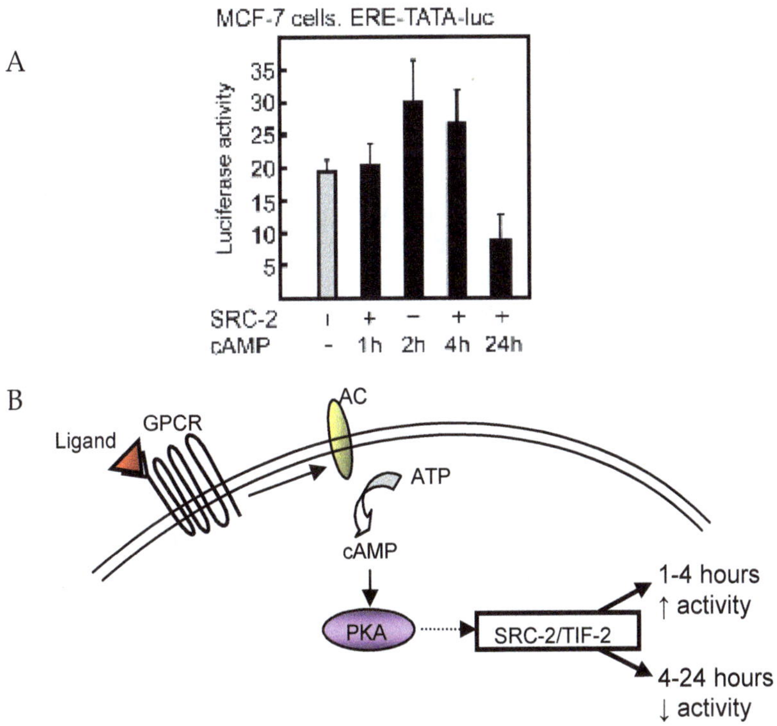

Fig. 4. cAMP-PKA signaling influence SRC-2/TIF-2 function in a time-dependent manner.

4.2 SRCs, growth factor signaling and response to endocrine therapy

The SRCs are regulated by post-translational modifications by kinases found downstream in growth factor signaling pathways often activated in cancers, such as the MAPKs operating downstream of HER-2/neu. Posttranslational modification can stabilize and functionally activate the SRC proteins, a mechanism which has been shown to contribute not only to ER-agonstic effects of tamoxifen, but also to estrogen hypersensitivity and resistance to aromatase inhibitors. *In vitro* it has been shown that tamoxifen resistance with loss of ER antagonistic effects develops when SRC-3/AIB1 is high and the transcriptional repressor PAX2 is low in breast cancer cells (Hurtado et al., 2008). Conversely, dissociation of SRC-3/AIB1 from ER restores tamoxifen's antagonistic effect in resistant breast cancer cells and inhibits further breast cancer cell growth (Planas-Silva et al., 2001; List et al., 2001).

Clinically, studies have shown an association between SRC-1 and reduced disease-free survival in breast cancer patients with locally advanced disease treated with endocrine therapy (Al-azawi et al., 2008; Redmond et al., 2009). During neoadjuvant treatment with aromatase inhibitors, we found higher levels of SRC-1 mRNA levels during treatment, especially in tumors that responded to treatment (Flågeng et al., 2009). Low expression of SRC-1 combined with high ERβ expression has been found to be a good prognostic indicator to endocrine treatment in breast cancers (Myers et al., 2004). However, the clearest association between high levels of SRCs and poor clinical outcome has been found in tumors also overexpressing HER-2/neu. Patients with tumors overexpressing HER-2/neu in combination with SRC-3/AIB1 or SRC-1 undergoing tamoxifen treatment show reduced sensitivity to endocrine therapy, greater risk of disease recurrence and reduced disease-free survival (Fleming et al., 2004b; Osborne et al., 2003). Overexpression of SRC-3/AIB1 and HER-2/neu in breast tumors is associated with disease recurrences and poor prognosis. This could be linked to the HER-2/neu-mediated activation of MAPK and Akt which causes phosphorylation of SRC-3/AIB1 and ER, resulting in transcriptional activation and cell proliferation. Activation of Akt has also been shown to stabilize SRC-3/AIB1 by inhibiting GSK3 (Wu et al., 2007) whereas PKA-induced resistance to tamoxifen is associated with an altered orientation between ER and SRC-1 (Zwart et al., 2007). Overall, the SRCs can be targeted by central growth factor pathways mediating pro-survival signals and stimulating proliferation. The SRCs close functional relationship with the ER makes posttranslational modifications of the SRCs important points of crosstalk between ER and growth factor signaling pathways during endocrine treatment in breast cancer (Fig. 5).

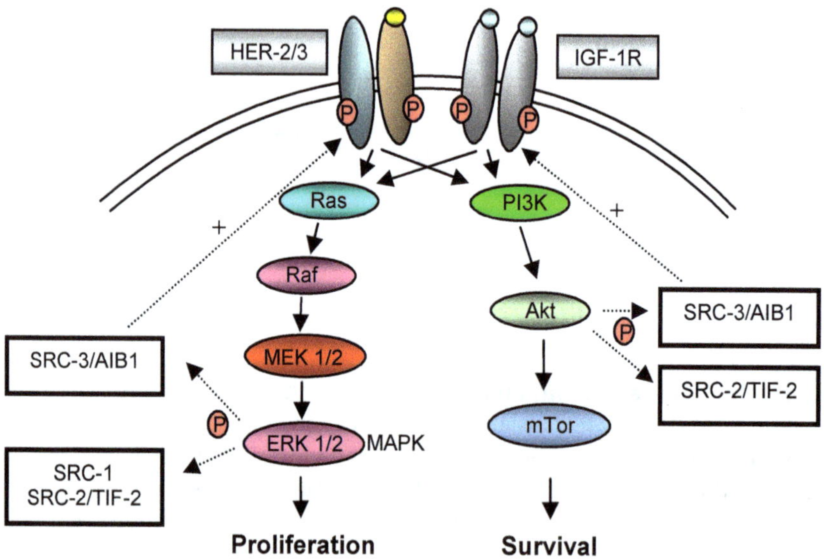

Fig. 5. Cross-talk between growth-factor signaling pathways and SRCs in breast cancer. Ligand-activated growth factor receptor dimers including the human epidermal growth factor receptor-2 and -3 (HER-2/3) and the insulin-like growth factor-1 receptor (IGF-1R) are phosphorylated at intracellular domains and signal both through the MAPK and the phosphatidyl-inositol 3-kinase (PI3K) signaling pathway. ERK 1 and 2 may phosphorylate SRC-1, SRC-2/TIF-2 and SRC-3/AIB1. Akt may phosporylate SRC-2/TIF-2 and SRC-3/AIB1. SRC-3/AIB1 is a modulator increasing the activity and signaling both through HER-2 and IGF-1R leading to cell growth.

5. Conclusion

Most human breast cancers express ER which belongs to the family of nuclear receptors and is a ligand-regulated transcription factor. Endocrine treatment involves blocking the ER with a selective ER modulator such as tamoxifen or inhibiting estrogen synthesis using aromatase inhibitors. The SRCs are crucial to ER mediated effects and their expression level and activity have been shown to dictate the effect of ER on gene expression to a large extent. SRC-1, SRC-2/TIF-2 and SRC-3/AIB1 are expressed in normal and malignant breast tissue where SRC-3/AIB1 is now considered to be an oncogene. SRC-1 and SRC-3/AIB1 may promote metastasis in mammary tumors by enhancing the transcriptional activation of regulators of metastasis such as Twist and MMPs. The expression levels of the SRCs are influenced by endocrine treatment, an observation which may be of relevance to the treatment response to endocrine therapy over time. We found the mRNA levels of the SRCs, especially SRC-3/AIB1, to be significantly upregulated in both normal and malignant breast tissue after 4 weeks of tamoxifen in the 1-20 mg dose range. The mRNA expression of SRC-1 has also been shown to increase significantly in a clinical study of neoadjuvant treatment with aromatase inhibitors for 14-16 weeks, especially in the subgroup of patients achieving an objective treatment response. This is in line with *in vitro* studies in MCF-7 cells showing that estrogens suppress the mRNA levels of SRC-3/AIB1 by suppressing SRC-3/AIB1 gene transcription whereas 4-hydroxytamoxifen increases the SRC-3/AIB1 mRNA expression level. The importance of the expression level and functional activation of the SRCs during endocrine treatment is evident from cellular assays on tamoxifen treatment. High levels of coactivators relative to corepressors may lead to ER agonistic effects by 4-hydroxytamoxifen. Further, posttranslational modification of both coactivators and ER can lead to altered molecular conformations, intracellular relocation, stabilization and ubiquitination which would influence the activity and stability of the SRCs, as shown for the PKA-mediated regulation of SRC-2/TIF-2. In several clinical trials the levels of coactivators have been found of relevance, not only to the response to endocrine treatment, but also to long term clinical outcome. High protein levels of SRC-1 have been shown to be associated with reduced disease-free survival, both in untreated and tamoxifen treated patients, whereas elevated mRNA expression levels of SRC-3/AIB1 have been associated with high tumor grade and shorter disease-free and overall survival. Tumors undergoing tamoxifen therapy and overexpressing HER-2/neu in combination with SRC-3/AIB1 are more likely to be tamoxifen resistant and are associated with reduced disease-free survival. High expression of HER-2/neu in combination with SRC-1 has also been associated with a greater risk of recurrence on endocrine treatment. In summary, SRCs are expressed in normal and malignant breast tissue and they have a crucial role in mediating the effect of endocrine treatment in breast cancer. The expression levels of SRCs are regulated by endocrine treatment and their functional role is modified by posttranslational modifications mediated by growth factor pathways involved in breast cancer development and endocrine resistance. Further research on SRCs and their role in the crosstalk between ER and growth factor pathways during endocrine treatment is important to improve breast cancer therapy.

6. References

Al-azawi, D., McIlroy, M., Kelly, G., Redmond, A.M., Bane, F.T., Cocchiglia, S., Hill, A.D.K. & Young, L.S. (2008). Ets-2 and p160 proteins collaborate to regulate c-Myc in endocrine resistant breast cancer. *Oncogene*, Vol. 27, No. 21, pp. 3021-3031.

Amazit, L., Alj, Y., Tyagi, R.K., Chauchereau, A., Loosfelt, H., Pichon, C., Pantel, J., Foulon-Guinchard, E., Leclerc, P., Milgrom, E. & Guiochon-Mantel, A. (2003). Subcellular localization and mechanisms of nucleocytoplasmic trafficking of steroid receptor coactivator-1. *J Biol Chem*, Vol. 278, No. 34, pp. 32195-32203.

Anzick, S. L., Kononen, J., Walker, R. L., Azorsa, D. O., Tanner, M. M., Guan, X. Y., Sauter, G., Kallioniemi, O. P., Trent ,J. M. & Meltzer, P.S. (1997). AIB1, a steroid receptor coactivator amplified in breast and ovarian cancer. *Science* , Vol. 277, No. 5328, pp. 965-968.

Baek, S.H. & Rosenfeld, M.G. (2004). Nuclear receptor coregulators: their modification codes and regulatory mechanism by translocation. *Biochem Biophys Res Commun,* Vol. 319, No. 3, pp. 707-714.

Bautista, S., Valles, H., Walker, R. L., Anzick, S., Zeillinger, R., Meltzer, P. & Theillet, C. (1998). In breast cancer, amplification of the steroid receptor coactivator gene AIB1 is correlated with estrogen and progesterone receptor positivity. *Clin Cancer Res,* Vol. 4, No. 12, pp. 2925-2929.

Bouras, T., Southey, M. C. & Venter, D.J. (2001). Overexpression of the steroid receptor coactivator AIB1 in breast cancer correlates with the absence of estrogen and progesterone receptors and positivity for p53 and HER2/neu. *Cancer Res,* Vol. 61, No. 3, pp. 903-907.

Brzozowski, A. M., Pike, A. C., Dauter, Z., Hubbard, R. E., Bonn, T., Engstrom, Ohman, O., L., Greene, G. L., Gustafsson, J. A. & Carlquist, M. (1997). Molecular basis of agonism and antagonism in the oestrogen receptor. *Nature,* Vol. 389, No. 6652, pp. 753-758.

Bulynko, Y.A. & O'Malley, B.W. (2011). Nuclear receptor coactivators: structural and functional biochemistry. *Biochemistry,* Vol. 50, No. 3, pp. 313-328.

Carapeti, M., Agular, R.C., Chase, A., Goldman, J.M. & Cross, N.C. (1998). Assignment of the steroid receptor coactivator-1 (SRC-1) gene to human chromosome band 2p23. *Genomics,* Vol. 52, No. 2, pp. 242-244.

Cavarretta, I.T., Mukopadhyay, R., Lonard, D.M., Cowsert, L.M., Bennett, C.F., O'Malley, B.W. & Smith, C.L. (2002). Reduction of coactivator expression by antisense oligodeoxynucleotides inhibits ERalpha transcriptional activity and MCF-7 proliferation. *Mol Endocrinol,* Vol. 16, No. 2, pp. 253-270.

Chauchereau, A., Amazit, L., Quesne, M., Guiochon-Mantel, A. & Milgrom, E. (2003). Sumoylation of the progesterone receptor and of the steroid receptor coactivator SRC-1. *J Biol Chem,* Vol. 278, No. 14, pp. 12335-12343.

Cuzick, J., Powles, T., Veronesi, U., Forbes, J., Edwards, R., Ashley, S. & Boyle, P. (2003). Overview of the main outcomes in breast-cancer prevention trials. *Lancet,* Vol. 361, No. 9354, pp. 296-300.

Dubik, D. & Shiu, R.P. (1992). Mechanism of estrogen activation of c-myc oncogene expression. *Oncogene,* Vol. 7, No. 8, pp. 1587-1594.

Fenne, I.S., Hoang, T., Hauglid, M., Sagen, J.V., Lien, E.A. & Mellgren, G. (2008). Recruitment of coactivator glucocorticoid receptor interacting protein 1 to an estrogen receptor transcription complex is regulated by the 3`,5`-cyclic adenosine 5`-monophosphate-dependent protein kinase. *Endocrinology,* Vol. 148, No. 9, pp. 4336-4345.

Fereshteh, M. P., Tilli, M.T., Kim, S.E., Xu, J., O'Malley, B.W., Wellstein, A., Furth, P.A. & Riegel, A.T. (2008). The nuclear receptor coactivator amplified in breast cancer-1 is required for Neu (ErbB2/HER2) activation, signaling, and mammary tumorigenesis in mice. *Cancer Res,* Vol. 68, No. 10, pp. 3697-3706.

Fleming, F. J., Hill, A. D., McDermott, E.W., O'Higgins, N. J. & Young, L. S. (2004a). Differential recruitment of coregulator proteins steroid receptor coactivator-1 and silencing mediator for retinoid and thyroid receptors to the estrogen receptor-estrogen response element by beta-estradiol and 4-hydroxytamoxifen in human breast cancer. *J Clin Endocrinol Metab,* Vol. 89, No. 1, pp. 375-383.

Fleming, F. J., Myers, E., Kelly, G., Crotty, T. B., McDermott, E.W., O'Higgins, N. J., Hill, A. D. & Young, L. S. (2004b). Expression of SRC-1, AIB1, and PEA3 in HER2 mediated endocrine resistant breast cancer; a predictive role for SRC-1. *J Clin Pathol,* Vol. 57, No. 10, pp. 1069-1074.

Flågeng, M.H., Haugan Moi, L.L., Dixon, J.M., Geisler, J., Lien, E.A., Miller, W.R., Lønning, P.E. & Mellgren, G. (2009). Nuclear receptor co-activators and HER-2/neu are upregulated in breast cancer patients during neo-adjuvant treatment with aromatase inhibitors. *Br J Cancer,* Vol. 101, No. 8, pp. 1253-1260.

Font de Mora, J. & Brown, M. (2000). AIB1 is a conduit for kinase-mediated growth factor signaling to the estrogen receptor. *Mol Cell Biol,* Vol. 20, No. 14, pp. 5041-5047.

Foster, J. S., Henley, D. C., Ahamed, S.& Wimalasena, J. (2001). Estrogens and cell-cycle regulation in breast cancer. *Trends Endocrinol Metab,* Vol. 12, No. 7, pp. 320-327.

Frigo, D.E., Basu, A., Nierth-Simpson, E.N., Weldon, C.B., Dugan, C.M., Elliott, S., Collins-Burow, B.M., Salvo, V.A., Zhu, Y., Melnik, L.I., Lopez, G.N., Kushner, P.J., Curiel, T.J., Rowan, B.G., McLachlan, J.A. & Burow M.E. (2006). p38 mitogen-activated protein kinase stimulates estrogen-mediated transcription and proliferation through the phosphorylation and potentiation of the p160 coactivator glucocorticoid receptor-interacting protein 1. *Mol Endocrinol,* Vol. 20, No. 5, pp. 971-983.

Gehin, M., Mark, M., Dennefeld, C., Dierich, A., Gronemeyer H. & Chambon, P. (2002). The function of TIF2/GRIP1 in mouse reproduction is distinct from those of SRC-1 and p/CIP. *Mol Cell Biol,* Vol. 22, No. 16, pp. 5923-5937.

Gianni, M., Parrella, E., Raska, I. Jr, Gaillard, E., Nigro, E.A., Gaudon, C., Garattini, E. &Rochette-Egly, C. (2006). P38MAPK-dependent phosphorylation and degradation of SRC-3/AIB1 and RARalpha-mediated transcription. *EMBO J,* Vol. 25, No. 4, pp. 739-751.

Gregory C.W., Fei, X., Ponguta, L.A., He, B., Bill, H.M., French, F.S. & Wilson, E.M. (2004). Epidermal growth factor increases coactivation of the androgen receptor in recurrent prostate cancer. *J Biol Chem,* Vol. 279, No. 8, pp. 7119-30.

Haugan Moi, L.L., Flågeng, M.H., Gandini, S., Guerrieri-Gonzaga, A., Bonanni, B., Lazzeroni, M., Gjerde, J., Lien, E.A., DeCensi, A. & Mellgren, G. (2010). Effect of low dose tamoxifen on Steroid Receptor Coactivator 3/Amplified in Breast Cancer 1 in normal and malignant human breast tissue. *Clin Cancer Res,* Vol. 16, No. 7, pp. 2176-2186.

Heery, D. M., Kalkhoven, E., Hoare S. & Parker, M.G. (1997). A signature motif in transcriptional co-activators mediates binding to nuclear receptors. *Nature,* Vol. 387, No. 6634, pp. 733-736.

Hoang, T., Fenne, I. S., Cook, C., Borud, B., Bakke, M., Lien, E.A. & Mellgren, G. (2004). cAMP-dependent protein kinase regulates ubiquitin-proteasome-mediated degradation and subcellular localization of the nuclear receptor coactivator GRIP1. *J Biol Chem,* Vol. 279, No. 47, pp. 49120-49130.

Hudelist, G., Czerwenka, K., Kubista, E., Marton, E., Pischinger, K. & Singer, C. F. (2003). Expression of sex steroid receptors and their co-factors in normal and malignant breast tissue: AIB1 is a carcinoma-specific co-activator. *Breast Cancer Res Treat,* Vol. 78, No. 2, pp. 193-204.

Hurtado, A., Holmes, K. A., Geistlinger, T. R., Hutcheson, I. R., Nicholson, R. I., Brown, M., Jiang, J., Howat, W. J., Ali, S. & Carroll, J. S. (2008). Regulation of ERBB2 by oestrogen receptor-PAX2 determines response to tamoxifen. *Nature,* Vol. 456, No. 7222, pp. 663-666.

Jeng, M. H., Shupnik, M. A., Bender, T. P., Westin, E. H., Bandyopadhyay, D., Kumar, R., Masamura, S. & Santen, R.J. (1998). Estrogen receptor expression and function in long-term estrogen-deprived human breast cancer cells. *Endocrinoloy,* Vol. 139, No.. 10, pp. 4164-4174.

Jeng, M. H., Yue, W., Eischeid, A., Wang, J. P. & Santen. R.J. (2000). Role of MAP kinase in the enhanced cell proliferation of long term estrogen deprived human breast cancer cells. *Breast Cancer Res Treat,* Vol. 62, No. 3, pp. 167-175.

Kalkhoven, E., Valentine, J. E., Heery,D. M. & Parker, M.G. (1998). Isoforms of steroid receptor co-activator 1 differ in their ability to potentiate transcription by the oestrogen receptor. *EMBO J,* Vol. 17, No. 1, pp. 232-243.

Karmakar, S., Foster, E. A. & Smith, C.L. (2009). Unique roles of p160 coactivators for regulation of breast cancer cell proliferation and estrogen receptor-alpha transcriptional activity. *Endocrinology,* Vol. 150, No. 4, pp. 1588-1596.

Kotaja, N., Karvonen, U., Jänne, O.A. & Palvimo, J.J. (2002). The nuclear receptor interaction domain of GRIP1 is modulated by covalent attachment of SUMO-1. *J Biol Chem,* Vol. 277, No. 33, pp. 30283-30288.

Kurebayashi, J., Otsuki, T., Kunisue, H., Tanaka, K., Yamamoto, S. & Sonoo, H. (2000). Expression levels of estrogen receptor-alpha, estrogen receptor-beta, coactivators, and corepressors in breast cancer. *Clin Cancer Res,* Vol. 6, No. 2, pp. 512-518.

Lauritsen, K. J., List, H. J., Reiter, R., Wellstein, A. & Riegel, A.T. (2002). A role for TGF-beta in estrogen and retinoid mediated regulation of the nuclear receptor coactivator AIB1 in MCF-7 breast cancer cells. *Oncogene,* Vol. 21, No. 47, pp. 7147-7155.

Li, C., Wu, R.C., Amazit, L., Tsai, S.Y., Tsai, M.J. & O'Malley, B.W. (2007). Specific amino acid residues in the basic helix-loop-helix domain of SRC-3 are essential for its nuclear localization and proteasome-dependent turnover. *Mol Cell Biol*, Vol. 27, No. 4, pp. 1296-1308.

Li, S. & Shang, Y. (2007). Regulation of SRC family coactivators by post-translational modifications. *Cell Signal,* Vol. 19, No. 6, pp. 1101-12.

List, H. J., Reiter, R., Singh, B., Wellstein, A. & Riegel, A. T. (2001). Expression of the nuclear coactivator AIB1 in normal and malignant breast tissue. *Breast Cancer Res Treat,* Vol. 68, No. 1, pp. 21-28.

Lonard, D. M. & O'Malley, B.W. (2005). Expanding functional diversity of the coactivators. *Trends Biochem Sci,* Vol. 30, No. 3, pp. 126-132.

Lonard, D.M., Tsai, S.Y. & O'Malley, B.W. (2004). Selective estrogen receptor modulators 4-hydroxytamoxifen and raloxifene impact the stability and function of SRC-1 and SRC-3 coactivator proteins. *Mol Cell Biol,* Vol. 24, No. 1, pp. 14-24.

Lopez, G. N., Turck, C. W., Schaufele, F., Stallcup, M.R. & Kushner, P.J. (2001). Growth factors signal to steroid receptors through mitogen-activated protein kinase regulation of p160 coactivator activity. *J Biol Chem,* Vol. 276, No. 25, pp. 22177-22182.

Louet, J. F., Chopra, A. R., Sagen, J. V., An, J., York, B., Tannour-Louet, M.,., Saha, P. K., Stevens, R. D., Wenner, B. R., Ilkayeva, O. R., Bain, J. R., Zhou, S., DeMayo, F., Xu, J., Newgard , C. B. & O'Malley, B.W. (2010). The coactivator SRC-1 is an essential coordinator of hepatic glucose production. *Cell Metab,* Vol. 12, No. 6, pp. 606-618.

Mangelsdorf, D. J., Thummel, C., Beato, M., Herrlich, P., Schutz, G., Umesono, K., Blumberg, B., Kastner, P., Mark, M., Chambon, P. & Evans, R.M. (1995). The nuclear receptor superfamily: the second decade. *Cell,* Vol. 83, No. 6, pp. 835-839.

Masamura, S., Santner, S. J., Heitjan, D. F. & Santen, R. J. (1995). Estrogen deprivation causes estradiol hypersensitivity in human breast cancer cells. *J Clin Endocrinol Metab,* Vol. 80, No. 10, pp. 2918-2925.

Metivier, R., Penot, G., Hubner, M. R., Reid, G., Brand, H., Kos M. & Gannon, F. (2003). Estrogen receptor-alpha directs ordered, cyclical, and combinatorial recruitment of cofactors on a natural target promoter. *Cell,* Vol. 115, No. 6, pp. 751-763.

Murphy, L. C., Simon, S. L., Parkes, A., Leygue, E., Dotzlaw, H., Snell, L., Troup, S., Adeyinka, A. & Watson. P.H. (2000). Altered expression of estrogen receptor coregulators during human breast tumorigenesis. *Cancer Res,* Vol. 60, No. 22, pp. 6266-6271.

Myers, E., Fleming, F. J., Crotty, G., Kelly, E.W., McDermott, J., O'Higgins N., Hill, A. D. & Young, L. S. (2004). Inverse relationship between ER-beta and SRC-1 predicts outcome in endocrine-resistant breast cancer. *Br J Cancer,* Vol. 91, No. 9, pp. 1687-1693.

Newman, S. P., Bates, N. P. , Vernimmen, D., Parker, M. G. & Hurst, H. C. (2000). Cofactor competition between the ligand-bound oestrogen receptor and an intron 1 enhancer leads to oestrogen repression of ERBB2 expression in breast cancer. *Oncogene,* Vol. 19, No. 4, 490-497.

Onate, S.A., Tsai, ., S. Y., Tsai M. J. & O'Malley, B. W. (1995). Sequence and characterization of a coactivator for the steroid hormone receptor superfamily. *Science,* Vol. 270, No. 5240, pp. 1354-1357.

Osborne, C. K., Bardou, V., Hopp, T. A., Chamness, G. C., Hilsenbeck, S. G., Fuqua, S. A., Wong, J., Allred, D. C., Clark, G. M. & Schiff, R. (2003). Role of the estrogen receptor coactivator AIB1 (SRC-3) and HER-2/neu in tamoxifen resistance in breast cancer. *J Natl Cancer Inst,* Vol. 95, No. 5, pp. 353-361.

Pearce, S. T. & Jordan, V.C. (2004). The biological role of estrogen receptors alpha and beta in cancer. *Crit Rev Oncol Hematol,* Vol. 50, No. 1, pp. 3-22.

Picard, F., Gehin, M., Annicotte, J., Rocchi, S., Champy, M. F., O'Malley, B. W., Chambon, P. & Auwerx, J. (2002). SRC-1 and TIF2 control energy balance between white and brown adipose tissues. *Cell,* Vol. 111, No. 7, pp. 931-941.

Planas-Silva, M. D., Shang, Y., Donaher, J. L., Brown, M. &. Weinberg, R. A. (2001). AIB1 enhances estrogen-dependent induction of cyclin D1 expression. *Cancer Res,* Vol. 61, No. 10, pp. 3858-3862.

Qin, L., Liao, L., Redmond, A., Young, L., Yuan, Y., Chen, H., O'Malley, B. W. & Xu, J. (2008). The AIB1 oncogene promotes breast cancer metastasis by activation of PEA3-mediated matrix metalloproteinase 2 (MMP2) and MMP9 expression. *Mol Cell Biol,* Vol. 28, No. 19, pp. 5937-5950.

Qin, L., Liu, Z., Chen, H. & Xu, J. (2009). The steroid receptor coactivator-1 regulates twist expression and promotes breast cancer metastasis. *Cancer Res*, Vol. 69, No. 9, pp. 3819-3827.

Redmond, A. M., Bane, F. T., Stafford, A. T., McIlroy, M., Dillon, M. F., Crotty, T. B., Hill, A. D. & Young, L.S. (2009). Coassociation of estrogen receptor and p160 proteins predicts resistance to endocrine treatment; SRC-1 is an independent predictor of breast cancer recurrence. *Clin Cancer Res*, Vol. 15, No. 6, pp. 2098-2106.

Rowan, B.G., Garrison, N., Weigel, N.L. & O'Malley, B.W. (2000a). 8-Bromo-cyclic AMP induces phosphorylation of two sites in SRC-1 that facilitate ligand-independent activation of the chicken progesterone receptor and are critical for functional cooperation between SRC-1 and CREB binding protein. *Mol Cell Biol*, Vol. 20, No. 23, pp. 8720-8730.

Rowan, B.G., Weigel, N.L. & O'Malley, B.W. (2000b). Phosphorylation of steroid receptor coactivator-1. Identification of the phosphorylation sites and phosphorylation through the mitogen-activated protein kinase pathway. *J Biol Chem*, Vol. 275, No. 6, pp. 4475-4483.

Sabbah, M., Courilleau, D., Mester, J. & Redeuilh, G. (1999). Estrogen induction of the cyclin D1 promoter: involvement of a cAMP response-like element. *Proc Natl Acad Sci U S A*, Vol. 96, No. 20, pp. 11217-11222.

Santen, R. J., Song R. X., Zhang, Z., Kumar, R., Jeng, M. H., Masamura, A., Lawrence Jr., J., Berstein, L. & Yue, W. (2005). Long-term estradiol deprivation in breast cancer cells up-regulates growth factor signaling and enhances estrogen sensitivity. *Endocr Relat Cancer*, Vol. 12, No. Suppl 1, pp. S61-73.

Shang, Y. & Brown, M. (2002). Molecular determinants for the tissue specificity of SERMs. *Science*, Vol. 295, No. 5564, pp. 2465-2468.

Shiau, A. K., Barstad, D., Loria, P. M., Cheng, L., Kushner, P. J., Agard, D. A. & Greene, G.L. (1998). The structural basis of estrogen receptor/coactivator recognition and the antagonism of this interaction by tamoxifen. *Cell*, Vol. 95, No. 7, pp. 927-937.

Shou, J., Massarweh, S., Osborne, C. K., Wakeling, A. E., Ali S., Weiss, H. & Schiff, R. (2004). Mechanisms of tamoxifen resistance: increased estrogen receptor-HER2/neu cross-talk in ER/HER2-positive breast cancer. *J Natl Cancer Inst*, Vol. 96, No. 12, pp. 926-935.

Tai, H., Kubota, N. & Kato, S. (2000). Involvement of nuclear receptor coactivator SRC-1 in estrogen-dependent cell growth of MCF-7 cells. *Biochem Biophys Res Commun*, Vol. 267, No. 1, pp. 311-316.

Takeshita, A., Cardona, G. R., Koibuchi, N., Suen C. S. & Chin, W.W. (1997). TRAM-1, A novel 160-kDa thyroid hormone receptor activator molecule, exhibits distinct properties from steroid receptor coactivator-1. *J Biol Chem*, Vol 272, No. 44, pp. 27629-27634.

Torres-Arzayus, M. I., Font de Mora, J., Yuan, J., Vazquez, F. , Bronson, R., Rue, M., Sellers W. R. & Brown, M. (2004). High tumor incidence and activation of the PI3K/AKT pathway in transgenic mice define AIB1 as an oncogene. *Cancer Cell*, Vol. 6, No. 3, pp. 263-274.

Ueda, T., Mawji, N. R., Bruchovsky, N. & Sadar, M.D. (2002). Ligand-independent activation of the androgen receptor by interleukin-6 and the role of steroid receptor coactivator-1 in prostate cancer cells. *J Biol Chem*, Vol. 277, No. 41, pp. 38087-38094.

Wang, S., Yuan, Y., Liao, L., Kuang, S. Q., Tien, J. C., O'Malley, B. W. & Xu, J. (2009). Disruption of the SRC-1 gene in mice suppresses breast cancer metastasis without affecting primary tumor formation. *Proc Natl Acad Sci U S A*, Vol. 106, No. 1, pp. 151-156.

Webb, P., Nguyen P. & Kushner, P. J. (2003). Differential SERM effects on corepressor binding dictate ERalpha activity in vivo. *J Biol Chem*, Vol. 278, No. 9, pp. 6912-6920.

Webb, P., Nguyen, P., Shinsako, J., Anderson, C., Feng, W., Nguyen, M.P., Chen, D., Huang, S.M., Subramanian, S., McKinerney, E., Katzenellenbogen, B.S., Stallcup, M.R. & Kushner, P.J. (1998). Estrogen receptor activation function 1 works by binding p160 coactivator proteins. *Mol Endocrinol*, Vol. 12, No. 10, pp. 1605-1618.

Whitmarsh, A.J. & Davis, R.J. (2000). Regulation of transcription factor function by phosphorylation. *Cell Mol Life Sci*, Vol. 57, No. 8-9; pp. 1172-1183.

Wu, H., Sun, L., Zhang, Y., Chen, Y., Shi, B., Li, R., Wang, Y., Liang, J., Fan, D., Wu, G., Wang, D., Li, S. & Shang, Y. (2006). Coordinated regulation of AIB1 transcriptional activity by sumoylation and phosphorylation. *J Biol Chem*, Vol. 281, No. 31, pp. 21848-21856.

Wu, R.C., Feng, Q., Lonard, D.M. & O'Malley, B.W. (2007). SRC-3 coactivator functional lifetime is regulated by a phospho-dependent ubiquitin time clock. *Cell*, Vol. 129, No. 6, pp. 1125-1140.

Wu, R. C., Qin, J., Yi, P., Wong, J.S., Tsai, Y., Tsai, M. J. & O'Malley, B.W. (2004). Selective phosphorylations of the SRC-3/AIB1 coactivator integrate genomic reponses to multiple cellular signaling pathways. *Mol Cell*, Vol. 15, No. 6, pp. 937-949.

Wu, R. C., Smith, C.L. & O'Malley, B.W. (2005). Transcriptional regulation by steroid receptor coactivator phosphorylation. *Endocr Rev*, Vol. 26, No. 3, pp. 393-399.

Xu, J. & Li, Q. (2003). Review of the in vivo functions of the p160 steroid receptor coactivator family. *Mol Endocrinol*, Vol. 17, No. 9, pp. 1681-1692.

Xu, J., Liao, L., Ning, G., Yoshida-Komiya, H., Deng, C. & O'Malley, B.W. (2000). The steroid receptor coactivator SRC-3 (p/CIP/RAC3/AIB1/ACTR/TRAM-1) is required for normal growth, puberty, female reproductive function, and mammary gland development. *Proc Natl Acad Sci U S A*, Vol. 97, No. 12, pp. 6379-6384.

Xu, J. & O'Malley, B.W. (2002). Molecular mechanisms and cellular biology of the steroid receptor coactivator (SRC) family in steroid receptor function. *Rev Endocr Metab Disord*, Vol. 3, No. 3, pp. 185-192.

Xu, J., Wu, R. C. & O'Malley, B.W. (2009). Normal and cancer-related functions of the p160 steroid receptor co-activator (SRC) family. *Nat Rev Cancer*, Vol. 9, No. 9, pp. 615-630.

Xu, J., Qiu, Y., DeMayo, F. J., Tsai, S. Y., Tsai, M. J. & O'Malley, B.W. (1998). Partial hormone resistance in mice with disruption of the steroid receptor coactivator-1 (SRC-1) gene. *Science*, Vol. 279, No. 5358, pp. 1922-1925.

Yi, P., Feng, Q., Amazit, L., Lonard, D.M., Tsai, S.Y., Tsai, M.J. & O'Malley, B.W. (2008). Atypical protein kinase C regulates dual pathways for degradation of the oncogenic coactivator SRC-3/AIB1. *Mol Cell*, Vol. 29, No. 4, pp. 465-476.

Zhao, C., Yasui, K., Lee, C. J., Kurioka, H., Hosokawa, Y., Oka, T. & Inazawa, J. (2003). Elevated expression levels of NCOA3, TOP1, and TFAP2C in breast tumors as predictors of poor prognosis. *Cancer*, Vol. 98, No. 1, pp. 18-23.

Zhou, G., Hashimoto, Y., Kwak, I., Tsai, S.Y. & Tsai, M.J. (2003). Role of the steroid receptor coactivator SRC-3 in cell growth. *Mol Cell Biol*, Vol. 23, No. 21, pp. 7742-7755.

Zwart, W., Griekspoor, A., Berno, V., Lakeman, K., Jalink, K., Mancini, M., Neefjes, J., Michalides, R. (2007). PKA-induced resistance to tamoxifen is associated with an altered orientation of ERalpha towards co-activator SRC-1. *EMBO J*, Vol. 26, No. 15, pp.3534-3544.

6

Adrenoceptors and Breast Cancer

Roisman Reuth[1], Alex Beny[2], Reznick Abraham Zeev[3], Klemm Ofer[1], Raphaeli Guy[1] and Roisman Isaac[1]
[1]*Carmel College, Haifa,*
[2]*Rambam Medical Center, Haifa,*
[3]*Rapapport Faculty of Medicine, Technion - Israel Institute of Technology, Haifa, Israel*

Dedicated to Mrs. Minka Klavins and Prof. Janis V. Klavins
Albert Einstein College of Medicine, New York, NY, USA

1. Introduction

The incidence of breast cancer has increased greatly in Israel over the past decade. It is estimated that in Israel in 2009 approximately 4800 new patients will suffer from breast cancer. Despite recent advances in the diagnosis and treatment of breast cancer, this disease continues to be a major cause of death. One of the biggest challenges in breast cancer treatment is bone metastasis. Breast cancer cells are capable of migrating to the bone marrow and utilizing the marrow microenvironment to remain quiescent. The preprotachykinin-1 (PPT-I) gene encodes for the tachykinin peptides, which interact with neurokinin (NK) receptors. Studies have correlated this interaction with breast cancer cells integration into the bone marrow and breast cancer progression [(1)].

Environmental and psychological stresses have been shown to be associated with an increased incidence of cancer in man and animals. Stress-induced neuron chemical hormonal and immunological changes have been shown to influence tumor development. Stress may promote mammary carcinogenesis by affecting the neuroendocrine system and I or immune function. Neuroendocrine affects may involve changes in adrenocortical steroids or opioid peptides which may exert their effects by altering immune functions [(2)].

One of the risk factors for breast cancer is the increased amount of adipose tissue after menopause which elevates estradiol production.

The adrenergic system plays a role in regulating energy balance through thermogensis and lipid mobilization from brown or white adipose tissues [(3)].

The human fat cells are equipped with adrenergic receptors (adreno receptors) β1, β2 (ADRB1/2) and β3 (ADRB3) [(4)].

2. Physiology

The degree of affinity for adrenaline (epinephrine) is $\beta 2 > \beta 1 > \beta 3$ and the noradrenaline (norephinephrine) it is $\beta 1 \geq \beta 2 > \beta 3$ [(5)].

Norepinephrine, epinephrine and dopamine are members of biogenic amines. They share a common precursor - tyrosine. It is converted to L-dopa by tyrosine hydroxylase and L-dopa is converted to dopamine by dopa decarboxylase. In the nerve terminal dopamine is converted to norepinepherine.
If phenylethanol - N - methyl transferase (PNMT) is present norepinephrine is methylated to epinephrine. Adrenergic neurons secrete norepinephrine because they contain dopamine β hydroxylase.
Adreno receptors may be activated by norepinephrine, which is released from adrenergic neurons, or by epinephrine, which is secreted into the circulation by the adrenal medulla. Among the sympathetic adrenoreceptors, receptor type is related to function [(6)].
In addition to their role as neurotransmitters and stress hormones, catecholamines play a trophic role in the control of cell replication and differentiation in target cells that express adrenergic receptors. In some cell lines, β -adrenergic stimulation elicits a small, promotional effect on cell replication, whereas in others, stimulation of these receptors and the consequent rise in intracellular cAMP levels inhibits mitosis. β -adrenoreceptors on cancer cells, thus, recapitulate both the promotional and inhibitory roles of these receptors in cell replication seen in the development of normal cells.

2.1 Location and mechanism of autonomic action

Adrenoreceptor type	Target organ	Mechanism of action
α1	Vascular smooth muscle, skin, renal and splanchnic gastrointestinal tract, bladder sphincter, iris, radial muscle, sphincters	IP_3, increase of intracellular [Ca^{2+}]
α2	Gastrointestinal tract wall, presynaptic adrenergic neurons	Inhibition of adenylyl cyclase, decrease cAMP
β1	Heart, salivary gland, adipose tissue, kidney	stimulation of adenylyl cyclase, increase cAMP
β2	Va Vascular smooth muscle of skeletal muscle, GI wall, GI bladder wall, bronchioles	stimulation of adenylyl cyclase, increase cAMP

The β -adrenergic agonist isoproterenol, stimulates mammary epithelial cell division in vitro, as well as the development of end bud structures in the mammary gland of ovary ectomized mice from which arise the mammary carcinoma induced by administration of dimethylbenz (α) anthracene (DMBA). Specific β -adrenergic receptors of the β2 subtype are present in epithelial cell membranes from lactating mammary gland tissue.
The hormonal modulations of receptors which affect uterine contractility correlates with the onset of psychological responses of the uterus such as contraction and relaxation. In analogy with the uterus the regulation of the physiological status of the mammary gland is achieved by modification of endocrine, autonomic and mechanical factors during adolescence, the menstrual cycle, pregnancy parturition and lactation. The mammary gland, as other paired endocrine glands (adrenals, ovaries and testes), receives sympathetic innervations.
High levels of β -adrenergic receptors are measured as palpable mammary tumors, reaching a maximal concentration well before the actual increase in tumor mass. The hormone

sensitivity of the tumoral β -adrenergic receptor is further confirmed by the high receptor concentration measured in progressing mammary tumors.
Stress effects may involve ACTH, glucocorticoids, catecholamines, prolactin, opioids and immunosuppression, all factors crucially involved in tumor growth.
Catecholestrogens, their receptors, together with their catabolizing enzyme, catecholo-methyltransferease(COMT), are locally formed in both normal and neoplastic mammary tissues. COMT levels are significantly increased in the cytosol of malignant tumor cells than in the cytosol of benign tumor or normal cells [(7)].

2.2 Adrenoceptors and cancer

Recent studies in human cancer cell lines in animal models have shown that the growth of adenocarcinomas of the lungs, pancreas and colon are under β -adrenergic control [(8-12)].
The expression of β -adrenergic receptors has been correlated with the over-expression of the arachidonic acid-metabolizing enzymes cyclooxygenase-2 (COX-2) and lipoxygenases (LOX) in adenocarcinomas of lungs, colon, prostate and pancreas. Inhibitors of these enzymes have been identified as cancer preventive agents in animal models.

2.3 Adrenoceptors and breast cancer

Many of breast adenocarcinomas over express COX-2 and / or LOX [(13)].
This may say that a subset of breast cancers may also be under β adrenergic control.
Studies have demonstrated that three estrogen-responsive and three non-estrogen responsive human cell lines derived from breast adenocarcinoma show a reduction in DNA synthesis in response to beta-blockers or inhibitors of the arachidonic acid- metabolizing enzymes COX-2 and 5-LOX.
Another study analysis by reverse transcription polymerase chain reaction (RT-PCR) revealed expression of β_2-adrenergic receptors in all six breast cancer cell lines tested (MDA-MB-361, ZR-75-I, MCF-7, MDA-MB-453, MDA-MB-468, MDA-MB-4355).
β_1 receptors were not found in two estrogen non-responsive cell lines (MDA-MB4355, MDA-MB-453 [(14)].
It was found that the second messenger cAMP may be a growth promoter for mouse, rat and human mammary epithelioma [(15, 16)].
The effects of cAMP observed in malignant cells are involved in redifferentiation amounting to renormalization of number of properties including morphology, adhesive properties, lectin agglutination, cell movement and biochemical functions [(17)].
A correlation between β adreno receptor (β -AR) stimulation and estrogen and progesterone receptor functions was found in human breast cancer [(18)].
β_2-adrenergic stimulation induced cell proliferation in hormone-dependent human breast cancer cell line (C6-5), but without involving the female steroid hormone receptor system [(18)].
In C6-5 cells, the presence of functional β -AR's could be reasonable related to cell proliferation when exposed to different concentrations of clenbuterol, a β_2-AR agonist showed increased cell proliferation without involving significantly lower than that induced by oestradiol β adreno receptor-mediated inhibition of DNA synthesis was not shared by another cancer cell line, C6 rat glioma, that expresses a different β -receptor subtype a lower levels whereas found that MDA-MB-231 cells express β_2-receptors exclusively, C6 cell express primarily the β_1 subtype [(19)].
In mammary tissue there are data that support a role of catecholamines in the control of many cellular activities. Initial experiments indicate epinephrine sensitive adenylate cyclase

activities in 7, 12 - dimethylbenz (α) anthracene - induced mammary carcinoma. Two groups have demonstrated the presence of β -adrenergic receptors (β -AR) from mammary glands of lactating rats. β -adrenergic compounds stimulated the enzyme leading to the generation of cAMP and its activation was completely abolished by the β -AR blocking drug propranolol.

β -adrenergic - related increases in cAMP formation undoubtedly influence lactose production by the acinar secretory end pieces. The initial response to β -AR is usually an increase in adenylate cyclase activity resulting in an increased cellular cAMP concentration.

Among the epithelial, endocrine, and secretory cancer cell lines that express adrenoreceptors, MDA-MB-231 human breast cancer cells exhibit comparatively high concentrations. It is thus of critical interest that stimulation of these receptors leads to immediate inhibition of DNA synthesis and, with prolonged exposure, reductions in the total number of cancer cells: inhibition of DNA synthesis is a reliable predictor of chemotherapeutic responses in breast cancer cells.

In prostate or breast cancer cells stimulated by EGF or androgen or estradiol, small peptides (6-10 amino acids) derived from ER or AR sequences involved in the receptor interaction with Src, prevent AR/ER/Src association, Src/Erk pathway stimulation, cyclin D1 expression and DNA synthesis. The peptide action is restricted to cells expressing the steroid receptors and to signals mediated by these receptors. Remarkably, the peptides do not modify. Although there has been no systematic screening of breast cancer cell lines for β -adrenergic expression these receptors have identified in both estrogen-dependent type and estrogen-independent type, including *C6-5*, BF 20, T47-D, VHB-1 and MCF-7. Regardless of the ancillary mechanisms involved in β -receptor — mediated inhibition of mitosis in MDA-MB-231 breast cancer cells, the fact that inhibition does not disappear with receptor down regulation and desensitization raises the possibility for therapeutic strategies employing receptor agonists, alone or in combination with glucocorticoids and phosphodiesterase inhibitors [(20)].

Screening of human cancers for the presence of β -adrenoreceptors or other cAMP —linked neurotransmitter receptors may establish new treatment strategies.

β -adrenergic receptors (β -AR's) were identified in CG-5 breast cancer cells using a radiometric assay. The total β -AR concentration was measured using the highly potent β -adrenergic antagonist CGP 12 177, and the densities of β -AR subtypes were discriminated in the presence of highly selective unlabelled ligands (CGP 207 12A and ICI 118551).

The second messenger cAMP was found to be a growth promoter for mouse, rat and human mammary epithelioma and its levels are elevated in several breast carcinomas.

The effects of cAMP observed in malignant cells are often involved in redifferentiation, amounting to apparent renormalization of a number of properties including morphology, adhesive properties, lectin agglutination, cell movement and biochemical functions. A correlation between β -AR stimulation and estrogen and progesterone receptor functions was found in human breast cancer.

It was observed that β_2-adrenergic stimulation induced cell proliferation in a hormone-dependent human breast cancer cell line (CG-5), but without involving the female steroid hormone receptor system.

CG-5 cells (mammary breast cell cancer cell line) contain measurable concentrations of specific β AR's coupled to adenylate cyclase. The characteristics of these β -AR's, identified by binding and competition assays, are those of β_1-AR and β_2 -AR subtypes. β_2-AR concentration is significantly higher than β_1-AR concentration in CG-5 cell membranes.

Negligible concentrations of β -AR's were found in MCF-7 breast cancer cells from which CG-5 cells are derived. In C6-5 cells the presence of functional β -AR's could be reasonably related to cell proliferation when exposed to different concentrations of clenbuterol, a β_2-AR agonist, showed increased cell proliferation without involving steroid hormone receptors.
Although the enhancement of CG-5 cell growth was significantly lower than that induced by estradiol the presence of functional β -AR's (with the prevalence of the β 2-AR subtype) in tumor cell line suggests that β -adrenergic stimulation and resulting cAMP production may be responsible for CG-5 cell proliferation.
Medroxyprogesterone acetate (MPA) is one of the most widely used compounds in the endocrine therapy of advanced breast cancer in women. The mechanisms underlying the antitumor activity of MPA are poorly understood. This steroid presents a high affinity for progesterone (PgR) as well as for androgen (AR) and glucocorticoid receptors (GR) in human mammary tumors.
The most easily explained effects of MPA are related to its glucocorticoid-like action.
Suppression of adrenal function by MPA is believed to be caused both by an inhibitory action at the pituitary level and by direct inhibition of steroidogenesis.
In addition to ER and PgR, which are the most widely used markers of differentiated endocrine functions in breast cancer; AR and GR (Glucocorticoid receptors) are present in a substantial number of mammary tumors and established cell lines. The ZR-75-1 human breast cancer cell line is an unusually appropriate system to study the direct effect of MPA on cell growth. ZR-75-1 cells contain functional receptors for estrogens, androgens, progestins and glucocorticoids. Progestins inhibit ZR-75-1 cell proliferation exclusively in presence of estrogens and in absence of insulin.
MPA further decreased the growth of ZR-75- 1 cells co-incubated with maximally inhibitory concentrations of either 5 alpha-dihydrotestosterone ((DHT) or dexamethasone (DEX) although at about 300-fold higher MPA concentrations with DHT-treated than with DEX-treated ZR-75-1 cells, thus demonstrating a highly predominant androgenic effect. The main action of MPA on ZR-75-1 human breast cancer cell growth is due to its androgen receptor-mediated inhibitory action.
The majority of breast cancer are adenocarcinomas and many of them over express cyclooxygenase - 2 (COX-2) [(9)] and/or lipoxygenases (LOX). This raises the possibility that comparable to findings in adenocarcinomas of the lungs, pancreas, colon and prostate, and a subset of breast cancer may also be under beta adrenergic control. Studies have demonstrated that three estrogen-responsive and three non-estrogen responsive human cell lines derived from breast adenocarcinomas demonstrated a significant reduction in DNA synthesis in response to beta-blockers or inhibitors of the arachidonic acid metabolizing enzymes COX-2 [(9)] and LOX-5.
Analysis by reverse transcription polymerase chain reaction (RT-PCR) revealed expression of β_2-adrenergic receptors in all six breast cancer cell tested (MDA-MB- 361, ZR-75-1, MCF-7, MDA-MB -453, MDA-MB-468, MDA-MB-435S) whereas β_1 receptors were not found in two estrogen non-responsive cell lines (MDA-MB-435S, MDA-MB-453).
Expression of mRNA that encodes a G-protein coupled inward by rectifying potassium channel 1 (GIRK1) [(7)] has been shown in 40% breast cancer samples. This expression of GIRK1 was associated with a more aggressive clinical behavior. Previous studies indicated that the beta-adrenergic agonist isoproterenol stimulates growth. GIRK currents have been shown to be increased in cells stimulated with the beta-adrenergic agonist isoproterenol in rat atrial myocytes transferred with β_1 or β_2 receptors. Two polymorphisms in the β_2 or β_3

adrenergic receptors were found to be correlated with decreased risk for breast cancer, suggesting an important role of this receptor family in the genesis of breast cancer.

In C6-5 cells [16, 19] the presence of functional β -AR's could be reasonable related to cell proliferation when exposed to different concentration of clenbuterol, a β_2-AR agonist showed increased cell proliferation without involving significantly lower than that induced by estradiol β adreno receptor-mediated inhibition of DNA synthesis was not shared by another cancer cell line, C6 rat glioma, that expresses a different β -receptor subtype a lower levels whereas [20] found that MOA-MB-23 1 cells express β_2-receptors exclusively, C6 cell express primarily the β_1 subtype.

There is increasing evidence that describes a histamine role in normal and cancer cell proliferation. To better understand the importance of histamine in breast cancer development, the expression of histamine H3 (H3R) and H4 (H4R) receptors and their association with proliferating cell nuclear antigen (PCNA), histidine decarboxylase (HDC) and histamine content were explored in mammary biopsies. Additionally, we investigated whether H3R and H4R were implicated in the biological responses triggered by histamine in MDA-MB-231[20] breast cancer cells.

Centrally assess estrogen receptor (ER) and progesterone receptor (PgR) levels by immunohistochemistry and investigate their predictive value for benefit of chemo-endocrine compared with endocrine adjuvant therapy alone in two randomized clinical trials for node-negative breast cancer.

Low levels of ER and PgR are predictive of the benefit of adding chemotherapy to endocrine therapy. Low PgR may add further predictions among pre-and perimenopausal but not postmenopausal patient whose tumors express ER.

The majority of all breast cancers are hormone responsive, traditionally defined by he expression of oestogen receptor (ER) alpha and/or progesterone receptors. In contrast to ERalpha, the clinical significance of the relatively recently identified ERbeta is still unclear.

ERalpha and ERbeta seem to be differentially associated to clinicopathological parameters, and this would support the fact that they might have different functions in vivo.

In prostate or breast cancer cells stimulated by EGF or androgen or estradiol, small peptides (6-10 amino acids) derived from ER or AR sequences involved in the receptor interaction with Src, prevent AR/ER/Src association, Src/Erk pathway stimulation, cyclin D1 expression and DNA synthesis. The peptide action is restricted to cells expressing the steroid receptors and to signals mediated by these receptors. Remarkably, the peptides do no modify!

Epidermal growth factor (EGF), transforming growth factor-alpha (TGFalpha), amphiregulin (AREG), betacellulin (BTC), heparin-binding EGF-like growth factor (HB-EGF),epiregulin (EREG) and neuregulins1-4 (NRG1-4) were quantified in 363 tumors by real-time reverse transcription-polymerase chain reaction using TaqMan probes.

Paget's disease (PD) of the breast as well as the vulva is a rare condition, therefore anti-hormonal therapy is not indicated. The high frequency of Her-2/neu and COX-2 overexpression, however, suggests that these molecules could be therapeutically relevant in patients with PD.

Epidemiological evidence indicates that the association between body weight and breast cancer risk may differ across menopausal status as well as the estrogen receptor (ER) and progesterone receptor (PR) tumor status.

The relation between body weight and breast cancer risk is critically dependent on the tumor's ER/PR status and the woman's menopausal status. Body weith control is the effective strategy for preventing ER+PR+ tumors after menopause.

ErbB3 transactivation can make tumor cells resistance to ErbB1/ErbB2 targeting drugs. This urges for a reliable method to determine cel surface ErbB3 levels, but their hands iodinated NRG1 beta is unstable and tends to underestimate the umber of ErbB3 receptors in a radio-receptor assay.

Furthermore, they show by differential competition with unlabled NRG/YYDLL and betacellulin that the number of ErbB3 and ErbB4 receptors can be quantified separately on cultured human breast cancer cells.

Esterogen receptor (ER) antagonists have been widely used for breast cancer treatment, but the efficacy and drug resistance remain to be clinical concerns. The purpose of this study was to determine whether the extracts of coptis, an anti-inflammatory herb, improve the anticancer efficacy of ER antagonists, Their results showed that the combined treatment of ER antagonists and the crude extract of coptis or its purified compound berberine conferred synergetic growth inhibitory effect on MCF-7 cells (ER+), but not on MDA-MB-231 cells (R-). Similar results were observed in the combined treatment of fulvestrant, a specific aromatase antagonist. Analysis of the expression of breast cancer related genes indicated the EGFR, HER2, bci-2, and COX-2 were significantly downregulated, while IFN-beta and p21 were remarkably upregulated by herberine.

The negative association between he oestrogen receptor (ER) and the human epidermal growth factor 2 (HER-2) in breast cancer travels in both directions. ER+ tumors are less likely HER-2+ and HER-2+ are less likely ER+. Studies the age-related immunohistochemical (IHC) expression of ER, HER-2 in 2,227 tumors using age as a continuous variable [(21)].

Estrogen receptors (ERs) are overexpressed in human breast cancers (BCs) and associated with differentiated tumors and with a more favorable prognosis [(22-34)].

Paradoxically, ERs mediate the mitogenic action of estrogens in human BC cells and the efficacy of antiestrogens in adjuvant therapy of primary tumors. The exact mechanism underlying the ER protection against cancer progression to metastasis remains to be investigated. They show that ERs decrease invasiveness of BC cells. Detailed studies revealed that the unliganded and the E2-activated ERs decrease cancer cell invasion in vitro through two distinct mechanisms. In the presence of ligand, ERalpha inhibits invasion through a mechanism requiring the functional ERalpha domains involved in the transcriptional activation of target genes.

Hormone receptors play important roles in breast cancer. The expression of hormone receptors in breast cancer was investigated to evaluate the importance of hormone receptors in the clinicopathology of breast cancer.

Androgen receptor (AR), estrogen receptor (ER) and progesterone receptor (PR) expression characteristics were evaluated using immunohistochemistry stain, comparing patient age, tumor size and axillary lymph node status for 23 pure mucinous and 105 non-mucinous infiltrating ductal carcinomas in the human female breast.

Findings revealed that mucinous carcinoma samples from the breast show distinct clinicopathologic and hormone receptor expression features compared to non-mucinous carcinoma.

There is increasing evidence that describes a histamine role in normal and cancer cell proliferations. To better understand the importance of histamine in breast cancer development, the expression of histamine H3 (H3R) nad H4 (H4R) receptors and their association with proliferating cell nuclear antigen (PCNA), histidine decarboxylase (HDC) and histamine content were explored in mammary biopsies. Additionally, we investigated whether H3R and H4R were implicated in the biological MDA-MB-231 breast cancer cells.

β -adrenergic receptors (β -AR's) were identified in C6-5 breast cancer cells using a radiometric assay. The total β -AR concentration was measured using the highly potent β - adrenergic antagonist CGP 12 177, and the densities of β -AR subtypes were discriminated in the presence of highly selective unlabelled ligands (CGP 20712A and ICI 118551).
The second messenger cAMP was found to be a growth promoter for mouse, rat and human mammary epithelioma and its levels are elevated in several breast carcinomas.
It was observed that β_2-adrenergic stimulation induced cell proliferation in a hormone dependent human breast cancer cell line (CG-5), but without involving the female steroid hormone receptor system. CG-5 cells (mammary breast cell cancer cell line) contain measurable concentrations of specific β AR's coupled to adenylate cyclase. The characteristics of these β -AR's, identified by binding and competition assays, are those of β_1-AR and β_2-AR subtypes. β_2-AR concentration is significantly higher than β_1-AR concentration in CG-5 cell membranes. Negligible concentrations of β –AR's were found in MCF-7 breast cancer cells from which CG-5 cells are derived.
Although the enhancement of CG-5 cell growth was significantly lower than that induced by estradiol the presence of functional β -AR's (with the prevalence of the β_2- subtype AR) in tumor cell line suggests that β -adrenergic stimulation and resulting cAMP production may be responsible for CG-S cell proliferation.
Medroxyprogesterone acetate (MPA) is one of the most widely used compounds in the endocrine therapy of advanced breast cancer in women.
The mechanisms underlying the antitumor activity of MPA are poorly understood.
This steroid presents a high affinity for progesterone (PgR) as well as for androgen (AR) and glucocorticoid receptors (GR) in human mammary tumors.
The most easily explained effects of MPA are related to its glucocorticoid-like action.
Suppression of adrenal function by MPA is believed to be caused both by an inhibitory action at the pituitary level and by direct inhibition of steroidogenesis.
In addition to ER and PgR, which are the most widely used markers of differentiated endocrine functions in breast cancer; AR and GR are present in a substantial number of mammary tumors and established cell lines. The ZR-75-1 human breast cancer cell line is an unusually appropriate system to study the direct effect of MPA on cell growth. ZR-75-1 cells contain functional receptors for estrogens, androgens progestins and glucocorticoids. Progestins inhibit ZR-75- 1 cell proliferation exclusively in presence of estrogens and in absence of insulin.
MPA further decreased the growth of ZR-75-1 cells co-incubated with maximally inhibitory concentrations of either 5 alpha-dihydrotestosterone (DHT) or dexamethasone (DEX) at about 300-fold higher MPA concentrations with DHT-treated than with DEX-treated ZR-75-1 cells, thus demonstrating a highly predominant androgenic effect. The main action of MPA on ZR-75-1 human breast cancer cell growth is due to its androgen receptor-mediated inhibitory action.

3. Summary

In normal and malignant mammary tissues there are data supporting a role for catecholeamines in the control of many cellular activities. The presence of functional β-AR's in human mammary cell lines has been described. All six breast cell lines express either GIRK2 or GIRK4 indicating that functional GIRK potassium channels are possible in these cancer cell lines. The direct control of cell proliferation shown in vitro could eventually open new avenues for adjuvant therapies in the treatment of breast diseases.

4. References

Reddy BY, Trzaska KA, Murthy RG, et al. Neurokinin receptors as potential targets in breast cancer treatment. Curr Drug Discov Technol, 2008; 5:15-19

Tejwani GA, Gudehithlu KP, Hanissian SH, et al. Facilitation of dimethylbenz[α] antracene- induced rat mammary tumorigensis by restraint stress: role of β-endorphin, prolactin and naltrexone. Carcinogenesis, 1991; 12:637-641.

Lafontan M, Berlan M. Fat cell adrenergic receptors and the control of white and brown fat cell function. J Lipid Res. 1993; 34:1057-1091.

Huang XE, Hamajima N, Sito T, et al. Possible association of beta2- and beta3-adrenergic receptor gene polymorphism with susceptibility to breast cancer. Breast Cancer Res. 2001; 3: 264-269. Epub 2001 Apr 26.

Arch JR, Kaumann AJ. Beta 3 and atypical beta-adrenoceptors. Med Res Rev. 1993; 13:663-729.

Marchetti B, Spinola PG, Pelletier G, et al. A potential role for catecholamines in the development and progression of carcinogen-induced mammary tumors: hormonal control of beta-adrenergic receptors and correlation with tumor growth. J Steroid Biochem Mol Biol. 1991; 38:307-320.

Plummer HK, Yu Q, Cakir Y, et al. Expression of inwardly rectifying potassium channels (GIRKs) and beta-adrenergic regulation of breast cancer cell lines. BMC Cancer. 2004;4:93

Schuller HM, Tithof PK, Williams M, et al. The tobacco-specific carcinogen 4-(methylnitrosamino)-1-(3-pyridyl)-1-butanone is a beta-adrenergic agonist and stimulates DNA synthesis in lung adenocarcinoma via beta-adrenergic receptor- mediated release of arachidonic acid. Cancer Res. 1999; 59:4510-4515.

Schuller HM, Plummer HK, Bochsler PN, et al. Co-expression of beta adrenergic receptors and cyclooxygenase-2 in pulmonary adenocarcinoma. Int J Oncol. 2001; 19:445-449.

Schuller HM, Porter B, Riechert A. Beta-adrenergic modulation of NNK-induced lung carcinogenesis in hamsters. J Cancer Res Clin Oncol.2000; 126:624-630.

Masur K, Niggemann B, Zanker KS, et al. Norepinephrine-induced migration of SW 480 colon carcinoma cells is inhibited by beta-blockers. Cancer Res. 2001; 61:2866-2869.

Weddle DL, Tithoff P, Williams M, et al. Beta-adrenergic growth regulation of human cancer cell lines derived from pancreatic ductal carcinoma. Carcinogenesis. 2001; 22: 473-479.

Parrett ML, Harris RE, Joarder FS, et al. Cyclooxygenase-2 gene expression in human breast cancer. Int J Oncology. 1997; 10:503-507.

Cakir Y, Plummer HK, Tithof PK, et al. Beta-adrenergic and arachidonic acid-mediated growth regulation of human breast cancer cell lines. Int J Oncol. 2002; 21:153-157.

Yang Y, Guzman R, Richards J, et al. Growth factor- and cyclic nucleotide-induced proliferation of normal and malignant mammary epithelial cells in primary culture. Endocrinology. 1980; 107:35-41.

Badino GR, Novelli A, Girardi C, et al. Evidence for functional beta-adenoceptors subtypes in CG-5 breast cancer cell. Pharmacol Res. 1996; 33:255-260.

Yabushita H, Sartorelli AC. Effects of sodium butyrate, dimethylsulfoxide and dibutyryl cAMP on the poorly differentiated ovarian adenocarcinoma cell line AMOC-2. Oncol Res.1993; 5:173-182.

Draoui A, Vandewalle B, Hornez L, et al. Beta-adrenergic receptors in human breast cancer: identification, characterization and correlation with progesterone and estradiol receptors. Anticancer Res. 1991; 11:677-680.

Re G, Badino P, Girardi C, et al. Effects of beta-2 agonist (clenbuterol) on cultured human (CG-5) breast cancer cells. Pharmacol Res. 1992; 26:377-384.

Slotkin TA, Zhang J, Dancel R, et al. Beta-adrenoceptor signaling and its control of cell replication in MDA-MB-231 human breast cancer cells. Breast Cancer Res Treat. 2000; 60:153-166.

Neven P, Van Calster B, Van den Bempt I, et al. Age interacts with the expression of steroid and HER-2 receptors in operable invasive breast cancer. Breast Cancer Res Treat. 2008; 110:153-159.

Maynadier M, Nirdé P, Ramirez JM, et al. Role of estrogens and their receptors in adhesion and invasiveness of breast cancer cells. Adv Exp Med Biol. 2008; 617: 485-489.

Cho LC, Hsu YH. Expression of androgen, estrogen and progesterone receptors in mucinous carcinoma of the breast. Kaohsiung Med Sci. 2008; 24: 227-232.

Medina V, Croci M, Crescenti E, et al. The role of histamine in human mammary carcinogenesis: H3 and H4 receptors as potential therapeutic targets for breast cancer treatment. Cancer Biol Ther. 2008; 7: 28-35.

Subbaramaiah K, Hudis C, Chang SH, et al. EP2 and EP4 receptors regulate aromatase expression in human adipocytes and breast cancer cells. Evidence of a BRCA1 and p300 exchange. J Biol Chem. 2008; 283: 3433-3444.

Viale G, Regan MM, Maiorano E, et al. Chemoendocrine compared with endocrine adjuvant therapies for node-negative breast cancer: predictive value of centrally reviewed expression of estrogen and progesterone receptors - International Breast Cancer Study Group. J Clin Oncol. 2008; 26: 1404-1410.

Borgquist S, Holm C, Stendahl M, et al. Oestrogen receptors alpha and beta show different association to clinicopathological parameters and their co-expression might predict a better response to endocrine treatment in breast cancer. Clin Pathol. 2008; 61: 197-203.

Auricchio F, Migliaccio A, Castoria G. Sex-steroid hormones and EGF signalling in breast and prostate cancer cells: targeting the association of Src with steroid receptors. Steroids. 2008; 73: 880-884.

Révillion F, Lhotellier V, Hornez L, et al. ErbB/HER ligands in human breast cancer; and relationships with their receptors the bio-pathological features and prognosis. Ann Oncol. 2008;19:73-80.

Horn LC, Purz S, Krumpe C, et al. COX-2 and Her-2/neu are overexpressed in Paget's disease of the vulva and the breast: results of a preliminary study. Arch Gynecol Obstet. 2008; 277: 135-138.

Dawood S, Broglio K, Kau SW, et al. Triple receptor-negative breast cancer: the effect of race on response to primary systemic treatment and survival outcomes. J Clin Oncol. 2009; 27:220-226.

Suzuki R, Orsini N, Saji S, et al. Body weight and incidence of breast cancer defined by estrogen and progesterone receptor status - a meta-analysis. Int J Cancer. 2009; 124: 698-712.

Van der woning SP and van Zoelen EJ. Quantification of ErbB3 receptor density on human breast cancer cells, using a stable radio-labeled mutant of NRG1beta. Biochem Biophys Res Commun. 2009; 378: 285-289.

Lui J, He C, Zhou K, et al. Coptis extracts enhance the anticancer effect of estrogen receptor antagonists on human breast cancer cells. Biochem Biophys Res Commun. 2009; 378: 174-178.

7

$1,25(OH)_2D_3$ and Cyclooxygenase-2: Possible Targets for Breast Cancer?

M. Thill[1], S. Becker[1], D. Fischer[1], K. Diedrich[1], D. Salehin[2] and M. Friedrich[2]
[1]*Department of Obstetrics and Gynecology, University Schleswig-Holstein, Campus Luebeck, Luebeck*
[2]*Department of Gynecology and Obstetrics, Helios Hospital Krefeld, Krefeld*
Germany

1. Introduction

Currently, breast cancer is the most common malignancy in women. In the U.S. in 2005, approximately 211.240 patients were newly diagnosed with primary breast cancer and 58.490 women were diagnosed with ductal carcinoma in situ (DCIS). Of these, 58.490 deaths are estimated. Therefore breast cancer takes second place following only behind lung cancer [1,2,3]. Because of this, it is necessary to develop new strategies and treatment options that may improve the prognosis.

Besides the classic histo-pathological parameters used to estimate the prognosis of malignant diseases, the identification of additional molecular prognostic parameters would be very helpful in planning treatment by evaluating protein or mRNA expression in tumor tissue. One of these potential molecular prognostic parameters might be the cyclooxygenase-2 (COX-2) [4, 5]. New treatment strategies using compounds that attack well defined proteins in the tumor require verification of the expression of these target proteins. Many similarities exist between tumor tissue and inflammatory modified tissue and normally, inflammatory reaction is self limiting, however, in tumor tissue the inflammatory reaction is persistent. An increased angiogenesis and an elevated production of cytokines, chemokines and proteases lead to good conditions for cell proliferation and invasion in the tumor tissue [6].

Targeted strategies might eliminate this inflammatory reaction that promotes tumor growth and tumorigenesis and there is already promising data around the use of COX-2-inhibitors. The antiproliferative effects of vitamin D may be another starting point; however the data on vitamin D intake or to the exertion of vitamin D analogs is occasionally inconsistent.

The important role that vitamin D and calcium adopt in the human metabolism was recognized as early as the nineteen-twenties as it was used to prevent the bone disease, rickets which was widespread in children at that time [7]. In the last 20 years non-classical effects of vitamin D and its influence on physiology followed because it's potentially anticarcinogen impacts made it more and more interesting. Besides stable calcium-homeostasis by the renal expressed 1-α-hydroxylase functionality, extra renal expressed 1-α-hydroxylase also is also known to have antiproliferative and immune-modulating features

[8-10]. This fact has led to the development of new treatment strategies in the clinical use of $1,25(OH)_2D_3$ (calcitriol). The goal was to affect and treat cancer, psoriasis, autoimmune diseases and host-graft-rejection [11-14]. Implementation of these new treatment options in vivo was conspicuously hindered as $1,25(OH)_2D_3$ has a potentially hypercalcaemic side effect. Finally the application of synthetic $1,25(OH)_2D_3$ analogs led to several successful results due to its less calciotropic effects [15, 16]. The implementation of vitamin D, primarily cancer and autoimmune diseases appears to play a more preventative role as opposed to therapeutic [17, 18].

Observational studies showed an association between vitamin D intake and $25(OH)_2D_3$ plasma levels as well as a reduced risk of breast cancer [19, 20]. Studies that tried to elucidate the correlation between sunlight and cancer prevention demonstrated that long sunlight exposure was associated with a low rate of primary breast cancer and consecutively a low mortality rate [21-24]. $1,25(OH)_2D_3$ is the biologically active form of vitamin D that binds as a ligand to the nuclear vitamin D receptor (VDR) of the genes that are important for vitamin D metabolism (1-α-hydroxylase, 24-hydroxylase) [25]. $1,25(OH)_2D_3$ and its analogs are able to inhibit the proliferation of breast cancer cells in vitro and in vivo [26-29].

2. Prostaglandin metabolism

The cyclooxygenase system consists of two different isoenzymes, COX-1 and COX-2. This system is an integral part of the prostaglandin syntethase complex and is involved controlling inflammatory processes (1). After transformation of arachidonic acid to prostaglandin G_2 (PGG_2), a glutathione dependent peroxidase converts PGG_2 to PGH_2 by an oxi- and peroxidation. PGH_2 acts as basic substrate for the synthesis of different prostaglandins by the microsomal and cytosolic prostaglandin synthase, which are tissue- and cell-specific. Based on the cellular enzyme setting, different prostaglandins are synthesized in different tissues where they act in an auto- or paracrine manner [30]. Prostaglandin E_2 (PGE_2) is one of the best known prostaglandins and is generated by the prostaglandin E synthase. These consist of three different forms: two microsomal prostaglandin E synthases and the cytosolic prostaglandin synthase E [31].

The 15-hydroxyprostaglandin dehydrogenase (15-PGDH) belonging to the oxidoreductases family, inactivates all generated prostaglandins by oxidation to 15-keto metabolites which then have greatly reduced biological activity [32].

3. PG-receptors

The physiological effects of many prostaglandins are mediated by binding to G protein coupled receptors. These effects regulate inflammatory mediations, control hormone regulation, constrict or dilate in vascular smooth muscle cells and regulate calcium movement and their specific receptors activate signal transduction pathways which could induce chronic processes like angiogenesis. For example, PGE_2 interacts with four cell surface receptors - $EP_{1\text{-}4}$ and the EP_2 receptor subtype is involved in the G_s/cAMP/proteinkinase which is a-signalling pathway leading to an increased VEGF expression. PGJ_2 and PGA_2 interact with nuclear receptors, belonging to the peroxisome proliferator-activated receptors (PPARs) family. After dimerization with the 9-cis-Retinoid receptor (RXR) and then binding to a sequence specific responsive element located at the promoter of its target gene, they directly induce gene expression [33].

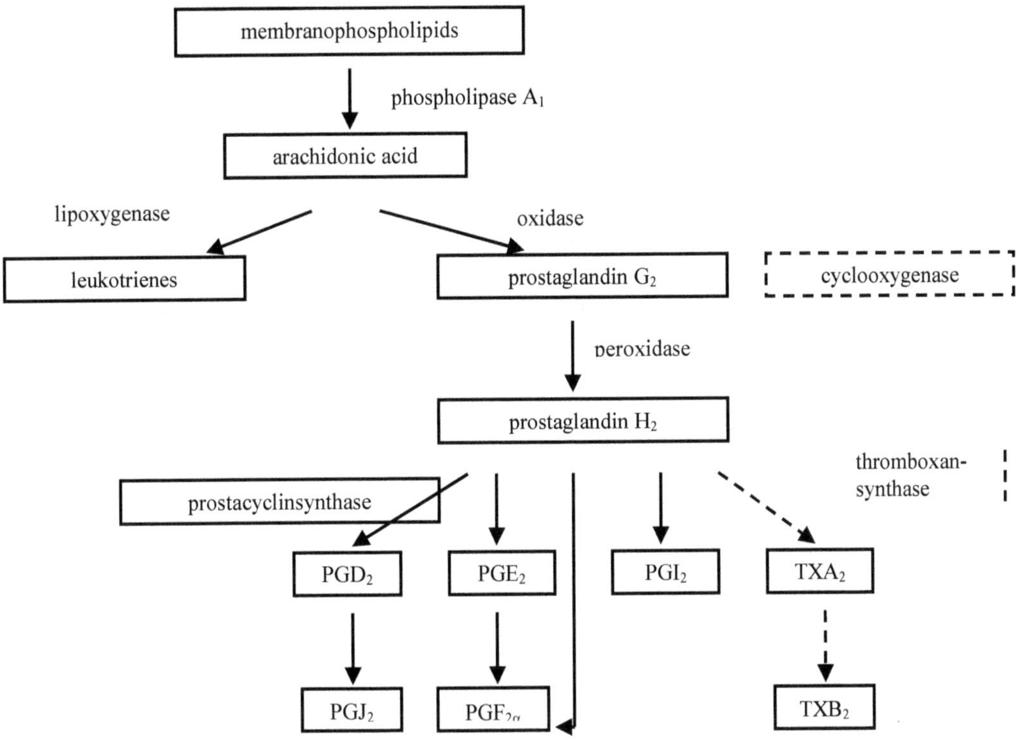

Fig. 1. Prostaglandin metabolism.

4. Isoenzymes COX-1 und COX-2

COX-1 is ubiquitary and not a relevant prognostic factor [34]. In contrast, the COX-2 enzyme is not constitutively expressed. The COX-2 gene expression is stimulated by many growth factors, cytokines and prostaglandins and is associated with inflammation [35]. COX-2 is predominantly a pro inflammatory enzyme but late in the inflammatory phase, the enzyme is involved in limiting inflammation.

Studies with COX-1 and COX-2 knockout mice lead to new consolidated findings about the function of these enzymes concerning ovarian functionality and reproduction as well as cardiovascular development [36 - 39]. The COX enzymes are the main target of non-steroidal anti inflammatory drugs (NSAID) where isoenzymes specifically inhibit the biological activity of COX enzymes. Celecoxib and rofecoxib are selective COX-2 inhibitors whereas acetylsalicylic acid, ibuprofen and indomethacin are non-specific and target both isoenzymes.

5. Role of COX-2 in carcinogenesis

The cyclooxygenases, especially COX-2, play an important role in the development and progression of malignant tumours. The over expression of COX-2 is associated with the differentiation of tumor cells by several mechanisms [40] and can be detected in various epithelial carcinomas such as in colon [41, 42], gastric [43] and esophageal cancers [44] as well as in prostate [45], liver, pancreas and lung cancers [46]. One of the mechanisms that are modulated during carcinogenesis is the neoangiogenesis [47 – 55].

Epidemiological studies have shown that a continuous intake of NSAIDs protects against the incidence of breast cancer [56-58].
Increased PGE_2 levels can be detected in cultivated human breast cancer cell lines as well as in invasive human breast cancer cells [59-62] and are associated with both a negative hormone receptor status and an escalated mestastic potential [59].
As mentioned previously, PGE_2 is the ligand for at least four cell surface receptors - EP_{1-4} and several studies have presented the impact of the EP_1-receptor in carcinogenesis of colon and breast cancer [63]. A blockage of the EP_2-receptor leads to a reduction and a diminishment of intestinal polyposis in $APC^{\Delta 716}$-knock-out mice [64]. There was an increased detection of EP_2- and EP_4-receptors in the breast tumors of COX-2-MMTV mice; therefore, it appears that the EP-receptors play an important role in mediating PG functions and in promoting carcinogenesis.

6. Role of 15-PGDH in carcinogenesis

Increased PGE_2 levels in context to mammary carcinomas are associated with an enhanced cell proliferation, invasiveness, resistance to apoptosis and angiogenesis [65, 66]. The regulation of plasma PGE_2 level results from its synthesis and its biological inactivation through 15-PGDH, the key enzyme for the biological inactivation of PGs [32]. Recent studies hypothesized 15-PGDH as a tumor suppressor gene in correlation to colon, bladder and bronchial carcinomas [67-69]. Wolf and co-workers [70] assumed antiproliferative effects of 15-PGDH in breast cancer cells. The estrogen receptor (ER) positive and well differentiated MCF-7 breast cancer cell line had an increased 15-PGDH expression compared to poorly differentiated, ER negative MDA-MB-231 cells, which express COX-2 and lead to primary breast cancer. Different studies reported that MCF-7 cells are the only breast cancer cell line with an enhanced 15-PGDH expression and low levels of 15-PGDH are accompanied by poorly prognostic factors [70]. This data attended by a microarray analysis of van't Veer and co-workers [71] supports the advice that a loss of 15-PGDH expression plays a pivotal role in the development of poorly differentiated mammary carcinomas. Data generated from genetically modified MDA-MB-231 cells that over express the enzyme and MCF-7 where 15-PGDH was knockout, corroborates the hypothesis that 15-PGDH acts as a tumor suppressor gene in breast cancer [70]. MDA-MB-231 cells showed a decreased invasiveness similar to studies in colon [67] and bronchial carcinomas [68]. Yan and co-workers [67] reported that 15-PGDH is naturally expressed in colon tissues and was dramatically reduced in colon carcinomas. The reconstitution of 15-PGDH in immunodeficiency mice prevented the colon cancer cells from generating tumors and so the authors concluded, that 15-PGDH acts as tumor suppressor and inhibits the angiogenic and proliferative effects of COX-2 in vivo.

7. COX-2 expression in breast cancer

Experimental immunochemical studies of COX-2 expression in breast cancer have produced varying and sometimes controversial and inconsistent data. Generally the consensus is that COX-2 is expressed by invasive ductal and lobular carcinoma and that the proportion of COX-2 positive tumors varies between studies (Table 1). In studies where poor prognostic tumor characteristics were examined, a correlation was found between prognostic parameters such as hormone receptor negativity, HER2 positivity, increased tumor size, high nuclear grade, development of distant metastases and a reduced survival rate (Table 1) [5]. Moreover COX-2 expression correlates with aromatase expression.

An explanation for the variable findings of COX-2 protein expression may be caused by the different scoring systems and cut-offs used for COX-2 immunoreactivity.

Half and co-workers [72] examined immonochemical human breast cell lines of normal and neoplastic breast tissue and detected a COX-2 expression in breast cancer cells in 43%, in DCIS in 62.5% and benign breast cells had a COX-2 expression in 81%. The more elevated COX-2 expression in DCIS in terms of a premalignant lesion might mean that an up-regulation or over-expression of COX-2 occurs relatively early in the carcinogenesis of breast cancer [72]. Contrary to Half and co-workers [72], Denkert and co-workers [73] could not detect a COX-2 expression in benign breast tissue and this may support the partially conflicting data. Denkert and co-workers [73] detected a COX-2 expression in 41% in invasive ductal breast cancer, however detected it in only 14% of invasive lobular tumors and 21% in other breast carcinomas (Table1). The COX-2 expression was associated with positive axillary lymph nodes (>50% node positive, just 16% in node negative breast cancer), extensive tumor growth (58% in tumors >20mm, in 24% in tumors <20mm), poor nuclear grading, vascular invasion and hormone receptor negativity.

Not all the studies have determined a correlation between COX-2 expression and clinicopathological parameters. Half and co-workers [72] could not demonstrate a significant correlation but Ristimäki and co-workers [74] certainly did show a significant correlation between COX-2 expression and hormone receptor negativity, extensive tumor growth, high nuclear grading and HER2 positivity. In a recently published paper by Singh-Ranger and co-workers [75], a correlation to distant metastases was described and Nassar and co-workers [76] demonstrated a correlation to nuclear grading and tumor size; however a correlation to important clinical goals such as eradicating the disease and enhancing overall survival rate have not yet been found.

Therefore COX-2 over-expression correlates in a different manner depending upon its aggressiveness the invasive potential of tumor cells, and then consequently exhibiting a higher incidence of distant metastases [40].

Reference	N =	COX-2 positive (%)			Correlation of COX-2 expression and clinicopathological parameters						
		Carcinoma	DCIS	Benign tissue	Angiogenesis	HR-status	HER2	Grading	Age	Node +	Big tumor
[77]	44	2/44 (4,5%)	-	-	Not examined						
[78]	27	7/17 (42%)	8/10 (80%)	-	Not examined						
[72]	106	18/42 (43%)	10/16 (63%)	39/48 (81%)	-	No	No	-	-	-	-
[73]	221	80/221 (36%)	-	0%	Yes	Yes	-	Yes	No	Yes	Yes
[79]	46	50%	-	-	Yes	No	No	No	No	Yes	
[74]	1576	589/1576 (37,4%)	-	-	-	Yes	Yes	Yes	-	Yes	Yes
[80]	106	90/106 (85%)	-	-	No	No	No	No	No	No	No
[81]	128	41%	-	-	Yes	-	-	Yes	-	Yes	Yes
[82]	192	40,6%	-	-	-	Yes	Yes	Yes	-	-	Yes
[83]	65	41/65 (63%)	-	-	-	Yes	Yes	-	-	-	-
[76]	43	41/43 (95%)	-	-	-	No	No	Yes	-	-	Yes

Table 1. Immunochemical examinations of COX-2 expression and correlation with selected clinicopathological parameters in breast tissue.

Transcriptional studies have also revealed a distinct variation in their results regarding COX-2 expression. The detection rate varies between 50 and 100% in the literature (Table 2). There is a comparable relationship between COX-2 immunoreactivity and mRNA expression in tumor tissue [77]. Zhao and co-workers [84] demonstrated an increased mRNA expression in hormone receptor positive breast cancer; a result that was confirmed by Singh and co-workers [85] in breast cancer with positive progesterone receptors. However, only a small number of studies have examined the correlation between mRNA expression and clinico-pathological parameters. These results are summarized in Table 2.

Reference	N =	COX-2-mRNA positive (%)	Clinicopathological correlation of COX-2 with						
			Angio-genesis	HR-status	HER2	Grading	Age	Node +	Big tumor
[86]	40	40/40 (100%)	Not examined						
[72]	9	9/9 (100%)	Not examined						
[87]	7	7/7 (100%)	-	-	-	-	-	-	-
[88]	20	10/20 (50%)	-	-	-	-	-	-	-
[85]	18	18/18 (100%)	Not examined	Yes (PR)	Not examined				
[84]	30	27/30 (90%)	-	Yes (ER+)	-	Not examined			

Table 2. COX-2 mRNA expression and correlation with selected clinicopathological parameters in breast cancer.

These results are contrary to the immunochemically evaluated data, which show an association to hormone receptor negative tumors. This could be explained because before the genetic information of COX-2 is translated into a biologically active protein, COX-2 mRNA is post transcriptionally modified in the nucleus. Thus, we speculate that the COX-2 mRNA is destabilised by its AU rich sequences and no COX-2 protein is generated. Therefore, the correlation between the hormone receptor status and COX-2 mRNA levels is not obvious in studies where the COX-2 protein expression was investigated [5]. There are some well known factors which affect the COX-2 mRNA levels like interleukin-1 stabilises the highly unstable COX-2 mRNA transcript [89], however steroids may destabilise the COX-2 mRNA [90]. Furthermore, it might be possible that genetically different subtypes of breast cancer express COX-2 and are then associated with both hormone receptor-negative and receptor-positive tumors [91]. Additionally, Ristimäki and co-workers [74] reported that hormone receptor-positive patients who express COX-2 had a poor survival rate.

7.1 COX-2 and hormone receptors

There is concurrent evidence about the interaction of PGE_2/COX-2 and the estrogen receptor signalling pathway. For example, COX-2 expression is correlated with the expression of the aromatase [92] and in vitro studies support this data. It has been shown that COX-2 promotes the aromatase transcription, whereas COX-2 inhibitors diminish it [93]. Based on the elevated synthesis of prostaglandins in cells that express COX-2, the aromatase expression and activity is increased in breast cells [94, 95]. Expression of aromatase leads to estrogen production and from cell line studies; we know that hormone receptor expression can be induced by sex steroid hormones [96]. All the data supports the

close correlation between COX-2 and hormone receptors. Wolf and co-workers [70] reported a link between the estrogen signalling pathway and 15-PGDH by a negative feedback mechanism. High levels of this hormone reduced the 15-PGDH expression but the activity of the ERE (estrogen responsive element) and the activity of the aromatase increased.
New studies suggest a synergism between selective COX-2 and aromatase inhibitors.

7.2 Results from in vivo studies

The impact of COX-2 in carcinogenesis of breast tumors has been shown in transgenic mice models [97]. It has been reported that the over-expression of COX-2 in breast tissues is associated with decreased BAX and Bcl-xL (pro apoptotic) and increased Bcl-2 (anti apoptotic) protein levels. Therefore, the author suggested that induction of carcinogenesis is COX-2 dependent [97]. In contrast, the resistance to apoptosis is associated with increased COX-2 levels [98]. The importance of COX-2 in correlation to the tumor formation has been investigated in COX-2 knockout mice. The COX-2 knockout mice lead to an 86% reduction of intestinal adenoids [99].

7.3 COX-2 and tumorigenesis

The expression of COX-2 is regulated by post-transcriptional and -translational mechanisms. Different cytokines, growth factors and oncogenes have been shown to induce the COX-2 expression which is associated with carcinogenesis [46, 100].

7.3.1 Influence of COX-2 on angiogenesis and apoptosis

Angiogenesis is the development of new blood vessels and is an important factor in tumor proliferation, invasion and metastasis. Davies and co-workers [101] showed a significant positive correlation between COX-2 expression and the endothelial surface marker CD31. Other reports confirmed a positive correlation between COX-2 and the vascular endothelial growth factor (VEGF) [102, 103]. During carcinogenesis COX-2 modulates the neoangiogenesis and seems to stimulate the production of proangiogenic factors such as VEGF, basic fibroblast growth factor (bFGF), transforming growth factor 1 (TGF1), platelet derived growth factor (PDGF) and endothelin [104, 105]. The application of selective COX-2 inhibitors decreased the angiogenesis in different vivo models [106]. Recently, an angiogenesis independent mechanism, so called Vasculogenic Mimicry (VM), was described where poorly differentiated breast cancer cells were nourished without the mechanisms of classic neoangiogenesis [107-109]. VM is a phenomenon of vessel formation of epithelial tumor cells without any participation of endothelial cells and itis a mechanism independent of or simultaneous to neoangiogenesis thus ensuring the tumor perfusion [110]. Hence, the VM might be an important factor for new antiangiogenic therapeutical approaches. The existence of VM in breast cancer patients is associated with a poor 5-year survival rate compared to patients without. [111]. Basu and co-workers [112] reported that highly invasive MDA-MB-231 breast cancer cells and the less invasive subtype MDA-MB-435 cells that over express COX-2, formed new micro vessels. In contrast, non-invasive MCF-7- and ZR-75-1-breast cancer cells which had a lower COX-2 expression did not. The application of the COX-2 inhibitor celecoxib (40 und 60 µmol/l, $p>0.001$), inhibits the formation of new vessels. This effect was restored with PGE_2. This data was confirmed by an in vivo xenograft model. VEGF, GRO, IL-6, IL-8, TIMP1, TIMP2 were the main angiogenic proteins which were inhibited by celecoxib [112].

7.4 Breast cancer and NSAIDs

The rationale for using NSAIDs is their non-selective (ASS, ibuprofen etc.) or selective (COX-2 inhibitors such as celecoxib) suppression of the COX-system. In a meta-analysis consisting of 14 epidemiological studies (6 cohort studies and 8 case control studies) breast cancer risk was reduced by 18% due to constant intake of NSAIDs [113]. An extensive Canadian study including 5882 patients reported a reduction of breast cancer incidence by 24% due to the NSAIDs intake for 2 - 5 years [58]. Another case control study demonstrated a 40% reduction after 5 years of NSAIDs intake [57]. These results seemingly justify the preventive use of NSAIDs, however, contrarian results were delivered by the Nurses Health Study. This trial showed no difference during the intake of ASS (100mg) in neither women with breast cancer nor in healthy women [114]. On the contrary it was in patients with colon cancer who led the continuous intake of NSAIDs to a reduction of incidence in 40-50% [56, 115, 116].

Data of animal models supports the use of selective COX-2 inhibitors both for the therapeutic and preventive uses. For instance, the use of celecoxib in rats led to an averaged downsizing of breast tumor volume by 32%, however, a tumor volume enlargement of 518% was observed in the control group [117]. Harris and co-workers [118] examined the influence of celecoxib in 120 rats. Three groups of rats were formed. In one group the food was enriched with celecoxib. The other two groups obtained either ibuprofen or nothing. After seven days 7,12-Dimethylbenz(a)anthracene (DMBA) was applied intragastrically and the described food was continued for another 105 days. A distinct reduction in tumor incidence, variety and tumor volume was shown in the celecoxib treated group [118]. In a recently published paper Barnes and co-workers [119] could induce breast tumors in mice by injecting estrogen-positive MCF7/HER2-18- and estrogen-negative MDAMB231 breast cancer cells. The application of celecoxib resulted in a significant growth reduction of the MCF7/HER-18 tumors (58.7%) and the MDAMB231 tumors (46.3%) in comparison to the control group. Therefore, celecoxib dropped the COX-2 expression and enhanced the apoptosis significantly [119]. Yoshinaka and co-workers [120] also showed that the use of celecoxib significantly reduced tumor sizes, increased apoptosis and that a reduced DNA synthesis in the tumor tissue of mice induced breast carcinomas. Moreover the neoangiogenesis was influenced as VEGF-A-mRNA levels were found to be reduced [120].

7.5 COX-2-inhibitors in systemic treatment

Several studies have evaluated the significance of COX-2 inhibitors in combination with systemic treatment. A phase II study observed a clinical benefit of 47.5% for the combination of capecitabine and celecoxib in patients with metastatic breast cancer. The combination was well tolerated [121].

Recently published data about COX-2 and its significance on the aromatase and influence on the female hormonal balance are of strong interest. Besides finding an increased effect on estrogen synthesis in malignant breast tissue, a strong correlation between COX-2 and aromatase mRNA expression were found. This data supports the assumption that COX-2 is able to regulate aromatase activity in breast tissue [92]. A possible synergism between COX-2 and aromatase-inhibitors is even more interesting and so a prospective randomised phase III multicenter trial (REACT-trial) was conducted that included primary breast cancer patients in order to evaluate the combination of celecoxib and exemestane, an aromatase

inhibitor, in an adjuvant setting. The combination of celecoxib and exemestane was already well tolerated and had shown a clinical benefit of 74% [122] or had led to a benefit extension (median 96.6 weeks vs. 49.1 weeks) in patients with metastatic breast cancer [123].
Other malignancies were also proven on the benefit of selective and non-selective COX-2 inhibitors in combination with other compounds such as chemotherapy [124, 125], tyrosinekinase inhibitors [126] and other new approaches [127]. Some of them are encouraging, like the results of the ASCENT trial [124] and some are disappointing. Further work is required to establish how NSAIDs can be best applied for therapeutic benefit.

8. Vitamin D

8.1 Vitamin D metabolism

Vitamin D, a secosteroid hormone, is assimilated by food (milk, fish, liver), multi-vitamin preparations and dietary supplements [128]. Vitamin D is also synthesised from 7-dehydrocholesterol and provitamin D3 after skin exposure with sunlight (ultraviolet spectrum 290-315nm) [129]. Based on its animal or herbal origin, there are two existing vitamin D metabolites: cholecalciferol (vitamin D_3) and ergocalciferol (vitamin D_2) [17], which is less efficient in increasing the 25-hydroxyvitaminD [$25(OH)_2D_3$] serum levels [130]. Cholecalciferol attains to the liver through the bloodstream and is transformed to $25(OH)_2D_3$ (25-hydroxyvitamin D_3, calcediol, 25-hydroxycholecalciferol) by a hydroxylation on the C25 position [131, 132]. $25(OH)_2D_3$, a circulating metabolite, correlates with the vitamin D balance. The hydroxylation of cholecalciferol on the C25 position is inadequately regulated. $25(OH)_2D_3$ level increased with the vitamin D intake, therefore, the $25(OH)_2D_3$ serum level is normally used as an indicator of the vitamin D balance [133]. The serum level range of $25(OH)_2D_3$ is between 10 and 50 ng/ml and round about 30pg/ml for $1,25(OH)_2D_3$ [134]. $25(OH)_2D_3$ is renally converted to the biologically active metabolite 1,25-dihydroxycholecalciferol [$1,25(OH)2D_3$] by the 1-α-hydroxylase (CYP27B1). $1,25(OH)_2D_3$ is 100-1000 fold more active than the other natural metabolites [135]. The 1-α-hydroxylase, a mitochondrial enzyme, which belongs to the P450 enzyme family is located in the renal proximal tubule. Besides the renal expression of the enzyme, many studies reported an extra renal expression of 1-α-hydroxylase and thus an extra renal synthesis of $1,25(OH)_2D_3$. This enzyme has been detected in many cell types and tissues, e.g. prostate, breast, lung, pancreas, parathyroid and monocytes [136]. The extra renal synthesised $1,25(OH)_2D_3$ has cell specific functions and as a result acts as local auto- and paracrine factors. In this context, many extra renal effects of $1,25(OH)_2D_3$, e.g. cell cycle arrest, induction of apoptosis and cell differentiation, have been reported [136]. The fine tuned activity of 1-α-hydroxylase correlates inversely with the calcium metabolism and thus the circulating levels of $1,25(OH)_2D_3$ correlates inversely with the ingested amount of calcium [137]. $1,25(OH)_2D_3$ Serum levels are maintained in pmol/l range by a classic negative feedback mechanism. The decrease of calcium or phosphate levels leads to an increase of the 1-α-hydroxylase activity and an enhanced synthesis of $1,25(OH)_2D_3$ which in turn promotes the intestinal resorption of calcium and phosphate and the calcium mobilisation from the bones. The activity of 1-α-hydroxylase decreased with increasing $1,25(OH)_2D_3$ levels, which leads to 24 hydroxylase activation. This enzyme degrades $1,25(OH)_2D_3$ to its inactive metabolite $24,25(OH)_2D_3$ [138, 139], which is subsequently converted to calcitroic acid and excreted. Hence, the nutritive intake of calcium directly regulates 1-α-hydroxylase activity and indirectly modifies parathormone levels. This hormone produced in the parathyroids increases the phosphate excretion in the proximal tubule but promotes the sodium, potassium and calcium resorbtion in the distal tubule. Under normocalcemic conditions, the activity of 1-α-hydroxylase is inhibited. These regulations are necessary to synthesize 1,25$(OH)_2D_3$ even though much is needed to cover the calcium and phosphate demand and to avoid a 1,25 $(OH)_2D_3$ intoxication [139]. The circulating vitamin D level depends on many different factors such as: the vitamin D content in either the ingested nutrition or the dietary supplements, and the endogenous production and degeneration via vitamin D metabolising enzymes. A simplified scheme of vitamin D metabolism is presented in figure (**2**).

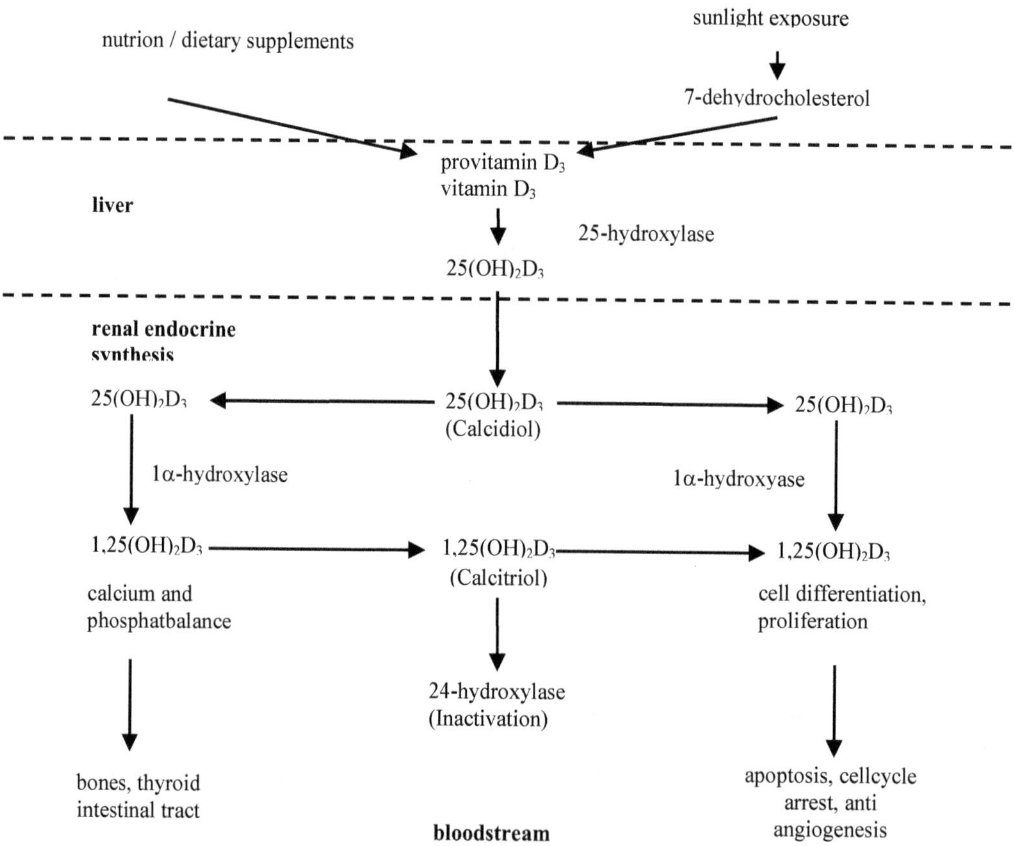

Fig. 2. Simplified scheme of the vitamin D metabolism. Vitamin D (food intake, synthesis in skin) is metabolised in liver to 25$(OH)_2D_3$, then via the renal 1-α-hydroxylase (endocrine signalling pathway or extra renal in tissues (autocrine/paracrine signalling pathway) to 1,25$(OH)_2D_3$.

8.2 Extrarenal vitamin D metabolizing enzymes

The biologically active metabolite is produced after a series of hydroxylations through cytochrome P450 enzymes which belong to the cytochrome p450 super family. The different enzymes are handled as follows:

8.2.1 1-α-hydroxylase (CYP27B1)

The 25-hydroxyvitamin-D_3-[25$(OH)_2D_3$]1-α-hydroxylase (1-α-hydroxylase) is encoded by the CYP27b1 gene and catalyzes the synthesis of 1,25$(OH)_2D_3$ from 25$(OH)_2D_3$. 1,25$(OH)_2D_3$ is the most important regulator of the enzyme that leads to a decreased enzyme expression. The regulation of the extra renal 1-α-hydroxylase depends on local factors like cytokines (interleukins, interferones and tumor necrosis) and growth. The optimal 1,25$(OH)_2D_3$-level tuning mechanism is not yet completely understood [139]. The reduced expression of the enzyme suggests the involvement of a negative vitamin D responsive element (VDRE) and Turunen and co-workers [140] showed that the enzyme's response to 1,25$(OH)_2D_3$ is a cell specific event with participation of many VDREs. The suppression of cell proliferation, the induction of apoptotic events and the modulation of immune responses are counted among the classical features of 1,25$(OH)_2D_3$. After binding to the vitamin D receptor, 1,25$(OH)_2D_3$ is able to arrest the cell cycle of a tumor cell in the G1-G0 phase via specific mechanisms [139]. In prostate and colon cancer the tumor protective effects of vitamin D is correlated to vitamin D deficiency [141]. Much data reports that both the renal and extra renal 1-α-hydroxylase are based on the expression of the same gene product. In contrast to the renal 1-α-hydroxylase, the extra renal enzyme is not subjected to the auto regulation as mentioned above [136, 142]. Therefore the enzyme's tissue specific expression might be a key mechanism in connecting the vitamin D metabolism to the anticarcinogenic effects of 1,25$(OH)_2D_3$.

Although the enzyme's cytokine and growth factor related regulation is not completely understood, it has been shown that different cytokines stimulate the 1-α-hydroxylase in different cell types [139, 143-146]. Another potential mechanism of gene regulation is the incidence of different gene polymorphisms [147] and inactive variants due to alternative splicing of the 1-α-hydroxylase mRNA. But this mechanism's function is not completely clarified. Alternative splicing within the post transcriptional modification is a normal process of gene expression in breast cancer cells and based on the pre mRNA, different mature mRNAs are generated when introns or exons are deleted or added. Thus, the translation of these mRNAs leads to different enzyme proteins, however, mis-spliced mRNAs are usually quickly degraded although it appears that this mechanism has failed in various cells. It has been reported that different protein variants of 1-α-hydroxylase might have diverse biological functions. Fischer and co-workers [148] showed 6 different variants of the enzyme in MCF10F via nested touchdown PCR, but in MCF-7, these variants appeared weakly expressed. Based on this data, the authors concluded that because alternative splicing regulates the level of the active enzyme extrarenaly it therefore regulates the local production of 1,25$(OH)_2D_3$ [149]. The activity of the extrarenally expressed 1-α-hydroxylase is an important factor of the tumor pathophysiology because of an accumulation of 1,25$(OH)_2D_3$ in many tissues. Studies of prostate [150, 151], colon [152-154] and breast cancer [148, 155, 156] have shown the expression of 1-α-hydroxylase in healthy as well as in malignant tissues. Thus, 1,25$(OH)_2D_3$, which is produced extrarenally might have autocrine behaviour to protect cells against transformation and supports the suggestion of its carcinoprotective effects. Accordingly, low 1-α-hydroxylase levels correlate with the risk of prostate-, colon- [157] or breast cancer [158, 159]. Moreover, the extra renal production of 1,25$(OH)_2D_3$ inhibits cell proliferation and promotes cell differentiation in xenograft models [160]. Besides the expression of the 1-α-hydroxylase in breast [155, 161], endometrial [162], cervical and ovarian carcinomas [163], the induction of the enzyme has also been shown in lymphomas [164] and dysgerminomas [165]. In these reports, the local synthesis of 1,25$(OH)_2D_3$ was mediated by the 1-α-hydroxylase expression of tumor associated macrophages. The expression of the enzyme mammary gland tissue occurs in lobules and ductus, primarily in the cancer tissue and invasive tumor cells and inflammatory infiltrate. Thus, it might be possible that the enzyme activity and the vitamin D receptor (VDR) expression are considerably higher than in the benign tissue compared to aggressive tumor cell lines (MCF-7res, MDA-MB231) [166]. Townsend and co-workers [166] compared breast cancer and benign tissue samples via reverse transcription PCR. They reported a 27-fold induction of the 1-α-hydroxylase expression and 7-fold induction of the VDR expression in tumor samples. Because 80% of the tumor tissues had an increased 1-α-hydroxylase und VDR, they concluded that there was a closed coupling of both gene products. These results are in compliance with Segersten and co-workers [161]. The capacity of 1-α-hydroxylase to synthesize 1,25$(OH)_2D_3$ within the mammary gland parenchyma results in, on the one hand, the available amount of 25$(OH)_2D_3$, and is dependent on sun light exposure and the season [167-170] - normally there is no definite correlation between 25$(OH)_2D_3$ and 1,25$(OH)_2D_3$ - yet on the other hand, the level of the extra renal production of 1,25$(OH)_2D_3$ is limited by the expression of the 1,25$(OH)_2D_3$- decomposing enzyme 24-hydroxylase, which is stimulated by 1,25$(OH)_2D_3$ in VDR expressing tissues. Based on the missing correlation of 24-hydroxylase and VDR or the 1-α-hydroxylase in breast cancer tissues, it seems that 24-hydroxylase is independently regulated. Kemmis and co-workers [171] demonstrated the expression of a functioning VDR and an inhibition of proliferation via 1,25$(OH)_2D_3$ in benign breast cells and MCF-7. The VDR expression in HMEC breast cells was higher than in MCF7 cells. Furthermore, the authors showed an expression of 25$(OH)_2D_3$ metabolizing 1-α-hydroxylase and 24-hydroxylase in these cell types, whereas the 1-α-hydroxylase expression was higher in MCF-7. In contrast to renal HKC8 cells, the expression of 1-α-hydroxylase was not inhibited by 1,25$(OH)_2D_3$. Based on the strong induction of the 24-hydroxylase through the 1,25$(OH)_2D_3$ application, the authors showed that MCF7 cells were more sensitive in response to 1,25$(OH)_2D_3$ compared to HKC-8 and HMEC cells. From this data, they concluded that there is a functional vitamin D receptor as well as intact signalling transduction pathways in MCF-7 cells. The data suggests that the synthesis of 1,25$(OH)_2D_3$ and the activation of the VDR inhibits the cell proliferation in breast cells. Thus, the treatment of benign breast cells with 25$(OH)_2D_3$ leads to an activation of the VDR transcription and the regulation of its target genes (CYP27B1, CYP24) and finally to an inhibition of cell proliferation. According to that, CYP27B1 lords it over CYP24 which means a transformation of 25$(OH)_2D_3$ to 1,25$(OH)_2D_3$. Kemmis and co-workers [171] have shown for the first time that physiological 1,25$(OH)_2D_3$ levels (30-100nmol/L) are able to inhibit cell proliferation in benign HMEC cells and in MCF7 breast cancer cells. Interestingly, aging process and the associated lack of estrogens correlate with decreased 25$(OH)_2D_3$ levels. The reason is that the ability of estrogen to stimulate the renal CYP27B1 activity [172]. Accordingly, the lack of estrogens leads to decreased 1,25$(OH)_2D_3$ levels and presents the highest risk for breast cancer in postmenopausal women [273].

8.2.2 24-hydroxylase (CYP24)

The 25-hydroxyvitamine D_3-24 hydroxylase (24-OHase, 24-hydroxylase) encoded by the CYP224 gene is induced by 1,25$(OH)_2D_3$ in breast cell lines where the enzyme is time and dose dependently stimulated by 1,25$(OH)_2D_3$ [174]. An increased enzyme expression in ovarian, cervical and breast cancer compared to healthy tissue samples has been shown by immunochemistry and real time PCR [163]. In contrast, Townsend and co-workers [166] showed a 4-fold increase of the enzyme expression in malignant breast tissues compared to healthy tissue samples using the same technique. Additionally, the expression of 24 hydroxylase increased in breast cancer cells foremost in hormone resistant MCF-7 Res and the aggressive MDA-MB231 cells compared to benign MCF-12A cells [166]. Kemmis and co-workers [171] reported the highest 24 hydroxylase expression in MCF-7 cells and Segersten and co-workers [161] showed a 2-fold enzyme expression in tumor tissues compared to benign tissue samples. The authors concluded that the conversion of $1,25(OH)_2D_3$ into the inactive metabolite $1,24,25(OH)_3D_3$ is significantly higher in malignant tissues. Furthermore Townsend and co-workers [166] detected the enzyme only in breast cancers with an increased 1-α-hydroxylase and VDR expression. Further analysis showed that in a healthy tissue sample expression of 24-hydroxylase correlated with both 1α-hydroxylase and VDR. There was not such a correlation in breast tumors. Hypothetically, the 24 hydroxylase acts as a part of a well organized feedback mechanism and is transcriptionally modulated to increase the local $1,25(OH)_2D_3$ and VDR level [166]. The synthesis of $1,25(OH)_2D_3$ via the 1-α-hydroxylase has been shown in benign and malignant mammary gland tissues but this mechanism's efficiency in tumor tissues might be affected by a dysregulated 24 hydroxylase expression.

8.3 Vitamin D-receptor (VDR / mVDR)

The vitamin D receptor (VDR) is an ubiquitary expressed steroid hormone receptor. Like other steroid, thyroid and retinoid receptors, the VDR is a member of the nuclear hormone receptor family. The receptor binds to its ligand $1,25(OH)_2D_3$, interacts with other receptors by dimerization and binds as homodimers or heterodimers to specific DNA sequences. So called vitamin D responsive elements (VDRE) recruit additional co-activators (such as SRC-1, GRIP-1/TIF2, ACTR) and interact with the transcriptional processing order to initiate or inhibit the transcription of its target genes [25]. It is well known, that steroid receptors consist of different variants with distinct specificities. Sunn and co-workers [175] described an N-terminal variant of the VDR. $1,25(OH)_2D_3$ mediates its genomic effects as a VDR ligand and via the directed binding to the VDRE [176]. Besides its function in bone metabolism and in the calcium/phosphate balance, the VDR interacts with different signalling pathways, e.g. with p21, a cyclin dependent kinase inhibitor which is involved in cell cycle regulation and inhibition of the cancer cell proliferation [26]. There are some suggestions about the existence of a membrane VDR (mVDR) [177]. The mVDR mediates its signals through the change of the intracellular calcium concentrations and through interactions with the protein kinase C and enzymes of the MAPK family [178-183]. Although the mVDR seems unrelated to the nuclear VDR, Marcinkowska and co-workers [184] reported an interaction of both receptors. The function of this mechanism is not clearly defined and the cloning of the mVDR has failed until today.

Many studies reported that extra renal VDR expression is associated with the non-classical effects of $1,25(OH)_2D_3$. The VDR expression has been shown in healthy breast tissues and in more than 80% of the breast cancer tissues [185]. The natural ligand of the VDR, $1,25(OH)_2D_3$ and many new developed synthetic vitamin D analogues inhibit cell proliferation and induce apoptosis in breast cancer cell lines [186, 187]. Furthermore, in animal models, vitamin D analogues retard the tumor growth and lead to a regression of breast tumors [12].

8.4 Vitamin D-receptor gene polymorphism

The gene that encodes the VDR has various polymorphisms. It has been hypothesised that the genetic VDR polymorphism influences the breast cancer risk due to its potential effects on VDR gene expression and protein function [188, 189]. Many polymorphisms of the VDR gene have been identified and several, such as FOK1, Bsm1, APA1, TAQ1 and Poly(A) are well analysed [190, 191]. The studies that were conducted had conflicting results [191]. Curran and co-workers [192] showed a significant association of the VDR polymorphism APA1 und TAQ with the breast cancer risk. A significant increased breast cancer risk in women with the ff genotype FOK1 was observed by Chen and co-workers [193]. Sinotte and co-workers [194] detected a significant link between familial breast cancer disposition and FOK1. Other data came from Trabert and co-workers [195] who found a correlation between a higher breast cancer risk and the genotype Bsm1 bb in postmenopausal women although there is also published data without any evidence for a link between VDR polymorphisms and breast cancer risk [196-199]. An analysis of the last 13 published studies in which different VDR polymorphisms and its relation to breast cancer were examined leads to the suggestion that the modification of breast cancer risk is associated with certain VDR polymorphisms and therefore $1{,}25(OH)_2D_3$ might modify the risk of breast cancer [200]. A recently published paper by McCullough and co-workers [201] presented certain VDR gene polymorphisms associated with a decreased breast cancer risk in women who ingested high doses of calcium (no calcitriol) concluding that nutritive influences might modify the link between gene polymorphisms and breast cancer. This data could shed light on breast cancer risk evaluation or could even be used in a predictive manner to answer the question about which women are strongly endangered to develop distant metastases.

9. Calcium

Like vitamin D, humans ingest calcium through food or dietary supplements. 99% of calcium is bound as hydroxyl phosphatide in bones and teeth [202]. Only 1% calcium is extracellularly located. Plasma levels of calcium (Ca^{2+}) are limited by the intestinal absorption, the renal secretion and the reabsorption. Additionally, the skeletal calcium storage and resorption keep the plasma levels of calcium in a closed range (3.5-5mmol/l) [202].

10. Vitamin D, calcium and breast cancer risk

10.1 Dietary and supplemental vitamin D intake

For $1{,}25(OH)_2D_3$ several studies have shown both an antiproliferative effect and an inhibition of angiogenesis in malignant and healthy breast cancer cells [17, 185, 203-206]. In mouse models, an increased intake of vitamin D led to the suppression of epithelial hyperproliferation and tumorigenesis of the mammary gland that was caused by rich nutrition [207, 208].

Last but not least, it has been proven by the First National Health and Nutrition Examination Survey Epidemiologic Follow-Up Study that sunlight exposure is inversely correlated with breast cancer risk [209, 210]. In this study, the female population in the north-eastern parts of the U.S. have a higher risk of contracting breast cancer compared to the other states of the U.S. This leads to the suggestion that sunlight induced vitamin D production has a positive influence in avoiding breast cancer [20].

In contrast, in the Nurses' Health Study, there was an inverse association between vitamin D intake and breast cancer risk among premenopausal women but no association among postmenopausal women [20]. Consistent with this observation, a study published a few years ago was based on the Cancer Prevention Study II Nutrition Cohort and observed no associations between breast cancer and total and dietary vitamin D intakes among postmenopausal women [211]. Another Italian study recently showed an inverse association between vitamin D intake (in the study >143 IU) and breast cancer in 2569 breast cancer patients [212]. Two other studies that concentrated on vitamin D deficiency and its susceptibility for breast cancer incidence approved that a deficiency conditional on nutrition in adolescence does not lead to an increased breast cancer risk [213, 214].

The proper dose of vitamin D remains unclear and a recommendation does not exist, however a meta-analysis gives evidence towards a dose of >400 IU per day to reduce breast cancer risk [213].

10.2 Role of vitamin D in breast cancer

To date, there have been several epidemiologic studies of the association between vitamin D and breast cancer risk, however, their results have not been consistent. Several studies observed an association between $25(OH)_2D_3$ plasma levels and breast cancer incidence [19, 215-217]. The predictive value of $25(OH)_2D_3$ plasma levels depends upon the time they have been measured. Plasma levels that have been measured within a few years before breast cancer diagnosis are less predictive than plasma level measured many years before [217]. Furthermore, plasma levels that have been measured around 15 years before diagnosis do not have any aetiological value for the genesis of breast cancer [216].

Bertone-Johnson and co-workers [217] found a marginally significant reduction of breast cancer risk in women >60 years who had elevated $25(OH)_2D_3$ and $1,25(OH)_2D_3$ plasma levels. In contrast, published data by Shin and co-workers [20] demonstrated a significantly decreased breast cancer incidence in premenopausal, but not in postmenopausal women, who had continuous vitamin D intake.

Furthermore, a case control study observed that women with plasma $25(OH)_2D_3$ concentration <50nmol/l had >5 times higher risk of breast cancer than those with plasma concentrations exceeding >150 nmol/l [158]. Janowsky and co-workers [19] also showed an inverse association between $1,25(OH)_2D_3$ plasma levels to the point of diagnosis and breast cancer risk in patients with breast cancer. However, there was no difference in $1,25(OH)_2D_3$ plasma levels between patients with breast cancer and those with DCIS. The authors suggested that the grade of invasion was not correlated with the extent of $1,25(OH)_2D_3$ level. Another nested case-control study with 96 breast cancer cases and 96 controls found no association between prediagnostic $1,25(OH)_2D_3$ levels and levels at the time of diagnosis and breast cancer risk among postmenopausal women [216].

The circulating concentration of $25(OH)_2D_3$ is considered to be an excellent measure of the availability of vitamin D from the diet, supplements and from synthesis in the skin [218]. Its potential importance in breast carcinogenesis is due to the fact that $25(OH)_2D_3$ can be metabolised to $1,25(OH)_2D_3$ by 1-α-hydroxylase in breast tissue [155]. Thus, $25(OH)_2D_3$ levels may be more representative of intracellular levels of $1,25(OH)_2D_3$ than circulating levels of $1,25(OH)_2D_3$ [217].

To date, no studies have been published investigating intracellular or tissue levels of $1,25(OH)_2D_3$ and $25(OH)_2D_3$ in association with breast cancer risk.

10.3 Dietary and supplemental calcium intake

Many studies about the importance of calcium and its association to breast cancer have already been published. Most of them are case-control studies and nearly all of them are relatively small and there is insufficient documentation regarding risk factors for breast cancer in multivariate analyses.

Calcium is participating on carcinogenesis via regulation of cell proliferation, differentiation and apoptosis [219-221]. Cell proliferation and differentiation of breast cells can be increased by elevated calcium levels [208, 222, 223]. Boyapati and co-workers [224] observed a non-significant inverse association between calcium intake and breast cancer risk among pre- and postmenopausal women but the Nurses' Health Study has shown this association only for premenopausal women [20].

The anti-carcinogenic effects of calcium are last but not least, mediated by vitamin D, therefore calcium is one of the key mediators of the vitamin D induced apoptosis in breast cancer cells [208].

11. Calcitriol and prostaglandins in cancer

The stimulation of the renal calcitriol [$1,25(OH)_2D_3$] synthesis in vitro is well known as well as the inhibition of acetysalicylic acid as a non-selective NSAID [225]. This justifies the clinical use of NSAIDs in treating arthritis for example. Hayes and co-workers [226] observed an inhibition of calcitriol synthesis caused by PGE_1 and PGE_2 in synovial fluid macrophages from arthritic joints and with that he proved the link between vitamin D and prostaglandin metabolism. Several published studies have proven the anti-carcinogenic effects shown in different signalling pathways on prostate cancer cells [227-229]. The team around David Feldman examined the influence of calcitriol in established human prostate cancer cell lines (androgen dependent LNCaP cells and androgen independent PC-3 cells) and in primary normal prostatic epithelial cells derived from normal and cancerous human prostate tissue. They showed that calcitriol regulates biologically active prostaglandin levels and prostaglandin actions by three mechanisms: calcitriol suppresses the COX-2 expression and moreover it up-regulates the expression of 15-PGDH. This dual influence of calcitriol was associated with a decrease of PGE_2 secretion in prostate cancer cells. Calcitriol reduces the mRNA expression of prostaglandin receptors EP_2 and FP, additionally a mechanism to inhibit the biological activity of prostaglandins.

The combination of calcitriol and NSAIDs led to a significant growth inhibition in prostate cancer cells via its synergistic effects. These findings might postulate that calcitriol and NSAIDs are definitely a useful combination in chemo preventive and/or therapeutic strategies in prostate cancer [230]. Unpublished own data support these results as we showed an inverse correlation between VDR- and COX-2 expression in breast cancer cells and a downregulation of COX-2 and an upregulation of 15 PGDH by calcitriol. Therefore we propose that these findings and suggest a possible link between VDR, associated target genes and the prostaglandin metabolism.

12. Concluding remarks

In conclusion, there is promising preclinical data inhibiting COX-2 in breast cancers, therefore the chance exists to innovatively disturb carcinogenesis of those gynecological oncological neoplasms Phase II trials have already been conducted to clear the safety of a celecoxib treatment in metastatic breast cancer. Furthermore, calcitriol and calcium have shown anti-carcinogenic effects in experimental studies and several epidemiological studies have demonstrated an inverse association between vitamin D and calcium intake and breast cancer. Other studies have detected an inverse association between plasma and serum levels and breast cancer risk. Experimental studies support the hypothesis that the reduction of breast cancer risk is more significant among premenopausal women than among postmenopausal women and mPGES-1 and EP receptors might be important targets for the development of new anti inflammatory and antiproliferative tumor therapies.

Questions that remain unanswered are: has calcitriol as antiproliferative effects in breast cancer as was proven in prostate cancer? Does a link exist between vitamin D and prostaglandin metabolism in breast cancers? These questions have to be answered as the increasing incidence of breast cancer have yet to be solved. Innovative treatment strategies fall on fruitful ground. Thus we need further studies that elucidate the importance of COX-2 inhibitors in the preventive as well as in the adjuvant settings in breast cancers and finally that will evaluate the promising importance in the neoangiogenesis in detail.

13. Acknowledgments

The authors declare no conflict of interest relevant to this article.

14. Abbreviations

bFGF	=	basic fibroblast growth factor
COX	=	cyclooxygenase
DCIS	=	ductal carcinoma in situ
DMBA	=	Dimethylbenz(a)anthracene
ER	=	estrogen receptor
ERE	=	estrogen responsive element
FIGO	=	Fédération Internationale de Gyneécologie et d'Obstétrique
GRO	=	growth related protein
HER2	=	human epidermal growth factor receptor 2
IL	=	interleukin
NSAID	=	non-steroidal anti-inflammatory drug
mPGES-1	=	microsomalmicrosomal prostaglandin E synthase-1
mRNA	=	messenger ribonucleic acid
PCR	=	polymerase chain reaction
PDGF	=	platelet derived growth factor
PG	=	prostaglandin
PGDH	=	prostaglandin dehydrogenase
PPAR	=	peroxisomes proliferator-activated receptor
TGF1	=	transforming growth factor 1
TIMP	=	tissue inhibitor of matrix metalloproteinase
VDR	=	vitamin D receptor
VDRE	=	vitamin D responsive element
VEGF	=	vascular endothelial growth factor
VM	=	vasculogenic mimicry

15. References

American Cancer Society. *Cancer facts and figures 2005*. Atlanta, American Cancer Society 2005, p. 9. (http://www.cancer.org/downloads/STT/CAFF2005f4PWSecured.pdf)

Ozols, R. F.; Rubins, S. C.; Dembo, A. J.; Robboy, S. In *Gynecologic oncology: Epithelial ovarian cancer*; Hoskins, W. J.; Perez, C. A.; Young, R. C.; Ed.; Lippincott Williams & Wilkins: Philadelphia, 1992 pp. 731–781.

FIGO (International Federation of Gynecology and Obstetrics) annual report on the results of treatment in gynecological cancer. *Int. J. Gynaecol. Obstet.* 2003, *83 Suppl 1: ix-xxii*, 1–229.

Ferrandina, G.; Lauriola, L.; Zannoni, G. F.; Fagotti, A.; Fanfani, F.; Legge, F.; Maggiano, N.; Gessi, M.; Mancuso, S.; Ranelletti, F. O.; Scambia, G. Increased cyclooxygenase-2 (COX-2) expression is associated with chemotherapy resistance and outcome in ovarian cancer patients. *Ann. Oncol.* 2002, *13*, 1205-1211.

Singh-Ranger, G.; Salhab, M.; Mokbel, K. The role of cyclooxygenase-2 in breast cancer: review. Breast Cancer Res. Treat. 2008, 109(2), 189-198.

Coussens, L. M.; Werb, Z. *Inflammation and cancer. Nature* 2002, *420(6917)*, 860-867.

Park, E. The etiology of rickets. *Physiol. Rev.* 1923 (Baltimore) iii, 106-163.

Deluca, H. F.; Cantorna, M. T. Vitamin D: its role and uses in immunology. *FASEB J.* 2001, *15*, 2579–2585.

Guyton, K. Z.; Kensler, T. W.; Posner, G. H. Vitamin D and vitamin D analogs as cancer chemopreventive agents. *Nutr. Rev.* 2003, *61*, 227–238.

Jones, G.; Strugnell, S. A.; Deluca, H. F. Current understanding of the molecular actions of vitamin D. *Physiol. Rev.* 1998, *78*, 1193–1231.

Adorini L. Immunomodulatory effects of vitamin D receptor ligands in autoimmune diseases. *Int. Immunopharmacol.* 2002, *2*, 1017–1028.

Colston, K. W.; Hansen, C. M. Mechanisms implicated in the growth regulatory effects of vitamin D in breast cancer. *Endocr. Relat. Cancer* 2002, *9(1)*, 45–59.

Johnson, C. S.; Hershberger, P. A.; Trump, D. L. Vitamin D-related therapies in prostate cancer. *Cancer Metastasis Rev.* 2002, *21*, 147–158.

Mathieu, C.; Adorini, L. The coming of age of 1,25-dihydroxyvitamin D3 analogs as immunomodulatory agents. *Trends Mol. Med.* 2002, *8*, 174–179.

O'Kelly, J.; Koeffler, H. P. Vitamin D analogs and breast cancer. *Recent Results Cancer Res.* 2003, *164*, 333–348.

van den Bemd, G. J.; Chang, G. T. Vitamin D and vitamin D analogs in cancer treatment. *Curr. Drug Targets* 2002, *3*, 85–94.

Welsh, J.; Wietzke, J. A.; Zinser, G. M.; Byrne, B.; Smith, K.; Narvaez, C. J. Vitamin D3 receptor as a target for breast cancer prevention. *J. Nutr.* 2003, *133*, 2425–2433S.

Garland, C. F.; Garland, F. C.; Gorham, E. D. Calcium and vitamin D. Their potential roles in colon and breast cancer prevention. *Ann. N. Y. Acad. Sci.* 1999, *889*, 107–119.

Janowsky, E. C.; Lester, G. E.; Weinberg, C. R.; Millikan, R. C.; Schildkraut, J. M.; Garrett, P. A.; Hulka, B. S. Association between low levels of 1,25- dihydroxyvitamin D and breast cancer risk. *Public Health Nutr.* 1999, *2*, 283–291.

Shin, M. H.; Holmes, M. D.; Hankinson, S. E.; Wu, K.; Colditz, G. A.; Willett, W. C. Intake of dairy products, calcium, and vitamin D and risk of breast cancer. J. *Natl. Cancer Inst.* 2002, *94*, 1301–1311.

Studzinski, G. P.; Moore, D. C. Sunlight—can it prevent as well as cause cancer? *Cancer Res.* 1995, *55*, 4014–4022.

Gorham, E. D.; Garland, F. C.; Garland, C. F. Sunlight and breast cancer incidence in the USSR. *Int. J. Epidemiol.* 1990, *19*, 820–824.

Garland, F. C.; Garland, C. F.; Gorham, E. D.; Young J. F. Geographic variation in breast cancer mortality in the United States: a hypothesis involving exposure to solar radiation. *Prev. Med.* 1990, *19*, 614–622.

Blot, W. J.; Fraumeni J. F. Jr.; Stone B. J. Geographic patterns of breast cancer in the United States. *J. Natl. Cancer. Inst.* 1977, *59*, 1407–1411.

Malloy, P. J.; Pike, J. W.; Feldman, D. The vitamin D receptor and the syndrome of hereditary 1,25-dihydroxyvitamin D-resistant rickets. *Endocr. Rev.* 1999, *20*, 156-188.

Liu, M.; Lee, M. H.; Cohen, M.; Bommakanti, M.; Freedman, L. P. Transcriptional activation of the Cdk inhibitor p21 by vitamin D3 leads to the induced differentiation of the myelomonocytic cell line U937. *Genes Dev.* 1996, *10*, 142–153.

Polly, P.; Carlberg, C.; Eisman, J. A.; Morrison, N. A. Identification of a vitamin D3 response element in the fibronectin gene that is bound by a vitamin D3 receptor homodimer. *J. Cell. Biochem.* 1996, *60*, 322–333.

Polly, P.; Carlberg, C.; Eisman, J. A.; Morrison, N. A. 1α,25-dihydroxyvitamin D3 receptor as a mediator of transrepression of retinoid signaling. *J. Cell. Biochem.* 1997, *67*, 287–296.

Berger, U.; Wilson, P.; McClelland, R. A.; Colston, K.; Haussler, M. R.; Pike, J. W.; Coombes, R. C. Immunocytochemical detection of 1,25-dihydroxyvitamin D receptors in normal human tissues. J. *Clin. Endocrinol. Metab.* 1988, *67*, 607–613.

Stack, E.; DuBois, R. N. Regulation of cyclo-oxygenase-2. *Best Pract. Res. Clin. Gastroenterol.* 2001, *15 (5)*, 787-800.

Murakami, M.; Kudo, I. Recent advances in molecular biology and physiology of the prostaglandin E2-biosynthetic pathway. *Prog. Lipid. Res.* 2004, *43(1)*, 3-35.

Anggard, E. The biological activities of three metabolites of prostaglandin E1. *Acta Physiol. Scand.* 1966, *66*, 509–510.

Tsuboi, K.; Sugimoto, Y.; Ichikawa, A. Prostanoid receptor subtypes. *Prostaglandins Other Lipid. Mediat.* 2002, *68-69*, 535–556.

Williams, C. S.; DuBois, R. N. Prostaglandin endoperoxide synthase: why two isoforms? *Am. J. Physiol.* 1996, *270*, 393-400.

Herschman, H. R. Prostaglandin synthase 2. *Biochim. Biophys. Acta.* 1996, *1299(1)*, 125-140.

Langenbach, R.; Morham, S. G.; Tiano, H. F.; Loftin, C. D.; Ghanayem, B. I.; Chulada, P. C.; Mahler, J. F.; Lee, C. A.; Goulding, E. H.; Kluckman, K. D.; Kim, H. S.; Smithies, O. Prostaglandin synthase 1 gene disruption in mice reduces arachidonic acid- induced inflammation and indomethacin-induced gastric ulceration. *Cell* 1995, *83(3)*, 483-492.

Lim, H.; Paria, B. C.; Das, S. K.; Dinchuk, J. E.; Langenbach, R.; Trzaskos, J. M.; Dey, S. K. Multiple female reproductive failures in cyclooxygenase 2-deficient mice. *Cell* 1997, *91(2)*, 197-208.

Davis, B.J.; Lennard, D. E.; Lee, C. A.; Tiano, H. F.; Morham, S. G.; Wetsel, W. C.; Langenbach, R. Anovulation in cyclooxygenase-2 deficient mice is restored by prostaglandin E2 and interleukin-1 beta. *Endocrinology* 1999, *140(6)*, 2685–2695.

Loftin, C. D.; Trivedi, D. R.; Tiano, H. F.; Clark, JA.; Lee, C. A.; Epstein, J. A.; Morham, S. G.; Breyer, M. D.; Nguyen, M.; Hawkins, BM. Failure of ductus arteriosus closure and remodelling in neonatal mice deficient in cyclooxygenase-1 and -2. *Proc. Natl. Acad. Sci. U.S.A.* 2001, *98(3)*, 1059–1064

Rozic, J. G.; Chakraborty, C.; Lala, P. K. Cyclooxygenase inhibitors retard murine mammary tumor progression by reducing tumor cell migration, invasiveness and angiogenesis. *Int. J. Cancer.* 2001, *93*, 497-506.

Eberhart, C. E.; Coffey, R. J.; Radhika, A.; Giardiello, F. M.: Ferrebach, S.; Dubois, R. N. Up-regulation of cyclooxygenase gene expression in human colorectal adenomas and adenocarcinomas. *Gastroenterology* 1994, *107*, 1183-1188.

Sinicrope, F. A.; Lemoine, M.; Xi, L.; Lynch, P. M.; Cleary, K. R.; Shen, Y.; Frazier, M. L. Reduced expression of cyclooxygenase 2 proteins in hereditary nonpolyposis colorectal cancers relative to sporadic cancers. *Gastroenterology* 1999, *117*, 350-358.

Ristimaki, A.; Honkanen, N.; Jankala, H.; Sipponen, P.; Harkonen, M. Expression of cyclooxygenase-2 in human gastric carcinoma. *Cancer Res.* 1997, *57*, 1276-1280.

Zimmermann, K. C.; Sarbia, M.; Weber, A.; Bochard, F.; Gabbert, H. E.; Schror, K. Cyclooxygenase-2 expression in human esophageal carcinoma. *Cancer Res.* 1999, *5*, 198-204.

Swami, S.; Krishnan, A. V.; Moreno, J.; Bhattacharyya, R. B.; Peehl, D.; Feldman, D. Calcitriol and enistein actions to inhibit the prostaglandin pathway: potential combination therapy to treat prostate cancer. *J. Nutr.* 2007, *137*, 205S-210S.

Subbaramaiah, K.; Dannenberg, A. J. Cyclooxygenase 2: a molecular target for cancer prevention and treatment. Trends. *Pharmacol. Sci.* 2003, *24*, 96–102.

Heinonen, P. K.; Metsa-Ketela, T. Prostaglandin and thromboxane production in ovarian cancer tissue. *Gynecol. Obstet. Invest.* 1984, *18(5)*, 225-229.

Ylikorkala, O.; Kauppila, A.; Viinikka, L. Prostacyclin and thromboxane in ovarian cancer: effect of cytostatics and prostaglandin synthesis inhibitors. *Gynecol. Oncol.* 1983, *16(3)*, 340-345.

Munkarah, A. R.; Morris, R.; Baumann, P.; Deppe, G.; Malone, J.; Diamond, M. P.; Saed, G. M. Effects of prostaglandin E(2) on proliferation and apoptosis of epithelial ovarian cancer cells. *J. Soc. Gynecol. Investig.* 2002, *9(3)*, 168-173.

Gupta, R. A.; Tejada, L. V.; Tong, B. J.; Das, S. K.; Morrow, J. D.; Dey, S. K.; DuBois, R. N. Cyclooxygenase-1 is overexpressed and promotes angiogenic growth factor production in ovarian cancer. *Cancer Res.* 2003, *63(5)*, 906-911.

Ali-Fehmi, R.; Morris, R. T.; Bandyopadhyay, S.; Che, M.; Schimp, V.; Malone, J.M. Jr.; Munkarah, A. R. Expression of cyclooxygenase-2 in advanced stage ovarian serous carcinoma: correlation with tumor cell proliferation, apoptosis, angiogenesis, and survival. *Am. J. Obstet. Gynecol.* 2005, *192(3)*, 819-825.

Daikoku, T.; Wang, D.; Tranguch, S.; Morrow, J. D.; Orsulic, S.; DuBois, R. N.; Dey, S. K. Cyclooxygenase-1 is a potential target for prevention and treatment of ovarian epithelial cancer. *Cancer Res.* 2005, *65(9)*, 3735-3744.

Dore, M.; Cote, L. C.; Mitchell, A.; Sirois, J. Expression of prostaglandin G/H synthase type 1, but not type 2, in human ovarian adenocarcinomas. *J. Histochem. Cytochem.* 1998, *46(1)*, 77-84.

Daikoku, T.; Tranguch, S.; Trofimova, I. N.; Dinulescu, D. M.; Jacks, T.; Nikitin, A. Y.; Connolly, D. C.; Dey, S.K. Cyclooxygenase-1 is overexpressed in multiple genetically engineered mouse models of epithelial ovarian cancer. *Cancer Res.* 2006, *66(5)*, 2527-2531.

Rodriguez-Burford, C.; Barnes, M; N.; Oelschlager, D. K.; Myers, R. B.; Talley, L. I.; Partridge, E. E.; Grizzle, W. E. Effects of nonsteroidal anti-inflammatory agents (NSAIDs) on ovarian carcinoma cell lines: preclinical evaluation of NSAIDs as chemopreventive agents. *Clin. Cancer Res.* 2002, *8(1)*, 202-209.

Schreinemachers, D. M., Everson, R. B. Aspirin use and lung, colon, and breast cancer. Incidence in a prospective study. *Epidemiology* 1994, *5*, 138-146.

Harris, R. E., Namboodiri, K. K., Farrar, W. B. Non-steroidal anti-inflammatory drugs and breast cancer. *Epidemiology* 1996, *7*, 203-205.

Sharp, C. R., Collet, J. P., McNutt, M., Belzile, E., Boivin, J. F., Hanley, J. A. Nested case control study of the effect of non-steroidal anti-inflammatory drugs on breast cancer risk and stage. *Br. J. Cancer* 2000, *83*, 112-120.

Liu, X.; Rose, D. Differential expression and regulation of cyclooxygenase-1 and -2 in two human breast cancer cell lines. *Cancer Res.* 1996, *56*, 5125-5127.

Schrey, M. P.; Patel, K. V. Prostaglandin E2 production and metabolism in human breast cancer cells and breast fibroblasts. Regulation by inflammatory mediators. *Br. J. Cancer* 1995, *72*, 1412-1419.

Rolland, P. H.; Martin, P. M.; Jacquemier, J.; Rolland, A.; Toga, M. Prostaglandins in human breast cancer: evidence suggesting that elevated prostaglandin production is a marker of high metastatic potential for neoplastic cells. *J. Natl. Cancer Inst. (Bethesda)* 1980, *64*, 1061-1070.

Karmali, R. A.; Welts, S.; Thaler, H. T.; Lefevre, F. Prostaglandins in breast cancer. Relationship to disease stage and hormone status. *Br. J. Cancer* 1983, *48*, 689-696.

Kawamori, T.; Wakabayashi, K. COX-2 and prostanoid receptors: good targets for chemoprevention. *J. Environ. Pathol. Toxicol. Oncol.* 2002, *21(2)*, 149-153.

Sonoshita, M.; Takaku, K.; Sasaki, N.; Sugimoto, Y.; Ushikubi, F.; Narumiya, S.; Oshima, M.; Taketo, M. M. Acceleration of intestinal polyposis through prostaglandin receptor EP2 in Apc(Delta 716) knockout mice. *Nat. Med.* 2001, *7*, 1048–1051.

Zha, S.; Yegnasubramanian, V.; Nelson, W. G.; Isaacs, W. B.; De Marzo, A. M. Cyclooxygenases in cancer: progress and perspective. *Cancer Lett.* 2004, *215*, 1–20.

Chang, S. H.; Liu, C. H.; Conway, R.; Han, D. K.; Nithipatikom, K.; Trifan, O. C.; Lane, T. F.; Hla, T. Role of prostaglandin E2-dependent angiogenic switch in cyclooxygenase 2-induced breast cancer progression. *Proc. Natl. Acad. Sci. U S A* 2004, *101*, 591–596.

Yan, M.; Rerko, R. M.; Platzer, P.; Dawson, D.; Willis, J.; Tong, M.; Lawrence, E.; Lutterbaugh, A.; Lu, S.; Lu, S.; Willson, J. K.; Luo, G.; Hensold, J.; Tai, H. H.; Wilson, K.; Markowitz, S. D. 15-Hydroxyprostaglandin dehydrogenase, a COX-2 oncogene antagonist, is a TGF-beta-induced suppressor of human gastrointestinal cancers. *Proc. Natl. Acad. Sci. USA* 2004, *101*, 17468–17473.

Ding, Y.; Tong, M.; Liu, S.; Moscow, J. A.; Tai, H. H. NAD+-linked 15-hydroxyprostaglandin dehydrogenase (15-PGDH) behaves as a tumor suppressor in lung cancer. *Carcinogenesis* 2005, *26*, 65–72.

Gee, J. R.; Montoya, R. G.; Khaled, H. M.; Sabichi, A. L.; Grossman, H. B. Cytokeratin 20, AN43, PGDH, and COX-2 expression in transitional and squamous cell carcinoma of the bladder. *Urol. Oncol.* 2003, *21*, 266–270.

Wolf, I.; O'Kelly, J.; Rubinek, T.; Tong, M.; Nguyen, A.; Lin, B. T.; Tai, H. H.; Karlan,

B. Y.; Koeffler, H. P. 15-hydroxyprostaglandin dehydrogenase is a tumor suppressor of human breast cancer. *Cancer Res.* 2006, *66(15)*, 7818-7823.

van 't Veer, L. J.; Dai, H.; van de Vijver, M. J.; He, Y. D.; Hart, A. A.; Mao, M.; Peterse, H. L.; van der Kooy, K.; Marton, M. J.; Witteveen, A. T.; Schreiber, G. J.; Kerkhoven, R. M.; Roberts, C.; Linsley, P. S.; Bernards, R.; Friend, S. H. Gene expression profiling predicts clinical outcome of breast cancer. *Nature* 2002, *415*, 530–536.

Half, E.; Tang, X. M.; Gwyn, K.; Sahin, A.; Wathen, K.; Sinicrope, F. A. Cyclooxygenase-2 expression in human breast cancers and adjacent ductal carcinoma in situ. *Cancer Res.* 2002, *62*, 1676–1681.

Denkert, C.; Winzer, K. J.; Müller, B. M.; Weichert, W.; Pest, S.; Köbel, M.; Kristiansen, G.; Reles, A.; Siegert, A.; Guski, H.; Hauptmann, S. Elevated expression of cyclooxygenase-2 is a negative prognostic factor for disease free survival and overall survival in patients with breast carcinoma. *Cancer* 2003, *97(12)*, 2978-2987.

Ristimäki, A.; Sivula, A.; Lundin, J.; Lundin, M.; Salminen, T.; Haglund, C.; Joensuu, H.; Isola, J. Prognostic significance of elevated cyclooxygenase-2 expression in breast cancer. *Cancer Res.* 2002, *62*, 632–635.

Singh Ranger, G.; Thomas, V.; Jewell, A.; Mokbel, K. Elevated cyclooxygenase-2 expression correlates with distant metastases in breast cancer. *Anticancer Res.* 2004, *24(4)*, 2349–2351.

Nassar, A.; Radhakishnan, A.; Cabero, I. A.; Cotsonis, G.; Cohen, C. COX-2 expression in invasive breast cancer: Correlation with prognostic parameters and outcome. Appl. Immunohistochem. *Mol. Morphol.* 2007, *15(3)*, 255-259.

Hwang, D., Scollard, D., Byrne, J., Levine, E. Expression of cyclooxygenase-1 and cyclooxygenase-2 in human breast cancer. *J. Natl. Cancer Inst.* 1998, *90*, 455-460.

Soslow, R., Dannenberg, A., Rush, D., Woerner, B. M., Khan, K. N., Masferrer, J., Koki, A. COX-2 is expressed in human pulmonary, colonic, and mammary tumors. *Cancer* 2000, 2637-2645.

Costa, C.; Soares, R.; Reis-Filho, J. S.; Leitão, D.; Amendoeira, I., Schmitt, F. C. Cyclooxygenase 2 expression is associated with angiogenesis and lymph node metastasis in human breast cancer. *J. Clin. Pathol.* 2002, *55*, 429-434.

Kelly, L. M.; Hill, A. D. K.; Kennedy, S.; Connolly, E. M.; Ramanath, R.; The, S.; Dijkstra, B.; Purcell, R.; McDermott, E. W.; O'Higgins, N. Lack of prognostic effect of COX-2 expression in primary breast cancer on short term follow-up. *Eur. J. Surg. Oncol.* 2002, *29*, 707–710.

Lim, S. C. Role of COX-2, VEGF and cyclin D1 in mammary infiltrating duct carcinoma. *Oncol. Rep.* 2003, *10 (5)*, 1241-1249.

Wülfing, P.; Diallo, R.; Müller, C.; Wülfing, C.; Poremba, C.; Heinecke, A.; Rody, A.; Greb, R. R.; Böcker, W.; Kiesel, L. Analysis of cyclooxygenase-2 expression in human breast cancer: high throughput tissue microarray analysis. *J. Cancer Res. Clin. Oncol.* 2003, *129*, 375-382.

Boland, G. P.; Butt, I. P.; Prasad, R.; Knox, W. F.; Bundred, N. J. COX-2 expression is associated with an aggressive phenotype in ductal carcinoma in situ. *Br. J. Cancer* 2004, *90*, 423–429.

Zhao, X. Q.; Pang, D.; Xue, Y. Expression of the cyclooxygenase-2 gene in human breast carcinoma. *Zhongua Wai Ke Za Zhi* 2003, *41(6)*, 427–429.

Singh Ranger, G.; Kirkpatrick, K. L.; Clark, G. M.; Mokbel, K. Cyclooxygenase-2 (COX-2) mRNA expression correlates with progesterone receptor positivity in human breast cancer. *Curr. Med. Res. Opin.* 2003, *19(2)*, 131–134.

Kirkpatrick, K.; Ogunkolade, W.; Bustin, S.; Jenkins, P.; Ghilchik, M.; Mokbel, K. The mRNA expression of cyclooxygenase-2 and vascular endothelial growth factor in human breast cancer. *Breast Cancer Res. Treat.* 2001, *69(3)*, 373.

Watanabe, O.; Shimizu, T.; Imamura, H.; Kinoshita, J.; Utada, Y.; Okabe, T.; Kimura, K.; Hirano, A.; Yoshimatsu, K.; Aiba, M.; Ogawa, K. Expression of cyclooxygenase-2 in malignant and benign breast tumours. *Anticancer Res.* 2003, *23(4)*, 3215–3221.

Yoshimura, N.; Sano, H.; Okamoto, M.; Akioka, K.; Ushogome, H.; Kadotani, Y.; Yoshimura, R.; Nobori, S.; Higuchi, A.; Ohmori, Y.; Nakamura, K. Expression of cyclooxygenase-1 and -2 in human breast cancer. *Surg. Today* 2003, *33*, 805–811.

Ristimäki, A.; Garfinkel, S.; Weesendorf, J.; Maciag, T.; Hla, T. Induction of cyclooxygenase-2 by interleukin-1 alpha. Evidence for post-transcriptional regulation. *J. Biol. Chem.* 1994, *269(16)*, 11769-11775.

Evett, G. E.; Xie, W.; Chipman, J. G.; Robertson, D. L.; Simmons, D. L. Prostaglandin GH Synthase isoenyme 2 expression in fibroblasts: regulation by dexamethasone, mitogens and oncogenes. *Arch. Biochem. Biophys.* 2003, *306*, 169–177.

Sorlie, T.; Perou, C. M.; Tibshirani, R. Gene expression patterns of breast carcinomas distinguish tumor subclasses with clinical implications. *PNAS USA* 2001, *98*, 10869– 10874.

Salhab, M.; Singh-Ranger, G.; Mokbel, R.; Jouhra, F.; Jiang, W.G.; Mokbel, K. Cyclooxygenase-2 mRNA expression correlates with aromatase expression in human breast cancer. *J. Surg. Oncol.* 2007, *96(5)*, 424-428.

Diaz-Cruz, E. S.; Shapiro, C. L.; Brueggemeier, R. W. Cyclooxygenase inhibitors suppress aromatase expression and activity in breast cancer cells. *J. Clin. Endocrinol. Metab.* 2005, *90*, 2563–2570.

Richards, J. A.; Petrel, T. A.; Brueggemeier, R. W. Signaling pathways regulating aromatase and cyclooxygenases in normal and malignant breast cells. *J. Steroid. Biochem. Mol. Biol.* 2002, *80*, 203–212.

Brueggemeier, R. W.; Richards, J. A.; Petrel, T. A. Aromatase and cyclooxygenases: enzymes in breast cancer. *J. Steroid. Biochem. Mol. Biol.* 2003, *86*, 501–507.

Vienonen, A.; Syvala, H.; Miettinen, S.; Tuohimaa, P.; Ylikomi, T. Expression of progesterone receptor isoforms A and B is differentially regulated by estrogen in different breast cancer cell lines. *J. Steroid. Biochem. Mol. Biol.* 2002, *80*, 307–313.

Liu, C. H., Chang, S., Narko, K., Trifan, O. C., Wu, M., Smith, E., Haudenschild, C., Lane, T. F., Hla, T. Overexpression of cyclooxygenase-2 is sufficient to induce tumorigenesis in transgenic mice. *J. Biol. Chem.* 2001, *276*, 18563-18569.

Tsujii, M.; DuBois, R. N. Alterations in cellular adhesion and apoptosis in epithelial cells overexpressing prostaglandin endoperoxide synthase 2. *Cell* 1995, *93*, 705-716.

Oshima, M., Dinchuk, J. E., Kargman, S. L., Oshima, H., Hancock, B., Kwong, E., Trzaskos, J. M., Evans, J. F., Taketo, M. M. Suppression of intestinal polyposis in Apc716 knockout mice by inhibition of cyclooxygenase-2 (COX-2). *Cell* 1996, *80*, 803-809.

Mestre, J. R.; Subbaramaiah, K.; Sacks, P. G.; Schantz, S. P.; Tanabe, T.; Inoue, H.; Dannenberg, A. J. Retinoids suppress epidermal growth factor-induced transcription of cyclooxygenase-2 in human oral squamous carcinoma cells. *Cancer Res.* 1991, *57(14)*, 2890–2895.

Davies, G.; Salter, J.; Hills, M.; Martin, L.-A.; Sacks, N.; Dowsett, M. Correlation between cyclooxygenase-2 expression and angiogenesis in human breast cancer. *Clin. Cancer Res.* 2003, *9*, 2651-2656.

Lim, S. C.; Park, S. Y.; Do, N. Y. Correlation of cyclooxygenase-2 pathway and VEGF expression in head and neck squamous cell carcinoma. *Oncol. Rep.* 2003, *10 (5)*, 1073-1079.

Chu, J.; Lloyd, F. L.; Trifan, O. C.; Knapp, B.; Rizzo, M. T. Potential involvement of the cyclooxygenase-2 pathway in the regulation of tumor-associated angiogenesis and growth in pancreatic cancer. *Mol. Cancer Ther.* 2003, *(1)*, 1-7.

Tsujii, M.; Kawano, S.; Tsujii, S.; Sawaoka, H.; Hori, M.; DuBois, N. Cyclooxygenase regulates angiogenesis induced by colon cancer cells. *Cell* 1998, *93*, 705-716.

Gately, S. The contributions of cyclooxygenase-2 to tumour angiogenesis. *Cancer Metastasis Rev.* 2001, *19(1–2)*, 19–27.

Daniel, T. O.; Liu, H.; Morrow, J. D.; Crews, B. C.; Marnett, L.J. Thromboxane A2 is a mediator of cyclooxygenase-2-dependent endothelial migration and angiogenesis. *Cancer Res.* 1999, *59*, 4574-4577.

Pezzella, F.; Pastorino, U.; Tagliabue, E.; Andreola, S.; Sozzi, G.; Gasparini, G.; Menard, S,.; Gatter, K. C.; Harris, A. L.; Fox, S.; Buyse, M.; Pilotti, S.; Pierotti, M.; Rilke, F. Non-small-cell lung carcinoma tumor growth without morphological evidence of neo-angiogenesis. *Am. J. Pathol.* 1997, *151*, 1417-1423.

Maniotis, A. J.; Folberg, R.; Hess, A.; Seftor, E. A.; Gardner, L. M.; Pe'er, J.; Trent, J. M.; Meltzer, P. S.; Hendrix, M. J. Vascular channel formation by human melanoma cells in vivo and in vitro: vasculogenic mimicry. *Am. J. Pathol.* 1999, *155*, 739-752.

Shirakawa, K.; Shibuya, M.; Heike, Y.; Takashima, S.; Watanabe, I.; Konishi, F.; Kasumi, F.; Goldman, C. K.; Thomas, K. A.; Bett, A.; Terada, M.; Wakasugi, H. Tumor-infiltrating endothelial cells and endothelial precursor cells in inflammatory breast cancer. *Int. J. Cancer* 2002, *99*, 344-351.

Hendrix, M. J.; Seftor, E. A.; Hess, A. R.; Seftor, R. E. Vasculogenic mimicry and tumour-cell plasticity: lessons from melanoma. *Nat. Rev. Cancer* 2003, *3*, 411-421.

Shirakawa, K.; Kobayashi, H.; Heike, Y.; Kawamoto, S.; Brechbiel, M. W.; Kasumi, F.; Iwanaga, T.; Konishi, F.; Terada, M;, Wakasugi, H. Hemodynamics in vasculogenic mimicry and angiogenesis of inflammatory breast cancer xenograft. *Cancer Res.* 2002, *62*, 560–566.

Basu, G. D.; Liang, W. S.; Stephan, D. A.; Wegener, L. T.; Conley, C. R; Pockaj, B. A.; Mukerjee, P. A novel role for cyclooxygenase-2 in regulating vascular channel formation by human breast cancer cells. *Breast Cancer Res.* 2006, *8(6)*, R69. Khuder, S.A.; Mutgi, A. B. Breast cancer and NSAID use: a metaanalysis. *Br. J. Cancer.* 2001, *84*, 1188–1192.

Egan, K., Stampfer, M., Giovannucci, E., Rosner, B., Colditz, G. Prospective study of regular aspirin use and the risk of breast cancer. *J. Natl. Cancer Inst.* 1996, (Bethesda), *88*, 988-993.

Rosenberg, L.; Palmer, J. R.; Zauber, A. G.; Warshaver, M. E.; Stolley, P.D.; Shapiro, S. A hypothesis: nonsteroidal anti-inflammatory drugs reduce the incidence of large- bowel cancer. *J. Natl. Cancer Inst.* 1991, *83*, 355-358.

Thun, M. J.; Namboodiri, M. M.; Heath, C. W. Jr. Aspirin use and reduced risk of fatal colon cancer. *N. Engl. J. Med.* 1991, *325*, 1593-1596.

Alshafie, G. A., Abou-Issa, H., Seibert, K., Harris, R. Chemotherapeutic evaluation of celecoxib, a cyclooxygenase-2 inhibitor, in rats mammary tumor model. *Oncol. Rep.* 2000, *7*, 1377-1381.

Harris, R. E.; Alshafie, G. A.; Abou-Issa, H.; Seibert, K. Chemoprevention of breast cancer in rats by celecoxib, a cyclooxygenase 2 inhibitor. *Cancer Res.* 2000, *60*, 2101- 2103.

Barnes, N. L.; Warnberg, F.; Farnie, G.; White, D.; Jiang, W.; Anderson, E.; Bundred, N. J. Cyclooxygenase-2 inhibition: effects on tumour growth, cell cycling and lymphangiogenesis in a xenograft model of breast cancer. *Br. J. Cancer* 2007, *96(4)*, 575-582.

Yoshinaka, R.; Shibata, M. A.; Morimoto, J.; Tanigawa, N.; Otsuki, Y. COX-2 inhibitor celecoxib suppresses tumor growth and lung metastasis of a murine mammary cancer. *Anticancer Res.* 2006, *26(6B)*, 4245-4254.

Fabi, A.; Metro, G.; Papaldo, P.; Mottolese, M.; Melucci, E.; Carlini, P.; Sperduti, I.; Russillo, M.; Gelibter, A.; Ferretti, G.; Tomao, S.; Milella, M.; Cognetti, F. Impact of celecoxib on capecitabine tolerability and activity in pretreated metastatic breast cancer: results of a phase II study with biomarker evaluation. *Cancer Chemother. Pharmacol.* 2008, *62(4)*, 717-725.

Canney, P. A.; Machin, M. A.; Curto, J. A feasibility study of the efficacy and tolerability of the combination of Exemestane with the COX-2 inhibitor Celecoxib in post-menopausal patients with advanced breast cancer. *Eur. J. Cancer* 2006, *42(16)*, 2751-2756.

Dirix, L. Y.; Ignacio, J.; Nag, S.; Bapsy, P.; Gomez, H.; Raghunadharao, D.; Paridaens, R.; Jones, S.; Falcon, S.; Carpentieri, M.; Abbattista, A.; Lobelle, J. P. Treatment of advanced hormone-sensitive breast cancer in postmenopausal women with exemestane alone or in combination with celecoxib. *J. Clin. Oncol.* 2008, *10, 26(8)*, 1253-1259.

Beer, T. M.; Ryan, C. W.; Venner, P. M.; Petrylak, D. P.; Chatta, G. S.; Ruether, J. D.; Chi, K. N.; Young, J.; Henner, W.D.; ASCENT(AIPC Study of Calcitriol ENhancing Taxotere) Investigators. Intermittent chemotherapy in patients with metastatic androgen-independent prostate cancer: results from ASCENT, a double-blinded, randomized comparison of high-dose calcitriol plus docetaxel with placebo plus docetaxel. *Cancer* 2008, *112(2)*, 326-330.

Dragovich, T.; Burris, H. 3rd, Loehrer, P.; Von Hoff, D. D.; Chow, S.; Stratton, S.; Green, S.; Obregon, Y.; Alvarez, I.; Gordon, M. Gemcitabine plus celecoxib in patients with advanced or metastatic pancreatic adenocarcinoma: results of a phase II trial. *Am. J. Clin. Oncol.* 2008, *31(2)*, 157-162.

Agarwala, A.; Fisher, W.; Bruetman, D.; McClean, J.; Taber, D.; Titzer, M.; Juliar, B.; Yu, M.; Breen, T.; Einhorn, L. H.; Hanna, N. Gefitinib plus celecoxib in chemotherapy- naïve patients with stage IIIB/IV non-small cell lung cancer: a phase II study from the Hoosier Oncology Group. *J. Thorac. Oncol.* 2008, *3(4)*, 374-379.

Xiao, H.; Zhang, Q.; Lin, Y.; Reddy, B. S.; Yang, C. S.; Combination of atorvastatin and celecoxib synergistically induces cell cycle arrest and apoptosis in colon cancer cells. *Int. J. Cancer* 2008, *122(9)*, 2115-2124.

Giovanucci, E. The epidemiology of vitamin D and cancer incidence and mortality: a review (United States). *Cancer causes control* 2005, *16*, 83-95.

Holick, M. F. Sunlight and vitamin D for bone health and prevention of autoimmune diseases, canc ers, and cardiovascular disease. *Am. J. Clin. Nutr.* 2004, *80*, 1678–1688S.

Trang, H. M.; Cole, D. E.; Rubin, L. A.; Pierratos, A.; Siu, S.; Vieth, R. Evidence that vitamin D3 increases serum 25-hydroxyvitamin D more efficiently than does vitamin D2. *Am. J. Clin. Nutr.* 1998, *68*, 854–858. Hollis, B. W.; Wagner, C. L. Normal serum vitamin D levels. *N. Engl. J. Med.* 2005, *352(5)*, 515-516.

Reichrath, J. Vitamin D and the skin: an ancient friend, revisited. *Experimental Dermatology* 2007, *16(7)*, 618-625

Holick, M. F. The cutaneous photosynthesis of previtamin D3: a unique photoendocrine system. *J. Invest. Dermatol.* 1981, *77*, 51-58.

Feskanich, D.; Ma, J.; Fuchs, C. S.; Kirkner, G. J.; Hankinson, S. E.; Hollis, B. W.; Giovannucci, E. L. Plasma vitamin D metabolites and risk of colorectal cancer in women. *Cancer Epidemiol. Biomarkers Prev.* 2004, *13(9)*, 1502-1508.

Ohyama, Y., Yamasaki, T. Eight cytochrome P450s catalyze vitamin D metabolism. *Front. Biosci.* 2004, *9*, 3007-3018.

Hewison, M.; Zehnder, D.; Chakraverty, R.; Adams, J. S. Vitamin D and barrier function: a novel role for extra-renal 1 α-hydroxylase. *Mol. Cell Endocrinol.* 2004, *215*, 31–38.

Bell, N. H. Renal and nonrenal 25-hydroxyvitamin D-1 α-hydroxylases and their clinical significance. *J. Bone Miner. Res.* 1998, *13*, 350–353.

Omdahl, J. L.; Morris, H. A.; May, B. K. Hydroxylase enzymes of the vitamin D pathway: expression, function, and regulation. *Annu. Rev. Nutr.* 2002, *22*, 139-166.

Dusso, A. S.; Brown, A. J.; Slatopolsky, E. Vitamin D. *Am. J. Physiol. Renal Physiol.* 2005, *289(1)*, F8-28.

Turunen, M. M.; Dunlop, T. W.; Carlberg, C.; Väisänen, S. Selective use of multiple vitamin D response elements underlies the 1 alpha,25-dihydroxyvitamin D3-mediated negative regulation of the human CYP27B1 gene. *Nucleic Acids Res.* 2007, *35(8)*, 2734-2747.

Zitterman, A. Vitamin D in preventive medicine: are we ignoring the evidence? *Br. J Nutr.* 2003, *89*, 552-572.

Hewison, M.; Zehnder, D.; Bland, R.; Stewart, P. M. 1 α -Hydroxylase and the action of vitamin D. *J. Mol. Endocrinol.* 2000, *25*, 141–148.

Zehnder, D.; Bland, R.; Chana, R. S.; Wheeler, D. C.; Howie, A. J.; Williams, M. C.; Stewart, P. M.; Hewison, M. Synthesis of 1,25-dihydroxyvitamin D(3) by human endothelial cells is regulated by inflammatory cytokines: a novel autocrine determinant of vascular cell adhesion. *J. Am. Soc. Nephrol.* 2002, *13(3)*, 621-629.

Stoffels, K.; Overbergh, L.; Giulietti, A.; Verlinden, L.; Bouillon, R.; Mathieu, C. Immune regulation of 25-hydroxyvitamin-D3-1alpha-hydroxylase in human monocytes. J. *Bone Miner. Res.* 2006, *21(1)*, 37-47.

Overbergh, L.; Stoffels, K.; Waer, M.; Verstuyf, A.; Bouillon, R.; Mathieu, C. Immune regulation of 25-hydroxyvitamin D-1alpha-hydroxylase in human monocytic THP1 cells: mechanisms of interferon-gamma-mediated induction. *J. Clin. Endocrinol. Metab.* 2006, *91(9)*, 3566-3574.

Stoffels, K.; Overbergh, L.; Bouillon, R.; Mathieu, C. Immune regulation of 1alpha-hydroxylase in murine peritoneal macrophages: unravelling the IFNgamma pathway. *J. Steroid. Biochem. Mol. Biol.* 2007, *103(3-5)*, 567-571.

Lopez, E. R,; Zwermann, O.; Segni, M.; Meyer, G.; Reincke, M.; Seissler, J.; Herwig, J.; Usadel K. H.; Badenhoop, K. A promoter polymorphism of the CYP27B1 gene is associated with Addison's disease, Hashimoto's thyroiditis, Graves' disease and type 1 diabetes mellitus in Germans. *Eur. J. Endocrinol.* 2004, *151*, 193–197.

Fischer, D.; Seifert, M.; Becker, S.; Ludders, D.; Cordes, T.; Reichrath, J.; Friedrich, M. 25-Hydroxyvitamin D3 1alpha-hydroxylase splice variants in breast cell lines MCF- 7 and MCF-10. *Cancer Genomics Proteomics* 2007, *4(4)*, 295-300.

Cordes, T.; Diesing, D.; Becker, S.; Fischer, D.; Diedrich, K.; Friedrich, M. Expression of splice variants of 1alpha-hydroxylase in mcf-7 breast cancer cells. *J. Steroid. Biochem. Mol. Biol.* 2007, *103(3-5)*, 326-329.

Barreto, A. M.; Schwartz, G. G.; Woodruff, R.; Cramer, S. D. 25-Hydroxyvitamin D3, the prohormone of 1,25-dihydroxyvitamin D3, inhibits the proliferation of primary prostatic epithelial cells. *Cancer Epidemiol. Biomarkers Prev.* 2000, *9*, 265–270.

Schwartz, G. G.; Whitlatch, L. W.; Chen, T. C.; Lokeshwar, B. L.; Holick, M. F. Human prostate cells synthesize 1,25-dihydroxyvitamin D3 from 25-hydroxyvitamin D3. *Cancer Epidemiol. Biomarkers Prev.* 1998, *7*, 391–395.

Tangpricha, V.; Flanagan, J. N.; Whitlatch, L. W.; Tseng, C. C.; Chen, T. C.; Holt, P. R.; Lipkin, M. S.; Holick, M. F. 25-Hydroxyvitamin D-1 α -hydroxylase in normal and malignant colon tissue. *Lancet* 2001, *357*, 1673–1674.

Bareis, P.; Bises, G.; Bischof, M. G.; Cross, H. S.; Peterlik, M. 25-hydroxy-vitamin D metabolism in human colon cancer cells during tumor progression. *Biochem. Biophys. Res. Commun.* 2001, *285*, 1012–1017.

Ogunkolade, B. W.; Boucher, B. J.; Fairclough, P. D.; Hitman, G. A.; Dorudi, S.; Jenkins, P. J.; Bustin, S. A. Expression of 25-hydroxyvitamin D-1- α -hydroxylase mRNA in individuals with colorectal cancer. *Lancet* 2002, *359*, 1831–1832.

Friedrich, M.; Diesing, D.; Cordes, T.; Fischer, D.; Becker, S.; Chen, T. C. Flanagan, J. N.; Tangpricha, V.; Gherson, I.; Holick, M. F.; Reichrath, J. Analysis of 25-hydroxyvitamin D3-1alpha-hydroxylase in normal and malignant breast tissue. *Anticancer Res.* 2006, *26(4A)*, 2615-2620.

Garland, C. F.; Comstock, G. W.; Garland, F. C.; Helsing, K. J.; Shaw, E. K.; Gorham, E. D. Serum 25-hydroxyvitamin D and colon cancer: eight-year prospective study. *Lancet* 1989, *2*, 1176–1178.

Holt, P. R.; Arber, N.; Halmos, B.; Forde, K.; Kissileff, H.; McGlynn, K. A.; Moss, S. F.; Kurihara, N.; Fan, K. Colonic epithelial cell proliferation decreases with increasing levels of serum 25-hydroxy vitamin D. *Cancer Epidemiol. Biomarkers Prev.* 2002, *11*, 113–119.

Lowe, L. C.; Guy, M.; Mansi, J. L.; Peckitt, C.; Bliss, J.; Wilson, R. G.; Colston, K. W. Plasma 25-hydroxy vitamin D concentrations, vitamin D receptor genotype and breast cancer risk in a UK Caucasian population. *Eur. J. Cancer* 2005, *41*, 1164–1169.

Berube, S.; Diorio, C.; Verhoek-Oftedahl, W.; Brisson, J. Vitamin D, calcium and mammographic breast densities. *Cancer Epidemiol. Biomarkers Prev.* 2004, *13*, 1466- 1472.

Huang, D. C.; Papavasiliou, V.; Rhim, J. S.; Horst, R. L.; Kremer, R. Targeted disruption of the 25-hydroxyvitamin D3 1alpha-hydroxylase gene in ras-transformed keratinocytes demonstrates that locally produced 1alpha,25-dihydroxyvitamin D3 suppresses growth and induces differentiation in an autocrine fashion. *Mol. Cancer Res.* 2002, *1*, 56–67.

Segersten, U.; Holm, P. K.; Björklund, P.; Hessman, O.; Nordgren, H.; Binderup, L.; Akerström, G.; Hellman, P.; Westin, G. 25-Hydroxyvitamin D3 1alpha-hydroxylase expression in breast cancer and use of non-1alpha-hydroxylated vitamin D analogue. *Breast Cancer Res.* 2005, *7(6)*, 980-986.

Agic, A.; Xu, H.; Altgassen, C.; Noack, F.; Wolfler, M. M.; Diedrich, K.; Friedrich, M.; Taylor, R. N.; Hornung, D. Relative expression of 1,25-dihydroxyvitamin D3 receptor, vitamin D 1 alpha-hydroxylase, vitamin D 24-hydroxylase, and vitamin D 25-hydroxylase in endometriosis and gynecologic cancers. *Reprod. Sci.* 2007, *14(5)*, 486-497.

Friedrich, M.; Rafi, L.; Mitschele, T.; Tilgen, W.; Schmidt, W.; Reichrath, J. Analysis of the vitamin D system in cervical carcinomas, breast cancer and ovarian cancer. *Recent Results Cancer Res.* 2003, *164*, 39-46.

Hewison, M.; Kantorovich, V.; Liker H. R.; van Herle, A. J.; Cohan, P.; Zehnder, D.; Adams, J. S. Vitamin D-mediated hypercalcemia in lymphoma: evidence for hormone production by tumoradjacent macrophages. *J. Bone Miner. Res.* 2003, *18*, 579-582.

Evans, K. N.; Taylor, H.; Zehnder, D.; Kilby, M. D.; Bulmer, J. N.; Shah, F.; Adams, J. S.; Hewison, M. Increased expression of 25-hydroxyvitamin D-1 α-hydroxylase in dysgerminomas: a novel form of humoral hypercalcemia of malignancy. *Am. J. Pathol.* 2004, *165*, 807–813.

Townsend, K.; Banwell, C. M.; Guy, M.; Colston, K. W.; Mansi, J. L.; Stewart, P. M.; Campbell, M. J.; Hewison, M. Autocrine metabolism of vitamin D in normal and malignant tissue. *Clin. Cancer Res.* 2005, *11(9)*, 3579-3586.

Ainsleigh, H. G. Beneficial effects of sun exposure on cancer mortality. *Prev. Med.* 1993, *22*, 132-140.

Gorham, E. D.; Garland, F. C.; Garland, C. F. Sunlight and breast cancer incidence in the USSR. *Int. J. Epidemiol.* 1990, *19*, 820–824.

Garland, F. C.; Garland, C. F.; Gorham, E. D.; Young, J. F. Geographic variation in breast cancer mortality in the United States: a hypothesis involving exposure to solar radiation. *Prev. Med.* 1990, *19*, 614–622.

Grant, W. B. An estimate of premature cancer mortality in the U.S. due to inadequate doses of solar ultraviolet-B radiation. *Cancer* 2002, *94*, 1867–1875.

Kemmis, C. M.; Salvador, S. M.; Smith, K. M.; Welsh, J. Human mammary epithelial cells express CYP27B1 and are growth inhibited by 25-hydroxyvitamin D-3, the major circulating form of vitamin D-3. *J. Nutr.* 2006, *136*, 887-892.

Holick, M. F.; Siris, E. S.; Binkley, N.; Beard, M. K.; Khan, A.; Katzer, J. T.; Petruschke, R. A.; Chen, E.; de Papp, A. E. Prevalence of vitamin D inadequacy among postmenopausal women. North American women receiving osteoporosis therapy. *J. Clin. Endocrinol. Metabo.* 2005, *90*, 3215-3224.

Sowers, M. R.; Wallace, R. B.; Hollis, B. W.; Lemke, J. H. Parameters related to 25-OH-D levels in a population-based study of women. *Am. J. Clin. Nutr.* 1986, *43*, 621–628.

Diesing, D.; Cordes, T.; Fischer, D.; Diedrich, K.; Friedrich, M. Vitamin D--metabolism in the human breast cancer cell line MCF-7. *Anticancer Res.* 2006, *26(4A)*, 2755-2759.

Sunn, K. L.; Cock, T. A.; Crofts, L. A.; Eismann, J. A.; Gardiner, E. M. Novel N-terminal variant of human VDR. *Mol. Endocrinol.* 2001, *15(9)*, 1599-1609.

Tsai, M. J.; O'Malley, B. W. Molecular mechanisms of action of steroid/thyroid receptor superfamily members. *Annu. Rev. Biochem.* 1994, *63*, 451–486.

Nemere, I.; Szego, C. M. Early actions of parathyroid hormone and 1,25-dihydroxycholecalciferol on istolated epithelial cells from rat intestine. *Endocrinology* 1981, *108*, 1450-1462.

Studzinski, G. P.; McLane, J. A.; Uskokovic, M. R. Signaling pathways for vitamin D-induced differentiation: implications for therapy of proliferative and neoplastic diseases. *Crit. Rev. Eukaryot. Gene Expr.* 1993, *4*, 279-312.

Marcinkowska, E.; Wiedlocha, A.; Radzikowsi, C. 1,25-dihydroxyvitamin D3 induced activation and subsequent nuclear translocation of MAPK is upstream regulated by PKC in HL-60 cells. *Biochem. Biophys. Res. Commun.* 1997, *241*, 410-426.

Marcinkowska, E.; Wiedlocha, A.; Radzikowski, C. Evidence that phosphatidylinositol

3-kinase and p70S6Kprotein are involved in differentiation of HL-60 cells induced by calcitriol. *Anticancer Res.* 1998, *18*, 3507-3514.

Marcinkowska, E. Evidence that activation of MEK1,2/erk1,2 signal transduction pathway is necessary for calcitriol-induced differentiation of HL-60 cells. *Anticancer Res.* 2001, *21*, 499-504.

Mehta, R. G.; Mehta, R. R. Vitamin D and cancer. *J. Nutr. Biochem.* 2002, *13*, 252–264.

Boland, R.; De Boland, A. R.; Buitrago, C.; Morelli, S.; Santillan, G.; Vazque, G.; Capiati, D.; Baldi, C. Non-genomic stimulation of tyrosine phosphorylation cascades by 1,25(OH)(2)D(3) by VDR-dependent and -independent mechanisms in muscle cells. *Steroids* 2002, *67*, 477-482.

Marcinkowska, E.; Wiedlocha, A. Steroid signal transduction activated at the cell membrane: from plants to animal. *Acta Biochimica Polonica* 2002, *49*, 735-745.

Colston, K. W.; Berger, U.; Coombes, R. C. Possible role for vitamin D in controlling breast cancer cell proliferation. *Lancet* 1989, *1*, 188–191.

James, S. Y.; Mackay, A. G.; Colston, K. W. Vitamin D derivatives in combination with 9-cis retinoic acid promote active cell death in breast cancer cells. *J. Mol. Endocrinol.* 1995, *14(3)*, 391-394.

Welsh, J. E. Induction of apoptosis in breast cancer cells in response to vitamin D and antiestrogens. *Biochem. Cell. Biol.* 1995, *72(11–12)*, 537-545.

Berger, U.; Wilson, P.; McClelland, R. A.; Colston, K.; Haussler, M. R.; Pike, J. W.; Coombes, R. C. Immunocytochemical determination of estrogen receptor, progesterone receptor, and 1,25-dihydroxyvitamin D3 receptor in breast cancer and relationship to prognosis. *Cancer Res.* 1991, *51*, 239–244.

Welsh, J. Targets of vitamin D receptor signaling in the mammary gland. *J. Bone Miner. Res.* 2007, *22 Suppl 2*, V86-90.

Uitterlinden, A. G.; Fang, Y.; Van Meurs, J. B.; Pols, H. A.; Van Leeuwen, J. P. Genetics and biology of vitamin D receptor polymorphisms. *Gene* 2004, *338(2)*, 143-156.

Guy, M.; Lowe, L. C.; Bretherton-Watt, D.; Mansi, J. L.; Peckitt, C.; Bliss, J.; Wilson, R. G.; Thomas, V.; Colston, K. W. Vitamin D receptor gene polymorphisms and breast cancer risk. *Clin. Cancer Res.* 2004, *15*, *10(16)*, 5472-5481.

Curran, J. E.; Vaughan, T.; Lea, R. A.; Weinstein, S. R.; Morrison, N. A.; Griffiths, L. R. Association of A vitamin D receptor polymorphism with sporadic breast cancer development. *Int. J. Cancer* 1999, *83*, 723–726.

Chen, W. Y.; Bertone-Johnson, E. R.; Hunter, D. J.; Willett, W. C.; Hankinson, S. E. Associations between polymorphisms in the vitamin D receptor and breast cancer risk. Cancer Epidemiol. *Biomarkers Prev.* 2005, *14(10)*, 2335-2339.

Sinotte, M.; Rousseau, F.; Ayotte, P.; Dewailly, E.; Diorio, C.; Giguere, Y.; Berube, S.; Brisson, J. Vitamin D receptor polymorphisms (FokI, BsmI) and breast cancer risk: association replication in two case-control studies within French Canadian population. *Endocr. Relat. Cancer.* 2008, *15(4)*, 975-83.

Trabert, B.; Malone, K. E.; Daling, J. R.; Doody, D. R.; Bernstein, L.; Ursin, G.; Marchbanks, P. A.; Strom, B. L.; Humphrey, M. C.; Ostrander, E. A. Vitamin D receptor polymorphisms and breast cancer risk in a large population-based case- control study of Caucasian and African-American women. *Breast Cancer Res.* 2007, *9(6)*, R84.

Lundin, A. C.; Soderkvist, P.; Eriksson, B.; Bergman-Jungestrom, M.; Wingren, S. Association of breast cancer progression with a vitamin D receptor gene polymorphism. South-East Sweden Breast Cancer Group. *Cancer Res.* 1999, *59*, 2332–2334.

Ruggiero, M.; Pacini, S.; Aterini, S.; Fallai, C.; Ruggiero, C.; Pacini, P. Vitamin D receptor gene polymorphism is associated with metastatic breast cancer. *Oncol. Res.* 1998, *10*, 43–46.

Dunning, A. M.; McBride, S.; Gregory, J.; Durocher, F.; Foster, N. A.; Healy, C. S.; Smith, N.; Pharoah, P. D.; Luben, R. N.; Easton, D. F.; Ponder, B. A. No association between androgen or vitamin D receptor gene polymorphisms and risk of breast cancer. *Carcinogenesis* 1999, *20*, 2131–2135.

Newcomb, P. A.; Kim, H.; Trentham-Dietz, A.; Farin, F.; Hunter, D.; Egan, K. M. Vitamin D receptor polymorphism and breast cancer risk. *Cancer Epidemiol. Biomarkers Prev.* 2002, *11*, 1503–1504.

Cui, Y.; Rohan, T. E. Vitamin D, Calcium, and breast cancer risk: A review. *Cancer Epidemiol. Biomarkers Prev.* 2006, *15(18)*, 1427-1437.

McCullough, M. L.; Stevens, V. L.; Diver, W. R.; Feigelson, H. S.; Rodriguez, C.; Bostick, R. M.; Thun, M. J.; Calle, E. E. Vitamin D pathway gene polymorphisms, diet, and risk of postmenopausal breast cancer: a nested case-control study. *Breast Cancer Res.* 2007, *9(1)*, R9.

Cashman, K. D. Calcium intake, calcium bioavailability and bone health. *Br. J. Nutr.* 2002, *87 Suppl 2*, S169–177.

Welsh, J. Vitamin D and breast cancer: insights from animal models. *Am. J. Clin. Nutr.* 2004, *80*, 1721–1724S.

Mantell, D. J.; Owens, P. E.; Bundred, N. J.; Mawer, E. B.; Canfield, A. E. 1α,25-Dihydroxyvitamin D(3) inhibits angiogenesis in vitro and in vivo. *Circ. Res.* 2000, *87*, 214–220.

Saez, S.; Falette, N.; Guillot, C.; Meggouh, F.; Lefebvre, M. F.; Crepin, M.; William, L. McGuire. Memorial Symposium. 1,25(OH)2D3 modulation of mammary tumor cell growth in vitro and in vivo. *Breast Cancer Res. Treat.* 1993, *27*, 69–81.

Eisman, J. A.; Sutherland, R. L.; McMenemy, M. L.; Fragonas, J. C.; Musgrove, E. A.; Pang, G. Y. Effects of 1,25-dihydroxyvitamin D3 on cell-cycle kinetics of T 47D human breast cancer cells. *J. Cell. Physiol.* 1989, *138(3)*, 611-616.

Jacobson, E. A.; James, K. A.; Newmark, H. L.; Carroll, K. K. Effects of dietary fat, calcium, and vitamin D on growth and mammary tumorigenesis induced by 7,12- dimethylbenz(a)anthracene in female Sprague-Dawley rats. *Cancer Res.* 1989, *49*, 6300–6303.

Xue, L.; Lipkin, M.; Newmark, H.; Wang, J. Influence of dietary calcium and vitamin D on diet-induced epithelial cell hyperproliferation in mice. *J. Natl. Cancer Inst.* 1999, *91*, 176–181.

John, E. M.; Schwartz, G. G.; Dreon, D. M.; Koo, J. Vitamin D and breast cancer risk: the NHANES I epidemiologic follow-up study, 1971-1975 to 1992. National Health and Nutrition Examination Survey. *Cancer Epidemiol. Biomarkers Prev.* 1999, *8*, 399–406.

Knight, J. A.; Lesosky, M.; Barnett, H.; Raboud, J. M.; Vieth, R. Vitamin D and reduced risk of breast cancer: A population-based control study. *Cancer Epidemiol. Biomarkers Prev.* 2007, *16*, 422-429.

McCullough, M. L.; Rodriguez, C.; Diver, W. R.; Feigelson, H. S.; Stevens, V. L.; Thun, M. J.; Calle, E. E. Dairy, calcium, and vitamin D intake and postmenopausal breast cancer risk in the Cancer Prevention Study II Nutrition Cohort. Cancer Epidemiol. *Biomarkers Prev.* 2005, *14*, 2898–2904.

Rossi, M.; McLaughlin, J. K.; Lagiou, P.; Bosetti, C.; Talamini, R.; Lipworth, L.; Giacosa,

A.; Montella, M.; Franceschi, S.; Negri, E.; La Vecchia, C. Vitamin D intake and breast cancer risk: a case-control study in Italy. *Ann. Oncol.* 2009, *20(2)*, 374-378.

Frazier, A. L.; Ryan, C. T.; Rockett, H.; Willett, W. C.; Colditz, G. A. Adolescent diet and risk of breast cancer. *Breast Cancer Res.* 2003, *5*, R59–64.

Frazier, A. L.; Li, L.; Cho, E.; Willett, W. C.; Colditz, G. A. Adolescent diet and risk of breast cancer. *Cancer Causes Control* 2004, *15*, 73–82.

Gissel, T.; Rejnmark, L.; Mosekilde, L.; Vestergaard P. Intake of vitamin D and risk of breast cancer--a meta-analysis. *J. Steroid. Biochem. Mol. Biol.* 2008, *111(3-5)*, 195-199.

Hiatt, R. A.; Krieger, N.; Lobaugh, B.; Drezner, M. K.; Vogelman, J. H.; Orentreich, N. Prediagnostic serum vitamin D and breast cancer. *J. Natl. Cancer Inst.* 1998, *90*, 461- 463.

Bertone-Johnson, E. R.; Chen, W. Y.; Holick, M. F.; Hollis, B. W.; Colditz, G. A.; Willett, W. C.; Hankinson, S. E. Plasma 25-hydroxyvitamin D and 1,25-dihydroxyvitamin D and risk of breast cancer. *Cancer Epidemiol. Biomarkers Prev.* 2005, *14*, 1991–1997.

Mawer, E. B.; Walls, J.; Howell, A.; Davies, M.; Ratcliffe, W. A.; Bundred, N. J. Serum 1,25-dihydroxyvitamin D may be related inversely to disease activity in breast cancer patients with bone metastases. *J. Clin. Endocrinol. Metab.* 1997, *82*, 118–122.

Whitfield, J. F.; Boynton, A. L.; MacManus, J. P.; Sikorska, M.; Tsang, B. K. The regulation of cell proliferation by calcium and cyclic AMP. *Mol. Cell Biochem.* 1979, *27*, 155–179.

Mathiasen, I. S.; Sergeev, I. N.; Bastholm, L.; Elling, F.; Norman, A. W.; Jaattela, M. Calcium and calpain as key mediators of apoptosis-like death induced by vitamin D compounds in breast cancer cells. *J. Biol. Chem.* 2002, *277*, 30738–30745.

Sergeev, I. N. Calcium as a mediator of 1,25-dihydroxyvitamin D3-induced apoptosis. *J. Steroid. Biochem. Mol. Biol.* 2004, *89–90*, 419–425.

McGrath, C. M.; Soule, H. D. Calcium regulation of normal human mammary epithelial cell growth in culture. *In Vitro* 1984, *20*, 652–662.

Russo, J.; Russo, I. H. The pathway of neoplastic transformation of human breast epithelial cells. *Radiat. Res.* 2001, *155*, 151–154.

Boyapati, S. M.; Shu, X. O.; Jin, F.; Dai, Q.; Ruan, Z.; Gao, Y. T.; Zheng, W. Dietary calcium intake and breast cancer risk among Chinese women in Shanghai. *Nutr. Cancer* 2003, *46*, 38–43.

Wark, J. D.; Larkins, R. G.; Eisman, J. A.; Wilson, K. R. Regulation of 25- hydroxyvitamin-D-la-hydroxylase in chick isolated renal tubules: effects of prostaglandin E2, frusemide and acetylsalicylate. Clin. Sci. 1981, 62, 53-59.

Hayes, M. E.; Rai, A.; Cooper, R. G.; Bayley, D.; Freemont, A. J.; Mawer, E. B. Inhibition by prostaglandin E1 and E2 of 1,25-dihydroxyvitamin D3 synthesis by synovial fluid macrophages from arthritic joints. *Ann. Rheum. Dis.* 1992, *51*, 632-637.

Miller, G. J. Vitamin D and prostate cancer: biologic interactions and clinical potentials. *Cancer Metastasis Rev.* 1998, *17*, 353–360.

Konety, B. R.; Getzenberg, R. H. Vitamin D and prostate cancer. Urol *Clin. North Am.* 2002, *29*, 95–106.

Zhuang, S. H.; Burnstein, K. L. Antiproliferative effect of 1α,25-dihydroxyvitamin D3 in human prostate cancer cell line LNCaP involves reduction of cyclin-dependent kinase 2 activity and persistent G1 accumulation. Endocrinology 1998, 139, 1197–1207.

Moreno, J.; Krishnan, A. V.; Swami, S.; Nonn, L.; Peehl, D. M.; Feldman, D. Regulation of prostaglandin metabolism by calcitriol attenuates growth stimulation in prostate cancer cells. *Cancer Res.* 2005, *65(17)*, 7917-7925.

8

Endocytic Trafficking of the Epidermal Growth Factor Receptor in Transformed Cells

Brian P. Ceresa
University of Oklahoma Health Sciences Center
United States of America

1. Introduction

The epidermal growth factor receptor (EGFR) is the prototypical receptor tyrosine kinase. It is localized to the plasma membranes of cells with an extracellular ligand binding domain and an intracellular kinase domain. Through the binding of extracellular ligands, the receptor undergoes a conformational change that alters the biochemical properties of proteins (effectors) within the cell. Ultimately, these changes result in modulation of the rate of cell growth, protein and DNA synthesis, cell motility, and cell proliferation. The EGFR is necessary for the proper development of organisms, as indicated by the fact that genetic knockout of the receptor results in animals that are embryonic lethal or die shortly after birth. This developmental role is also observed in adult animals, as pharmacological inhibition of the EGFR disrupts tissue homeostasis.

In addition to these developmental roles, there is a strong association between overexpression and/or hyperactivation of the EGFR and cancer. Currently, there are several small molecule inhibitors and neutralizing, humanized antibodies against the EGFR that successfully treat EGFR-positive cancers (*i.e.* non-small cell lung carcinomas, colon, and head and neck cancers). Breast cancer is among those cancers that are characterized by enhanced EGFR levels and activity. However, the aforementioned pharmacologic agents have been of little success in the treatment of breast cancers. Therefore, a more detailed understanding of the cellular and molecular biology of EGFR function is required in order to successfully attenuate the growth and metastasis of EGFR-positive cells.

Cells have numerous endogenous mechanisms to that regulate the specificity and duration of EGFR signaling. Endogenous regulatory mechanisms are logical pharmacological targets to inhibit EGFR activity because of their intrinsic ability to modulate signaling. One of the most important regulators of EGFR signaling is the endocytic pathway. The endocytic pathway can control both the duration of signaling and the spatial placement of the receptor. Historically, endocytosis has been considered a mechanism for the negative regulation of EGFR, as it decreases the number of cell surface receptors and inactivates the ligand:receptor complex by targeting it for lysosomal degradation. More recently, it has been appreciated that signaling of the EGFR varies based on the subcellular localization of the receptor. Specifically, in a given cell, the liganded EGFR can promote cell proliferation at some cellular locations (*i.e.* plasma membrane), whereas at others (*i.e.* the limiting membranes of endosomes) the receptor can induce apoptosis. Thus, a potential molecular etiology of EGFR overexpression in transformed cells is disrupted normal endocytic trafficking of the EGFR. Slowed kinetics of receptor degradation will increase the steady-state levels of the EGFRs over time. If this hypothesis holds true, the endocytic pathway is a logical target for pharmacological manipulation to prevent the progression of such cells.

This chapter will explore the basic cell biology of the EGFR and the endocytic mechanisms that regulate its signaling. To be discussed are the workings of the endocytic pathway, strategies used to understand the relationship between endocytic trafficking and EGFR signaling, and data indicating how trafficking regulates signaling. These mechanisms will be dissected and potential points for attenuating the enhanced EGFR activity will be discussed.

2. The EGFR

The EGFR is an approximately 180 kDa transmembrane protein that is oriented on the plasma membrane such that the amino terminus half of the protein is extracellular and the carboxyl terminus portion is intracellular. Thus, by virtue of its orientation, the amino terminus of the EGFR detects and binds ligands; the carboxyl terminal kinase domain converts the conformational change induced through ligand binding into intracellular, biochemical signals. The EGFR is also known as ErbB1, and is part of the larger ErbB family of receptor tyrosine kinases that is comprised of ErbB1, ErbB2, ErbB3 and ErbB4. This family shares many features such as membrane topology, mechanism of activation and signaling, and downstream effectors. However, each member is unique in its tissue expression, its activating ligands, magnitude and duration of effector signaling, and membrane trafficking (Hynes and MacDonald, 2009).

There have been seven ligands that have been reported to be able to activate the EGFR - epidermal growth factor (EGF), heparin binding epidermal growth factor (HB-EGF), betacellulin (BTC), transforming growth factor-α (TGF-α), amphiregulin (AR), epiregulin, and epigen (Harris *et al.*, 2003). The regulated secretion of these ligands is an important determinant of when a receptor gets activated. Further, overexpression of certain ligands, namely TGF-α, has been associated with an increase in receptor activity and enhanced cell proliferation (Matsui et al., 1990; Sandgren et al., 1993).

Based on the available data, it is commonly held that all ligands initiate signaling in the same fundamental manner (Figure 1). Briefly, ligand binding to an EGFR monomer induces a conformation change in the receptor that exposes a dimerization motif (cysteine rich domain). Through association with another EGFR or related family member (ErbB2, ErbB3, or ErbB4), a dimeric receptor forms, and initiates activation of the intracellular kinase domain (Dawson et al., 2005). In turn, the kinase domain phosphorylates tyrosine residues on the very carboxyl terminus of the protein. These newly formed phosphotyrosines serve as docking site for downstream signaling molecules (effectors). The EGFR-stimulated effector activity alters the intracellular biochemistry and results in cellular changes, such as cell proliferation, differentiation, and migration.

There is a long list of effector molecules reported to be downstream of the activated EGFR. Two of the major questions for scientists that study EGFR biology and pathology are 1) to identify which receptor:effector interactions occur under physiological and pathological conditions and which ones are an artifact of cell culture models and 2) to determine which effectors are necessary and sufficient for a specific cell physiology/pathology. Asking these questions is confounded by the fact that receptor:effector interactions can arise as an unintended consequence of receptor overexpression. This is true in model systems that are generated by the scientist as well as naturally occurring cell transformation. As discussed

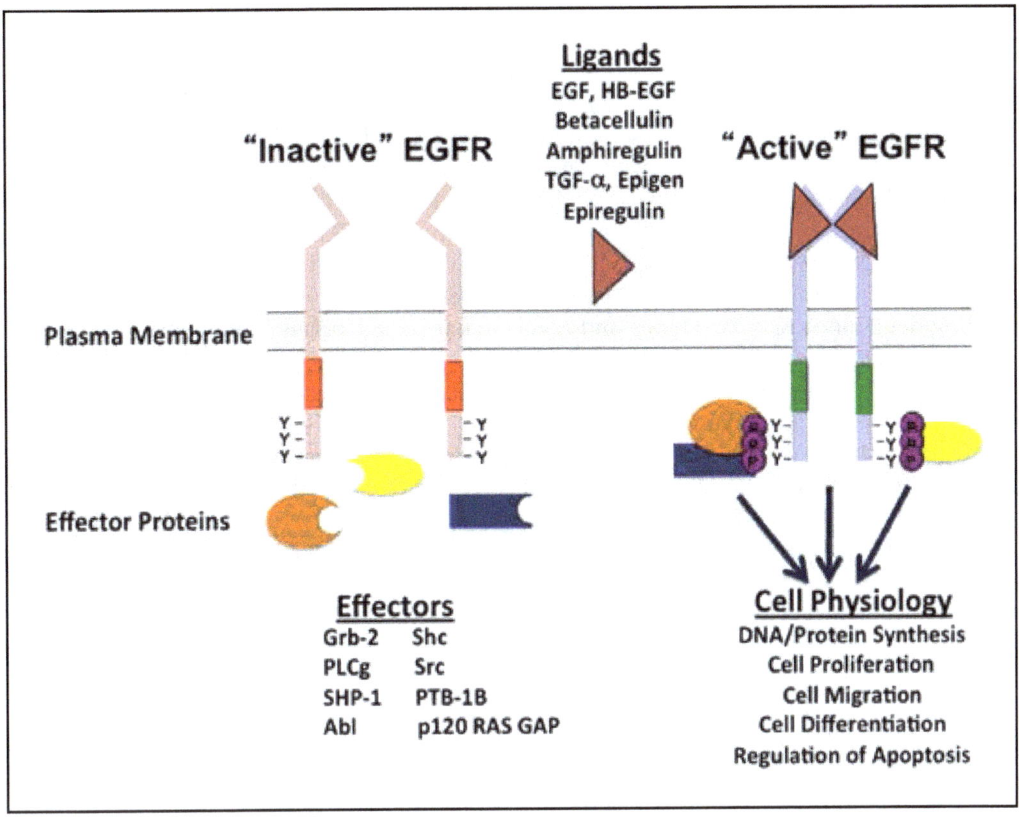

Fig. 1. Schematic of EGFR Activation. Binding of one of the EGFRs endogenous ligands induces a conformational change in the receptor that permits dimerization and kinase activity. Kinase active receptor than transphosphorylates the receptor with which it is associating. The resulting phosphotyrosines serve as docking sites for down stream signaling molecules.

below, many cancers are characterized by overexpression of the EGFR. Therefore, interactions that do not occur in a biological setting may be very relevant in a pathological condition.

There are numerous lines of evidence that indicate the EGFR plays important physiological roles in tissue development and homeostasis (Jorissen *et al.*, 2003). It is expressed on the surface of virtually every cell in the body. Mice that have been engineered to knock out the EGFR gene are either embryonic lethal or die shortly after birth, indicating its role in pre-natal development (Miettinen *et al.*, 1995; Sibilia and Wagner, 1995; Threadgill *et al.*, 1995). Patients taking EGFR inhibitors as part of an anti-cancer chemotherapeutic regimen, experience complications such as colitis, dermatitis, and corneal abrasions, indicating the receptor contributes to the homeostasis of those tissues (Tullo et al., 2005; Zhang et al., 2007). This is supported by the genetically engineered deletion of EGFR ligands (*i.e.* EGF, transforming growth factor-α (TGF-α), or amphiregulin) have revealed roles in maintaining development of tissue, such as mammary glands, eyes, hair, and epidermis (Luetteke *et al.*, 1999) and provide evidence of the receptors' role in tissue homeostasis.

3. EGFRs in cancer

In addition to roles in tissue development and homeostasis, the driving force behind the study of the EGFR has been its role in cancer. The EGFR is overexpressed and/or hyperactivated in many cancers including, but not limited to, cancers of the breast, ovary, colon, lung, head and neck, pancreas, and brain (Rowinsky, 2004). Further, overexpression of the EGFR in many cancers correlates with poor patient prognosis (Nicholson *et al.*, 2001).

There are a number of events that can cause the increase in EGFR activity that is associated with cancer. These include gene amplification, activating mutations of the receptor's kinase domain, and deletions of the extracellular domain that regulate the receptor's ligand-binding dependent activity (Hynes and MacDonald, 2009; Uberall et al., 2008). Despite this strong association, it remains unclear whether overexpression/hyperactivation of the EGFR is the root cause of cell transformation or a cell becoming transformed is what leads to the overexpression/hyperactivation of the EGFR.

Regardless of the cause of increased EGFR activity, there are several anti-cancer therapies that specifically target the EGFR that have been approved by the United States Food and Drug Administration (FDA). These drugs fall in two classes. First, humanized monoclonal antibodies target the extracellular portion of the receptor and antagonize the binding of endogenous EGFR ligands. These antibodies are 528 mouse IgG_{2a}, the 225 mouse IgG_1, and the C225 humanized monoclonal antibody. The second class of drugs are small molecule inhibitors of the EGFR kinase domain [Iressa (gefitinib) and Tarceva (erlotinib)]. Both classes of drugs are able to prevent the progression of cancer by inducing apoptosis specifically in those cells with increased EGFR activity. Therapeutic use of these drugs has been approved for non-small-cell lung cancer, squamous cell carcinoma of the head and neck, and colorectal cancers (Baselga and Arteaga, 2005).

One issue that remains unresolved is the limited therapeutic efficacy of EGFR inhibitors in the treatment of breast cancers. This is true, despite the fact that EGFR overexpression is associated with some breast cancers. To date, only Tykerb (lapatinib) is approved for the treatment of breast cancer. However, it should be noted that Tykerb inhibits both the EGFR and its receptor tyrosine kinase family member, ErbB2, and is only approved for use in conjunction with the aromatase inhibitor Femara (letrozole) (Cameron et al., 2010). Despite the limited success of EGFR inhibitors in treating breast cancers, the evidence from other cancers indicates the receptor still has potential as a therapeutic target. In order to develop better anti-cancer chemotherapeutic agents that target the EGFR in breast cancer, a more detailed understanding of EGFR signaling is required.

4. EGFR endocytic pathway

Not only are the effectors with which the EGFR interacts important, but also the quality of interaction. Both the duration and magnitude of effector activity are what determine how cell physiology is modified. A tremendous body of literature supports the idea that the regulation of signaling is the critical determinant in how receptor specific signals are produced. This is the most logical explanation for how a number of different cell surface receptor (*i.e.* EGFR, insulin receptor, and platelet derived growth factor receptor) can share an overlapping set of effector molecules, yet each produces a receptor-specific change in cell physiology.

One of the principle mechanisms by which EGFR signaling is regulated is ligand-mediated endocytosis. Internalization of the EGF:EGFR complex can be either clathrin-dependent or clathrin-independent. Clathrin-dependent endocytosis is the most well studied as it is the predominant route of receptor internalization in response to physiological concentrations of ligand.

By all accounts, all of the endogenous EGFR ligands can promote internalization of the EGFR, through a series of well-defined steps (Figure 2). Following binding of ligand, the ligand:receptor complex translocates along the plasma membrane to a domain that is enriched on the intracellular face with clathrin. The clathrin lattice invaginates to form a clathrin-coated pit that pinches off generating an intracellular clathrin-coated vesicle. Once inside the cell, clathrin is shed from the vesicle, giving rise to an intermediate vesicle. The intermediate vesicle fuses with and delivers the ligand:receptor complex to the early endosome. This compartment is where sorting of the cargo occurs. The predominant route of trafficking of the EGF:EGFR complex is into a late endosome/multivesicular body, by way of vesicle maturation. Alternative routes include recycling to the plasma membrane, trafficking to the nucleus, and delivery to the endoplasmic reticulum (Liao and Carpenter, 2007; Masui et al., 1993; Wang et al., 2010). For those receptors that get delivered to the late endosome/multivesicular body, that compartment fuses with the lysosome that degrades the ligand and receptor in the protease rich environment.

Each endocytic compartment has a number of distinguishing features. First, as the compartments get further away from the plasma membrane, they become more acidic and increase in density. In addition, each endocytic location has a unique protein composition. These three features have proven to be important in understanding ligand:receptor interactions, receptor trafficking, and receptor signaling. Further, researchers continue to utilize these features to distinguish one compartment from another. For instance, the different densities of the endosomes can be use to separate compartments by sedimentation centrifugation (Vanlandingham and Ceresa, 2009). Endosome specific proteins can be used as markers to identify which intracellular compartment the receptor resides (Vanlandingham and Ceresa, 2009).

It is important to note that following endocytosis, not all ligands target the EGFR for lysosomal degradation. A recent, comprehensive study of the trafficking of EGFR ligands was performed using human laryngeal carcinoma (Hep2) cells as a model (Roepstorff et al., 2009). In this study, six of the endogenous EGFR ligands were analyzed for their ability to induce receptor internalization, lysosomal degradation, and recycling. Following ligand treatment, the authors used indirect immunofluorence to monitor receptor co-localization with early and late endosome markers [early endosome autoantigen 1 (EEA1) and Lysosome associated membrane protein 1 (Lamp1)]. In addition, biochemical assays were used to assess the kinetics of ligand stimulated EGFR degradation and recycling. The data from the manuscript indicate that two ligands TGF-α and epiregulin lead to receptor recycling. HB-EGF and betacellulin, like EGF, target the receptor for degradation. Interestingly, amphiregulin treatment yields a phenotype that is somewhere in between - recycling with slower kinetics.

While the molecular basis for these differences in receptor trafficking are not entirely clear for all ligands, one ligand has been particularly well studied, particularly in the context of cancer. As stated above, treatment with TGF-α induces EGFR internalization and recycling to the plasma membrane. Once back at the plasma membrane, the receptor can be re-stimulated with available ligand and another round or signaling can occur (McClintock and Ceresa, 2010). The question becomes: what are the properties of TGF-α that promote

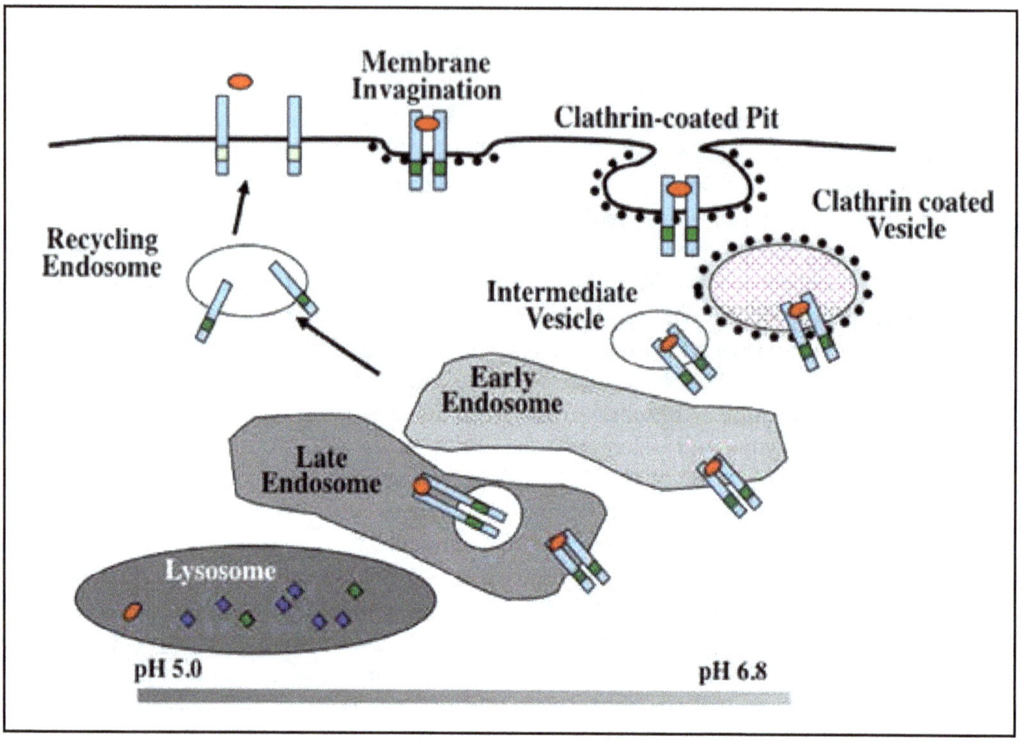

Fig. 2. Schematic of EGFR Endocytic Trafficking.

receptor recycling, whereas EGF (and others) does not? It is widely held that the difference lies in the pH sensitivity of ligand binding. Both EGF and TGF-α bind the EGFR with comparable affinity at neutral, physiological pH (pH 7.3-7.4). At pH 6.8, 50% of TGF-α will dissociate from the receptor. EGF requires a pH of 5.9 for 50% of ligand dissociation (Rutten et al., 1996). This is biologically important because the pH of the early endosome is ~6.8 (Gruenberg and Maxfield, 1995), therefore significant dissociation occurs. The loss of ligand likely converts the receptor back into a kinase-inactive conformation and is accompanied by dephosphorylation of the receptor. This would prevent association with the c-Cbl ubiquitin ligase that ubiquitylates the receptor, thereby targeting it to the lysosome for degradation.

Since EGFR endocytosis frequently culminates in the targeted destruction of the ligand:receptor complex in the lysosome, it is logical to assume this route of membrane trafficking would negatively regulate signaling. However, the role of endocytosis is more complex. Data exist that support the endocytic pathway positively regulating EGFR signaling, as well. It is clear that endocytic trafficking provides temporal regulation of receptor signaling.

4.1 Endocytosis as a negative regulator of EGFR signaling

Formal proof that endocytosis negatively regulates EGFR signaling came from the laboratory of Michael Rosenfeld (Wells *et al.*, 1990). In order to understand the role of endocytosis in signaling, Wells et al. generated mutant EGFRs that were deficient in the ability to internalize. They stably expressed these receptors in NR6 cells (derived from NIH3T3 cells) that are devoid of endogenous EGFRs. Once they established that ligand mediated endocytosis of these receptors was blocked, they examined EGF-mediated cell transformation using a colony formation assay. A dose response curve of EGF-mediated cell transformation revealed the EGFRs defective in the ability to internalize required lower doses of EGF to undergo transformation and produced more transformed cells. From these data, it was generally accepted that endocytosis is a negative regulator of EGFR signaling.

There have been numerous of additional lines of evidence to support this model, particular in cancer models. Importantly, several come from naturally occurring cancers. For instance, one common EGFR mutation, EGFRvIII, demonstrates the relationship between receptor internalization and signaling. EGFRvIII is associated with cancers of the brain, lung, prostate, and ovary. The receptor itself is a truncation mutant that is devoid of amino acids 6-273, which encompasses the ligand binding domain and dimerization arm (Wikstrand et al., 1995). Grandal et al. compared the levels of internalization and receptor phosphorylation in NR6 cells expressing either EGFRvIII or wild type EGFR (Grandal et al., 2007). While EGFRvIII can be internalized, its rate of degradation is much slower than the EGFR. These delayed kinetics correspond to prolonged signaling. While the authors do not perform a detailed analysis of signaling, there is clearly enhanced signaling based on their association with cancer.

A second example demonstrates how other ErbB family members can both delay EGFR degradation and enhance its signaling. Like the EGFR, ErbB2 is frequently overexpressed in cancers, notably breast cancers (Guerin et al., 1988). Several groups have examine how ErbB2 (and other ErbB family members) impinge on EGFR trafficking. Worthylake et al. performed a detailed biochemical characterization of EGFR ligand binding, cell surface expression, recycling and degradation with and without ErbB2 present (Worthylake et al., 1999). Using mammary epithelial cells (MTSV1 and derivative lines) as a model, they examined the EGFR and ErbB2 when the two receptors were expressed at a 9:1 and 1:1 ratio. One of their major findings was that ErbB2 inhibits the downregulation of the EGFR.

Similarly, Offterdinger and Bastiaens examined if expression of ErbB2 affected the signaling of the EGFR (Offterdinger and Bastiaens, 2008). Using Chinese Hamster Ovary (CHO) cells that express EGFRs, but low levels of ErbB2, the authors stably transfected the cells with ErbB2. Using single cell assays, the two cells line were transiently transfected with an EGFR that had been tagged with green fluorescent protein (GFP). With this model, they observed expression of ErbB2 attenuated the rate of EGFR-GFP internalization, it also prolonged the phosphorylation of the EGFR. Since kinase dead ErbB2 had similar affects on trafficking and signaling, the authors concluded that the increased phosphorylation was not due to ErbB2 kinase activity, but rather decreased EGFR degradation/phosphorylation in the presence of ErbB2.

Additionally, there are a number of cancers that have been associated with defects in the endocytic trafficking of the EGFR and other cell surface receptors. Mutations and deletions of proteins involved in trafficking have been reported to be associated with acute myeloid leukemia (AML), hepatocellular carcinomas (HCC), breast and prostate cancer (Mosesson et al., 2008). It general, these protein aberrations result in a delay in the kinetics of receptor degradation and yield a higher level of receptor signaling, consistent with endocytosis negatively regulating signaling.

4.2 Endocytosis as a positive regulator of EGFR signaling

In the last fifteen years, a second role for the endocytic pathway to regulate EGFR signaling has come to light. This secondary mechanism is the spatial regulation conferred by placing the active receptor in the same microenvironment as downstream signaling molecules (or effectors). The first evidence for this came from the laboratory of Sandra Schmid. Vieira et al, expressed a dominant negative mutant of the large guanine nucleotide-binding protein, dynamin, in HeLa cells, which prevents endocytosis of the EGFR via clathrin-coated pits. EGFR stimulation of cells expressing this dominant negative protein retains the liganded EGFRs at the plasma membrane (Vieira *et al.*, 1996). This approach removes the potential confounding effects of receptor mutagenesis or differences in expression levels in stable cell lines. The data from this study revealed that the activity from some effectors was enhanced when endocytosis blocked (EGFR phosphorylation, Shc, Grb2). Conversely, other effectors required endocytosis for maximal activity, namely, mitogen activating protein kinase (MAPK) and phosphatidyl inositol 3′-kinase (PI3K). This finding introduced the idea that endocytosis could be a positive regulator of signaling.

This finding was not without controversy. Subsequent groups reported that the expression of dominant negative dynamin inhibited MAPK activity. Thus, it was suggested that the attenuated MAPK activity was not due to a failure of the active EGFR to reach the endosome and stimulate MAPK, but rather a dynamin-dependent activation of MAPK (Johanessen et al., 2000). In addition, it has been suggested that blocking normal endocytic trafficking may affect the ligand binding properties to the EGFR (Ringerike et al., 1998).

However, since the initial report, there have been several additional lines of evidence that endocytosis provides spatial regulation to EGFR signaling. Two separate studies from the Lauffenburger's group provide compelling support. To examine the spatial regulation of EGFR:effector interactions, the authors exploited the different trafficking itineraries used by TGF-α as compared to EGF. By comparing the effects of the two ligands, they were able to alter the ratio of active EGFR at the plasma membrane and within the cell. They discovered that EGFRs at the plasma membrane preferentially activated phospholipase Cγ1 (Haugh et al., 1999b). Although these data indicate that endocytosis negatively regulates PLCγ1 activity, it also supports the idea that receptor:effector interactions are spatially regulated . Evidence that the spatial regulation of signaling is a positively regulator came from the follow-up publication. Using a similar approach, the authors were able to demonstrate that p21ras was actively activated from within the cell (Haugh et al., 1999a).

The detailed kinetic analysis performed in these studies is not trivial. One of the strengths of this work is that the signaling is studied in the context of wild type EGFRs that are expressed at the physiological concentrations receptors (Chen et al., 1996). Further, there was not perturbation of the endocytic pathway. Thus, these data likely provide the most accurate snapshot of what occurs physiologically.

Regardless of exactly how endocytic trafficking affects EGFR signaling, it is clearly an important mechanism. Understanding this process will undoubtedly generate important insights regarding the etiology of cancer and, potentially, the treatment of cancers.

4.3 Deciphering the role of endocytosis in EGFR signaling

There is plenty of direct and indirect evidence to indicate the endocytic trafficking regulates EGFR signaling, but a deeper understanding of the molecular mechanism is necessary. For instance, elucidating the molecular mechanism(s) will provide insight into how to specifically manipulate the pathway and modulate signaling as desired. There are a number of fundamental questions that need to be answered. Does endocytosis regulate EGFR signaling spatially, temporally, or both? Are the regulatory processes unique for individual cells and tissues? Do variations in receptor expression (as often occur in cancers) affect the regulation?

Temporal regulation of signaling refers to the duration of signaling, and would be consistent with endocytosis serving strictly as a negative regulator. How this might occur is not entirely clear. There has been much speculation in the literature whether this occurs by: 1) promoting receptor dephosphorylation, thereby eliminating its ability to interact with downstream effectors, 2) sequestration into the intraluminal vesicles of the late endosome/multivesicular body which prevents interactions with cytosolic effector proteins, or 3) degradation of the receptor. Alternatively, it may be that a combination of the three events (or possibly others) may contribute to signal attenuation.

In contrast, if endocytosis provides spatial regulation to signaling, it could either positively or negatively regulate signaling, depending of the effector protein and its subcellular location. Spatial regulation suggests the co-localization of the receptor and effector. Since this could occur at any point along the pathway (*i.e.* plasma membrane, early endosome, late endosome), its effect on signaling could be positive or negative. If receptor:effector communication is occurring at the plasma membrane, then endocytosis negatively regulate those interactions; conversely, receptor:effector interaction at intracellular locales, such as the early endosome, would be positively regulated by endocytosis.

It is important to note that the model of spatial regulation of EGFR signaling is predicated on the fact that there is compartmentalization of effector proteins. Only if an effector is concentrated at a given subcellular locale will endocytosis be able to confer specificity. If an effector is ubiquitously expressed throughout the cell, either in normal or pathological conditions, then spatial regulation cannot be achieved. This is an important consideration when examining cancer cells with aberrant protein expression. The unregulated signaling may be a consequence of lost spatial regulation of signaling.

As mentioned above, it cannot be ruled out that the endocytic pathway plays both positive and negative roles, depending on the effector. In fact, such a model may help explain the diversity in the cell biology that can be mediated by the receptor. For instance, signals that promote cell migration may be negatively regulated by endocytosis whereas those that control cell proliferation may require endocytosis.

Understanding the contribution of the endocytic pathway to EGFR signaling has important implications for a number of reasons. First, it will reveal the fundamental mechanisms of cell surface receptor signaling. It is likely this regulatory process is not unique to the EGFR or receptor tyrosine kinases. Thus, understanding this regulatory process has implications for other cell surface receptors and may guide the development of novel therapeutic agents for diseases other than cancer. Second, understanding the molecular mechanisms that regulate EGFR signaling will provide potentially useful clues to how the EGFR contributes to the pathology that underlies many cancers. These findings may provide new insights into the causes and potential prevention of cancer. Finally, the intricacies of signaling need to be appreciated in order to develop novel therapeutics that target the EGFR. Currently, the EGFR inhibitors (antibodies and tyrosine kinase inhibitors) are only effective against a subset of EGFR-positive cancers. A better of understanding of EGFR signaling will aid in the targeted design of therapeutics for a broader spectrum of cancers.

5. Strategies for deciphering the role of endocytic trafficking in EGFR signaling

Membrane trafficking and signal transduction are two very dynamic processes. Studying these events in real time has proven difficult. As a result, most investigators use a strategy of disrupting endocytic trafficking or at least dramatically slowing it, and determining how signaling is affected. To this end, investigators have relied heavily on two fundamentally different strategies: mutagenesis of the receptor itself or perturbation of the endocytic pathway. Here we discuss the basic components of these strategies and the strengths and weaknesses of each approach.

5.1 Receptor mutagenesis to inhibit EGFR endocytic trafficking

Endocytosis-deficient, mutant EGFRs allows one to examine the EGFR directly, without disrupting proteins that are also used by other receptors that share the endocytic pathway. Therefore, the effects seen in response to EGF treatment are truly from the EGFR and do not represent a change in the fundamental properties of the cell. One technical limitation to this approach is that in order to accurately study two different receptor populations (*i.e.* wild type and an endocytosis-deficient mutant), the two receptors need to be stably expressed in cells that are devoid of the EGFRs. First, all cell line are not amenable to stable transfection, therefore the repertoire of cell lines can be limited. Second, in making stable cell lines, it is difficult to control the level of protein expression. Differences in receptor expression will affect the total level of activated receptor in response to ligand as well as number of effectors that are activated downstream. Thus, it could be hard to determine if the difference in signaling reflect changes in endocytic trafficking or receptor expression. Finally, as with all mutagenesis strategies, there is the potential that mutation of the receptor inhibits one function (such as endocytosis), there will an unexpected change in another (for instance, signaling).

In addition to the technical limitations to using mutant EGFRs, there is an even greater biological limitation. The molecular mechanisms the regulate EGFR endocytic trafficking are complex and multi-faceted. Despite the EGFR being arguably the most studied receptor in the field of endocytic trafficking, there are constantly new mechanisms of internalization being identified. Often newly discovered mechanisms are redundant with a previously identified mechanisms. The multiple mechanisms for regulating internalization are consistent with the notion EGFR endocytosis is critical to the proper function of the cell.

The complexity of EGFR endocytosis is illustrated by a recent study by Goh et al. (Goh et al., 2010). In this study, the authors used a combination of receptor mutagenesis and RNA interference (RNAi) to completely block EGFR endocytosis in porcine aortic endothelial (PAE) cells. PAE cells were chosen because they do not express the EGFR or any of its ErbB family members. Ultimately, the authors demonstrate that there are at least four completely redundant or partially interrelated mechanisms for EGFR endocytosis. When all four processes were targeted, the result was a signaling-capable EGFR with normal kinetics of kinase activation and tyrosine phosphorylation.

5.2 Disruption of endocytic trafficking by inhibition of stage-specific regulatory proteins

An alternative approach for understanding how the endocytic pathway affects EGFR signaling is to disrupt the machinery that guides the ligand:receptor complex through the endocytic pathway. Entry and exit from each endocytic location is highly regulated by a set of proteins that are unique for that endocytic stage. Knock down or expression of dominant negative forms of those proteins can be used to alter EGFR trafficking. For instance, as described above, internalization of the receptor is regulated by the large GTPase dynamin. Expression of dominant negative dynamin (Damke et al., 1994) or knock down of dynamin expression by RNAi (Huang et al., 2004) prevents EGFR endocytosis.

It should be noted that there are several proteins that are required for the internalization of the EGFR. Expression of dominant negative mutants or knock down of many of these proteins of proteins will impair the kinetics of EGFR endocytosis. For instance, work by the Sorkin laboratory has shown that knock down of clathrin heavy chain, Grb2, and dynamin II will all cause a decrease in EGFR endocytosis to some extent (Huang *et al.*, 2004). Further, since each step along the endocytic pathway is regulated by a variety of small molecular weight G-proteins, endosomal sorting complex required for transport (ESCRT), and adaptor proteins, the activity and expression of these proteins can also be targeted to inhibit intracellular trafficking. Considerable work has been done analyzing how the RAB family of proteins contributes to EGFR trafficking; therefore modulation of RAB expression or activity can alter movement of the receptor into and out of various endocytic compartments (Ceresa, 2006).

While this approach eliminates the complications like variable levels of receptor expression and potential conformational changes in the receptor, there are other caveats. First, many of the proteins used to regulate EGFR endocytic trafficking are shared with other receptors. Therefore, knocking down at protein to prevent EGFR endocytosis, will likely affect the internalization of other receptors. This likely will not be a problem if the focus is on receptor:effector communication, because the basal activity can be established by examining cells in the absence of an EGFR ligand. However, the analysis of whole cell physiology may be more complex, depending on what receptors are present in the cell, their basal activity, and the cell physiology that is being examined. Second, one must keep in mind that disrupting endocytic trafficking, only inhibits the kinetics of the pathway. It is not an absolute block. Therefore, receptors may accumulate at one endocytic stage, but in all likelihood, still be able to proceed to the next compartment, albeit at a dramatically slowed rate.

The third issue is more likely to be a problem. Disrupting endocytic trafficking can alter the steady-state distribution of the receptor . It is often under appreciated that the EGFR internalizes in the absence of ligand, albeit at a much slower rate than in the presence of ligand. Approximately, 2-3% of the EGFR constitutively internalizes every minute. Following internalization, these unliganded receptors recycle back to the plasma membrane (Herbst *et al.*, 1994).

The cause of unliganded EGFR internalization has not been determined experimentally, but may reflect receptors that spontaneously form an "active" conformation in the absence of ligand or receptors that randomly localize to a clathrin enriched membrane domain as the clathrin-coated pit forms. While the molecular determinants guiding unliganded receptors to internalize is not fully understood, it is clear that unliganded and liganded EGFRs trafficking through the same endocytic machinery. Therefore, when the endocytic trafficking is disrupted, receptors that constitutively internalize will accumulate within the endocytic pathway where the block is in place. This may, or may not, affect the total number of EGFRs in the cell. However, it has been shown for mutants of RAB5 to change the amount of cell surface EGFR (Dinneen and Ceresa, 2004).

This caveat is particularly important when using strategies that block receptor internalization (*i.e.* knock down of dynamin, clathrin heavy chain, Grb2), as an increase in cell surface receptors may result. In this case, one would need to be cautious when enhanced signaling is observed to determine whether it is the result of the block in endocytosis or increased number of ligand:receptor complexes. Similarly, if reagents were used to block

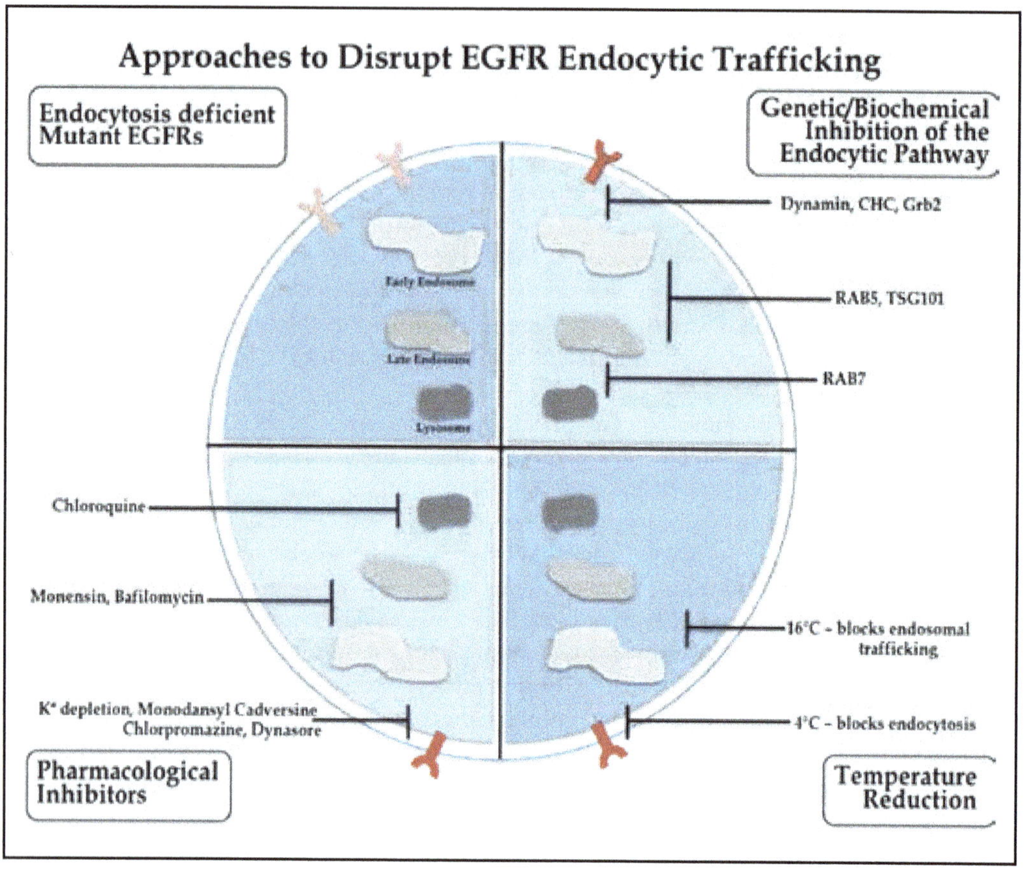

Fig. 3. Summary of Different Strategies Used to Study the Relationship between EGFR Endocytic Trafficking and Signaling.

endocytic trafficking within the cell (*i.e.* knock down of RAB5, RAB7, or TSG101), there may be an intracellular accumulation of receptors and a decrease in cell surface receptors. Under this scenario, the challenge is to understand whether decreases in signaling are due to the endocytic trafficking or decreased ligand:receptor complexes.

5.3 Pharmacological inhibitors of the endocytic machinery

Pharmacological inhibitors of the endocytic pathway offer an alternative strategy for studying EGFR endocytic trafficking. There are a limited number of such agents available. To date, these compounds have been primarily used for studying endocytic trafficking. Only recently have they been used to study how trafficking affects signal transduction.

As with most aspects of the endocytic pathway, the knowledge and reagents are greatest at the plasma membrane and decrease as one progresses to the lysosome. This is true for pharmacological inhibitors as well. At the plasma membrane, there are a number of pharmacological options available. One of the earliest strategies was intracellular potassium depletion. Work by Larkin et al. demonstrated that depletion of intracellular potassium reduced the formation of clathrin-coated pits and dramatically reduce low density lipoprotein internalization (Larkin et al., 1983). This strategy is particularly attractive because the technique is relatively easy to perform and the endocytic inhibition is readily reversible. Since that report, other agents have been used including, chlorpromazine (inhibitor of clathrin assembly/disassembly) (Feugaing et al., 2007), monodansyl cadversine (Ray and Samanta, 1996), and most recently the dynamin inhibitor, dynasore (Hill et al., 2009).

One of the most well described inhibitors of intracellular trafficking is the ionophore, monensin. Monensin functions by inhibiting early endosome acidification. When monensin-treated cells are incubated with EGF, the receptor accumulates in the early endosome, and rates of receptor degradation and recycling are dramatically reduced (King, 1984). A similar drug, bafilomycin, disrupts trafficking in a similar manner (Presly et al., 1997). Intracellular endocytic trafficking can also be inhibited by the anti-malarial drug, chloroquine. Due to its properties as a weak base, it accumulates in the lysosome and inhibits trafficking to that compartment (Anderson et al., 1984).

5.4 Temperature reduction to inhibit endocytic trafficking

Membrane trafficking is temperature dependent. Exploiting this property can be a useful, non-invasive strategy for disrupting endocytic trafficking. Carrying out experiments at 4°C will effectively reduce all endocytosis, whereas a 16°C incubation prevents movement out of the early endosome. Both inhibitions are reversible by restoring cells to physiological temperatures (37°C). Further, temperature reduction is readily applicable to all cells.

Many of the same advantages of pharmacological inhibitors are seen with temperature reduction. The effects on membrane trafficking are rapid and reversible, which minimizes the changes in the steady-state distribution of the receptor. The biggest disadvantage is in studying EGFR-signaling. Most receptor:effector communication is temperature dependent. While receptor:effector interactions would likely still occur at lower temperature (although it would take longer to reach steady-state), the kinetics of activation would be altered, thereby making the interpretation of signaling difficult.

As with most of cell biology, the best approach is multiple approaches. Complementing receptor mutagenesis and endocytic inhibitors will provide the strongest case that differences in signaling are due to changes in trafficking.

6. Ligand based strategies for studying EGFR endocytosis

Given the limitations of using a receptor based and a cell-based strategies, an alternative approach is to use a modified ligand to disrupt trafficking. An emerging strategy is to conjugate EGF (or another EGFR ligand) to an immobilized matrix. For instance, EGF can be covalently bound to polystyrene beads that are too large to internalize or a tissue culture dish. This strategy allows the ligand to bind and activate the receptor, but the conjugated matrix (polystyrene bead or tissue culture dish) physically impedes receptor internalization.

There are several advantages to this approach. First, there is no limitation to what EGFR-expressing cell type can be studied. This is particularly important since often times cell lines that are good models for studying EGFR endocytic trafficking are not good models for studying receptor signaling. In addition, previous methods favored the used of cell lines that are receptive to the introduction of cDNA, siRNA, and viral transduction. Second, since the endocytic inhibitor affects only liganded receptors, a homogenous population of

Approach	Advantages	Disadvantages
Endocytosis Deficient, Mutant EGFR	• Specific for the EGFR	• Requires stable cell line • Difficulty getting comparable receptor numbers • Numerous endocytic processes
Biochemical/Genetic Disruption of Endocytic Machinery	• Can examine endogenous receptors at physiological levels • Can examine an array of endocytic locations	• Other cell surface receptors are affected • Can change the steady-state distribution of EGFRs • Difficult to define endocytic compartments
Pharmacological Inhibitors	• Act Quickly • Can Use in a range of cell lines	• Questions of specificity on endocytic location • Disrupt trafficking of multiple receptors
Temperature Reduction	• Act Quickly • Can Use in a range of cell lines	• Disrupt trafficking of multiple receptors • Decreases Receptor and Effector enzyme activity
Tethered Ligands	• Can Use in a range of cell lines • Specific for activated EGFR	• May select for high affinity receptors

Table 1. Advantages and Disadvantages to Various Methods for Studying EGFR Endocytic Trafficking.

receptors is being examined, and there are no concerns that some receptors have escaped the endocytic inhibition. Finally, since the endocytic inhibitor is the ligand, there are no changes in the steady-state distribution of the receptor or compensatory mechanisms developed by the cell.

The use of EGF-beads has some limitations as well. First, by design, the EGF-beads have multiple molecules of EGF bound to them. Therefore, there could be multiple ligand:receptor interactions with one EGF-bead. While this will not likely affect the kinetics of ligand association, the increased stability may affect the kinetics of ligand dissociation. This may affect the duration of ligand binding. Second, it is unknown how the conjugation process affects ligand binding and subsequent biological activity. As illustrated in Figure 4, the EGF molecule is conjugated to a carboxylate modified polystyrene bead via zero length crosslinker. Depending on which amino group is the site of conjugation that may affect the ability of the ligand to bind to the receptor. Although all studies using modified EGF clearly demonstrate at least some of the immobilized ligand retains its biological activity, it is not always clear to what extent. Finally, the bead itself has unintended consequences. While the large physical size of the bead provides a means for blocking entry through clathrin-coated pits, it may also sterically hinder the formation of EGF:EGFR complexes within a subdomain of the cell.

At this point it is difficult to discern which issues are theoretical and which are practical. From a biochemical perspective, we attempted to circumvent these issues by comparing

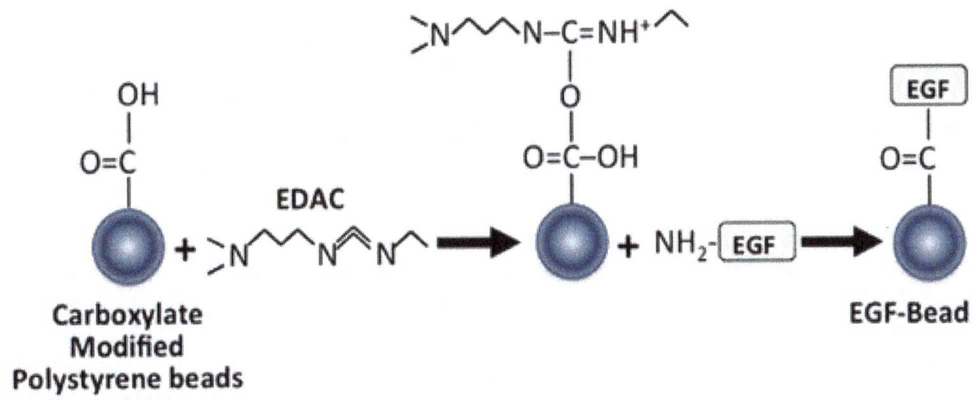

Fig. 4. Schematic of the Synthesis of EGF-beads. 900 nm polystyrene beads modified with carboxylate groups are reacted with 1-Ethyl-3-[3-dimethylaminopropyl]carbodiimide hydrochloride (EDAC) to form an active O-acylisourea intermediate that readily couples to the terminal amino group in EGF (Verveer *et al.*, 2000).

cells that had comparable levels of EGFR phosphorylation. Therefore, the basis for comparison was activated receptors at the cell surface (stimulated by EGF-beads) or within the cell (EGF stimulated).

6.1 Studying of EGFR-mediated cell signaling with immobilized EGF

The initial studies with immobilized EGF were not designed to study differences in EGFR signaling from the plasma membrane as compared to inside the cell. They were designed to understand how signaling was propagated at the plasma membrane. A study by Verveer et al. demonstrated that a liganded EGFR could propagate phosphorylation along the plasma membrane to other EGFRs that were not bound to a ligand (Verveer *et al.*, 2000).

The authors of this study used a microscopy-based assay that allowed the measure of receptor phosphorylation in real time. Briefly, cells expressing a green fluorescence protein (GFP)-tagged EGFR were microinjected with a Cyanine 3 (Cy3) labeled anti-phosphotyrosine antibody. When the receptor is phosphorylated, the anti-phosphotyrosine antibody binds and places the Cy3 in close enough proximity (nanometers) to the GFP conjugated to EGF for fluorescent energy transfer (FRET). From these studies, it was concluded that both soluble EGF and EGF-beads could propagate signaling along the plasma membrane of cells.

Secondary to the authors intent, this study demonstrated that EGF-beads could: 1) bind to the EGFR and 2) be retained at the plasma membrane. In addition to the insights about EGFR signal propagation provided by this study, it also provided an important foundation for future studies analyzing the temporal and spatial basis of EGFR signaling.

A second study using EGF-beads, also took a single cell approach (Kempiak *et al.*, 2003). The goal of this study was to assess the localized signaling of the EGFR using chemotaxis as the physiological readout. The authors demonstrate that EGF beads, like EGF, can induce a chemotactic response as visualized by video microscopy. Further, cell surface receptors could initiate the cell migration by triggering cytoskeletal reorganization as measured by staining with rhodamine phalloidin. The authors examined selected signaling pathways and found that phosphorylation of Akt was about three time greater following treatment with EGF-beads as compared to EGF.

It is worth re-stating that the goal of these two studies was not to distinguish cell surface versus intracellular EGFR signaling. Rather, both studies set up out to examine localized EGFR signals initiated from the plasma membrane. Therefore, they provide important information regarding cell surface receptor signaling, but are limited in what they reveal about what occurs within the cell.

6.2 Using EGF immobilized to a solid support to study EGFR-mediated cell migration

Although the EGF-beads are a useful way to study EGFR from the plasma membrane, variations on this theme have proven useful as well. Most notably, EGF that has been immobilized to the bottom of tissue culture dishes has proven to be an effective tool in studying cell migration. Bioengineering groups seeking to develop new methods for drug delivery performed these studies. Although EGFR is closely associated with the development of cancer, it has also been shown to be instrumental in wound healing and tissue homeostasis as well. Thus, cancer biologists should take notice of these engineering studies, as the tools developed for *in vitro* models of wound healing may provide important mechanistic insights into EGFR-mediated changes in cell biology and well as useful tools for studying the fundamental cell biology of the EGFR.

Early studies by Chen et al. used covalently linked EGF to a polystyrene dish using photo irradiation. Briefly, EGF was coupled with N-(4-azidobenzoyloxy)succinimide and the resulting solution was coated on a polystyrene dish, and the water was allowed to evaporate. Ultraviolet light was used to crosslink the modified EGF to the dish (Chen *et al.*, 1997).

To test the new ligand, Chinese Hamster Ovary (CHO) cells or mouse fibroblasts were plated on top of the immobilized EGF and monitored for cell growth by ^{3}H-thymidine incorporation. The rate of cell growth was approximately three fold higher with the immobilized EGF as compared to soluble EGF.

A modification of this approach was used by Stefonek and Masters (Stefonek and Masters, 2007). While these authors used the same basic model of immobilizing EGF to the bottom of a tissue culture dish, they did so with a concentration gradient. Using photo-patterning, precise control of the spatial localization of the EGF was achieved. Human keratinocytes (HaCaT cells) were plated on this EGF matrix and monitored for cell migration over the course of 16 days. These studies demonstrated that cells migrated toward the higher concentrations of immobilized EGF. Migration was approximately five fold greater than the control conditions. Both groups considered their findings to support the model that endocytosis negatively regulates EGFR signaling. Restricting endocytosis, prevents receptor degradation, and prolongs signaling, thereby enhancing cell migration.

Our understanding of EGFR signaling is enhanced by these studies for several reasons. First, in both studies with immobilized EGF are looking at EGFR-mediated responses in large populations of cells, rather than events in one cell. In doing so, these studies lay the groundwork for providing a biochemical analysis of changes in signaling. Second, they examine changes in cell biology that are of interest to a cancer biologist. Cell migration and proliferation are two key EGFR-mediated signaling events that need to be attenuated in the successful treatment of cancer. Finally, as bioengineering groups, the authors introduce the biologists to ways of modifying ligands in a manner that does not compromise their biologic activity.

However, in terms of understanding the spatial and temporal regulation of signaling, these studies are limited in their scope. These studies provide evidence, at least in these physiological assays that indicate endocytosis is a negative regulator of signaling. This finding supports the original report by Wells et al, in which mutant, endocytosis resistant EGF were more potent and efficacious activator of cell transformation (Wells *et al.*, 1990). However, it is not clear from these experiments whether all signaling pathways are enhanced or just a subset. Further, since all physiological responses being analyzed are enhanced, it is unclear whether some responses are positively regulated by endocytosis.

6.3 A biochemical analysis of EGFR signaling using EGF-beads

Work done by Hyatt and Ceresa combined the flexibility of EGF-beads with the biochemical analysis provided by immobilized EGF, to analyze EGFR signaling (Hyatt and Ceresa, 2008). This study, in contrast to the previous ones, specifically seeks to understand 1) whether EGFR signaling was spatially regulated, and 2) if so, how? Thus, in this work, the authors used EGF-beads to stimulate cells and examined cell physiology in response to activated EGFRs at the plasma membrane and within the cell.

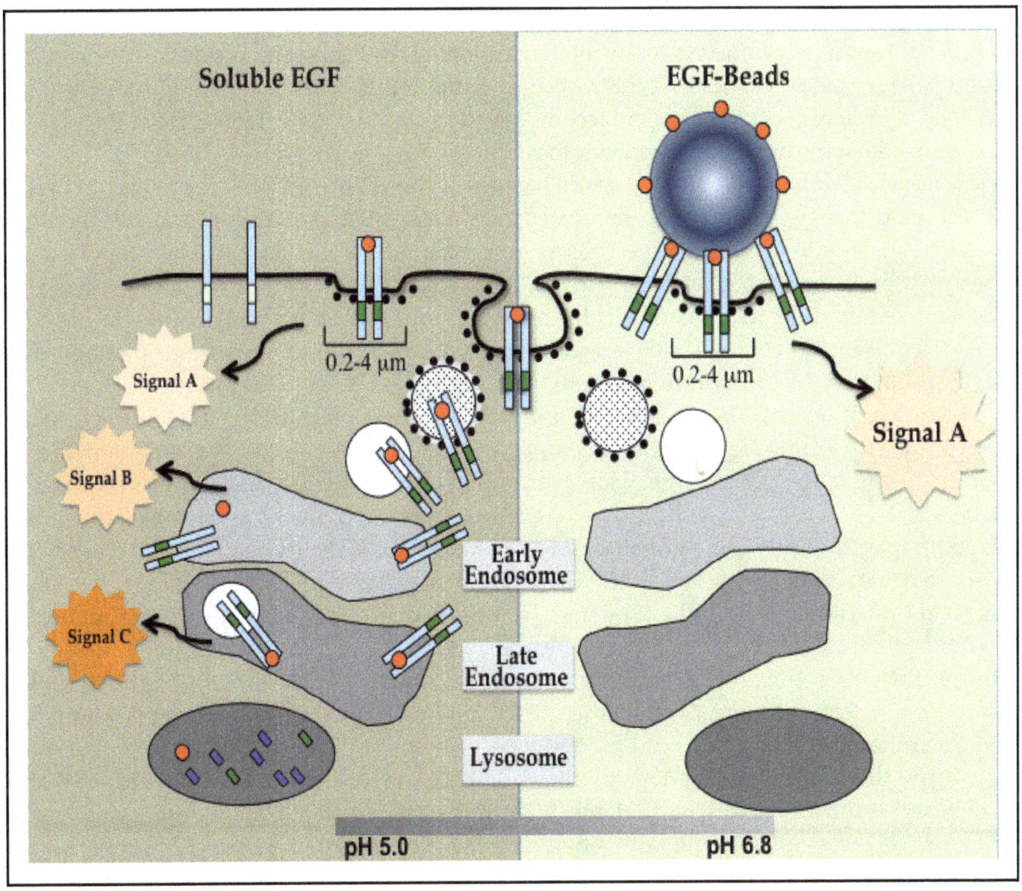

Fig. 5. Depiction of How Soluble EGF and EGF-beads elucidate Differences in EGFR Signaling.

MDA-MB-468 cells were used to study signaling by cell surface and intracellular receptors. MDA-MB-468 cells were first described by Cailleau et al, as part of a series of metastatic breast cancer cell lines derived at the MD Anderson Cancer Center in Houston, Texas (Cailleau *et al.*, 1978). Cell lines derived from metastatic breast cancer tumors were examined for common features as well as for developing model systems for studying the cell biology of transformed cells. Despite a number of similarities, each cell line has some unique features. In the case of the MDA-MB-468 cells, one of its distinguishing features is the overexpression of EGFR. It is reported that MDA-MB-468 cells express ~ 1.3 x 10^6 EGFRs/cell (Filmus *et al.*, 1985). This is about 15-25 times what is regarded as a physiological level of receptors (50-100,000 EGFRs/cell).

The high level of EGFRs makes it amenable for studying the spatial regulation of signaling for a number of reasons. First, the high levels of receptors provide a dynamic range of response following stimulation with ligand. This increases the signal-to-noise ratio. Second, cell lines with high levels of EGFR have slowed kinetics of endocytic trafficking. This has been demonstrated both in cell lines that naturally overexpress EGFR (*i.e.* cancer cell lines), as well as cells that have by stably transfected with receptors to increase their expression (French et al., 1994; Stoscheck and Carpenter, 1984). It is commonly held that the delay in trafficking is the result of saturation of the machinery that moves the ligand:receptor complex through the endocytic pathway. Regardless of the cause, the absence of appreciable receptor degradation facilitates analyzing the spatial regulation of signaling. In MDA-MB-468 cells, any changes signaling that accompany retaining the activated EGFR at the plasma membrane must be due to the receptor's location.

In this paper, the first apparent difference in signaling by EGF and EGF-beads was a change in cell morphology. Cells were incubated with either ligand and examined by light microscopy. The differences in the cells were readily apparent. As had been reported by numerous other groups, treatment with EGF caused the induction of apoptosis that was characterized by the transition of cells from spread-out cobblestone morphology to one that was rounded up. In contrast, cell treated with EGF-beads, maintained a morphology that was indistinguishable from untreated cells.

It is worth noting that EGF-mediated apoptosis is not is something that is commonly associated with EGFR signaling in the context of developmental biology, maintenance of healthy tissue, or cancer biology. However, among cell lines that overexpress the EGFR, such as MDA-MB-468 cells and A431 cells, EGF-mediated apoptosis has been well described (Armstrong et al., 1994; Gill and Lazar, 1981; Kottke et al., 1999; Tikhomirov and Carpenter, 2004). Further, indirect evidence for the role of apoptosis in cancer biology has been suggested by Tikhomirov and Carpenter. They note that in the literature, more moderate levels of ErbB receptor tyrosine kinases are associated with more invasive carcinomas. They suggest that the induction of apoptosis in cell lines with higher levels of ErbB receptor expression generates a cancer cell whose growth and metastasis is self limiting (Tikhomirov and Carpenter, 2004).

Of course, the easiest explanation for the differences in cell survival following EGF and EGF-bead treatment would be that the EGF-beads were not adequately stimulating the receptor. This was tested using both single cell and biochemical approaches. A time course of EGF-bead stimulation resulted in cells with anti-phosphoEGFR staining along the plasma membrane of the cell. This is evidence that 1) the EGFR was activated and 2) the EGFR was retained at the plasma membrane, two key features of the EGF-beads if a meaningful analysis of signaling is to be made. Further, when cell lysates were prepared from EGF-beads treated dishes of cells, a comparable level of EGFR phosphorylation was observed as seen with treatment with soluble EGF.

These data provide evidence that endocytosis is required for the induction of apoptosis, however, it does not determine whether distinct signals are occurring at the plasma membrane. To answer this question, the authors measured cell proliferation as a function of ^{3}H-thymidine incorporation. In cells treated with soluble EGF, there was a dose dependent decrease in ^{3}H-thymidine incorporation, which likely reflects the fact that the cells are undergoing apoptosis in response to EGF. Cells treated with EGF-beads had an approximately three-fold increase in ^{3}H-thymidine incorporation.

In addition, the authors demonstrate that intracellular, but not cell surface, EGFRs activate the caspase-3, an executioner caspase in the apoptotic pathway. Further, inhibition of caspase-3 prevents the induction of apoptosis, but does not enhance the proliferative effects of the cell surface EGFRs.

Together, these data provide evidence that cell surface and intracellular EGFRs, not only signal differently, but the induce reciprocal effects. Often such reciprocal effects indicate an important regulatory mechanism in biology. This work stimulates a number of important questions. Can the induction of the EGFR-mediated apoptosis be engineered into a therapeutic treatment for cancer? What are the effector proteins being activated at the cell surface versus inside the cell? How are these differences in signaling manifest in cell lines with physiological levels of receptors?

7. Future studies in the temporal and spatial regulation of EGFR signaling

Over the last approximately 25 year, the complex relationship between EGFR signaling and membrane trafficking has been increasingly exposed. While it is widely accepted that endocytic trafficking can both positively and negatively regulate EGFR signaling, it remains unclear exactly to what extent. The field has faced technical limitations that accompany studying two dynamic processes. Further, since both processes branch out into multiple directions, the complexity increases. Through normal, physiological membrane trafficking, the EGFR can be found on the plasma membrane, in endosomes, lysosomes, the nucleus, and endoplasmic reticulum. Similarly, the activated EGFR can signal to multiple downstream effectors. Therefore, identifying which signaling events occur at which subcellular locations is anything but a trivial undertaking.

Thus far, the most fruitful approaches have been ones that have attempted to disrupt or at least dramatically slow down endocytic trafficking. The myriad approaches have been discussed in this chapter. Essentially, these approaches allow the investigator to take a snapshot of signaling. Despite the caveats of such approaches, to date, it has proven to be the most effective strategy.

Although tremendous progress has been made, it appears that we have only begun to understand how these processes come together much more needs to be done. For example, a more comprehensive map of EGFR:effector communication at the cell surface and within the cell. Definitively proving that a receptor:effector interaction occurs is a major undertaking, and requires substantial experimentation to establish such a model. To date, there are only a limited number of effectors whose activity has been studied. Although many of these effectors have well-established roles in EGFR signaling, this does not preclude the need to study other effectors. Further, a systematic analysis of plasma membrane versus intracellular signaling for a large cohort of known EGFR effectors would be helpful for developing a model that predicts how receptor:effector communication occurs.

Once cell surface versus intracellular EGFR signaling is established, signaling from various locations within the cell needs to be understood. At this point, the most effective strategy is to disrupt membrane trafficking at discrete endocytic stages, despite the aforementioned caveats. Geographically, it does not seem likely that receptors in early endosomes and on the limiting membrane of the late endosome, would have access to different subsets of cytosolic effectors. However, the effectors may differentially associate with the various endocytic compartments either directly or through adaptor proteins. Together this analysis will generate a temporal and spatial map of EGFR:effector interactions that may be useful for anticipating how cell physiology is regulated.

In addition to delineating the receptor:effector interactions, another important question is whether the temporal/spatial regulation of EGFR:effector interaction is universal among all cell lines. This is a critical question because the EGFR mediates such a diverse array of physiological responses, endocytic regulation of EGFR signaling may provide important insight to explain the EGFR-dependent cell responses that are unique to a given cell line. This is particularly likely to be important in cancer cells that overexpress the EGFR. It is established that overexpression of the EGFR alters the endocytic trafficking of the EGFR and decreases the rate of receptor degradation. Since this effects both the duration and spatial placement of the activated receptor, it is reasonable to predict that there would be changes in signaling as well.

Ultimately, our goal for understanding the molecular basis of EGFR signaling is rooted in developing strategies for the pharmacological manipulation of signalling pathways. Knowing how the signaling pathways are regulated has a number of uses. First, understanding how each effector is activated will provide a better understanding of its contribution to a give cell physiology. Thus, the effector activity can be modulated downstream of the effector. Second, the endocytic pathway itself may be a useful target. Disrupting or accelerating endocytic trafficking may be sufficient to achieve desired changes in cell biology. Finally, an effort to study this regulation of signaling *in vivo* is necessary. Dissecting the *in vivo* regulation will not only help in develop anti-cancer therapeutics but also in other EGFR-mediated physiologies, such as wound healing.

8. Conclusion

Overexpression and hyperactivation of the EGFR as associated with many cancers. While inhibitors against the EGFR are effective for some EGFR-positive cancers, they are not effective in the treatment of breast cancers. In order to develop therapeutic agents to treat EGFR-positive breast cancers, a more thorough analysis of EGFR is needed, in particular, insight into how its signaling is regulated. Discussed here is the role of the endocytic pathway in controlling the duration and specificity of EGFR signaling. This field has made grade strides in understanding the relationship between the two processes. The basic science that underlies these studies has important implications in developing new tools for the detection, diagnosis, and treatment of breast cancers with elevated levels of the EGFR.

9. Acknowledgements

We apologize to our colleagues whose work was unable to be included due to space limitations. The author acknowledges support through NIH grant 1R01GM092874-01A1 and OCAST grant HR10-012.

10. References

Anderson, R.G., J.R. Falck, J.L. Goldstein, and M.S. Brown. 1984. Visualization of acidic organelles in intact cells by electron microscopy. *Proc Natl Acad Sci U S A*. 81:4838-4842.

Armstrong, D.K., S.H. Kaufmann, Y.L. Ottaviano, Y. Furuya, J.A. Buckley, J.T. Isaacs, and N.E. Davidson. 1994. Epidermal growth factor-mediated apoptosis of MDA-MB-468 human breast cancer cells. *Cancer Res*. 54:5280-5283.

Baselga, J., and C.L. Arteaga. 2005. Critical update and emerging trends in epidermal growth factor receptor targeting in cancer. *J Clin Oncol*. 23:2445-2459.

Cailleau, R., M. Olive, and Q.V. Cruciger. 1978. Long-term human breast carcinoma cell lines of metastatic origin: preliminary characterization. *In Vitro*. 14:911-915.

Cameron, D., M. Casey, C. Oliva, B. Newstat, B. Imwalle, and C.E. Geyer. 2010. Lapatinib plus capecitabine in women with HER-2-positive advanced breast cancer: final survival analysis of a phase III randomized trial. *Oncologist*. 15:924-934.

Ceresa, B.P. 2006. Regulation of EGFR endocytic trafficking by rab proteins. *Histol Histopathol*. 21:987-993.

Chen, G., Y. Ito, and Y. Imanishi. 1997. Photo-immobilization of epidermal growth factor enhances its mitogenic effect by artificial juxtacrine signaling. *Biochim Biophys Acta*. 1358:200-208.

Chen, P., J.E. Murphy-Ullrich, and A. Wells. 1996. A role for gelsolin in actuating epidermal growth factor receptor-mediated cell motility. *J Cell Biol*. 134:689-698.

Damke, H., T. Baba, D.E. Warnock, and S.L. Schmid. 1994. Induction of Mutant Dynamin Specifically Blocks Endocytic Coated Vesicle Formation. *J Cell Biol*. 127:915-934.

Dawson, J.P., M.B. Berger, C.C. Lin, J. Schlessinger, M.A. Lemmon, and K.M. Ferguson. 2005. Epidermal growth factor receptor dimerization and activation require ligand-induced conformational changes in the dimer interface. *Mol Cell Biol*. 25:7734-7742.

Dinneen, J.L., and B.P. Ceresa. 2004. Constitutive activation of rab5 results in a ligand independent redistribution of the EGFR and attenuates its ability to signal. *Traffic*. 5:606-615.

Feugaing, D.D., R. Tammi, F.G. Echtermeyer, H. Stenmark, H. Kresse, M. Smollich, E. Schonherr, L. Kiesel, and M. Gotte. 2007. Endocytosis of the dermatan sulfate proteoglycan decorin utilizes multiple pathways and is modulated by epidermal growth factor receptor signaling. *Biochimie*. 89:637-657.

Filmus, J., M.N. Pollak, R. Cailleau, and R.N. Buick. 1985. MDA-468, a human breast cancer cell line with a high number of epidermal growth factor (EGF) receptors, has an amplified EGF receptor gene and is growth inhibited by EGF. *Biochem Biophys Res Commun*. 128:898-905.

French, A.R., G.P. Sudlow, H.S. Wiley, and D.A. Lauffenburger. 1994. Postendocytic Trafficking of Epidermal Growth Factor-Receptor Complexes is Mediated through Saturable and Specific Endosomal Interactions. *J Biol Chem*. 269:15749-15755.

Gill, G.N., and C.S. Lazar. 1981. Increase phosphotyrosine content and inhibition of proliferation in EGF-treated A431 cells. *Nature*. 293:305-307.

Goh, L.K., F. Huang, W. Kim, S. Gygi, and A. Sorkin. 2010. Multiple mechanisms collectively regulate clathrin-mediated endocytosis of the epidermal growth factor receptor. *J Cell Biol*. 189:871-883.

Grandal, M.V., R. Zandi, M.W. Pedersen, B.M. Willumsen, B. van Deurs, and H.S. Poulsen. 2007. EGFRvIII escapes down-regulation due to impaired internalization and sorting to lysosomes. *Carcinogenesis*. 28:1408-1417.

Gruenberg, J., and F.R. Maxfield. 1995. Membrane Transport in the endocytic pathway. *Curr Opin Cell Biol*. 7:552-563.

Guerin, M., M. Barrois, M.J. Terrier, M. Spielmann, and G. Riou. 1988. Overexpression of either c-myc or c-erbB-2/neu proto-oncogenes in human breast carcinomas: correlation with poor prognosis. *Oncogene Res*. 3:21-31.

Harris, R.C., E. Chung, and R.J. Coffey. 2003. EGF Receptor ligands. *Exp Cell Res*. 284:2-13.

Haugh, J.M., A.C. Huang, H.S. Wiley, A. Wells, and D.A. Lauffenburger. 1999a. Internalized epidermal growth factor receptors participate in the activation of p21(ras) in fibroblasts. *J Biol Chem*. 274:34350-343560.

Haugh, J.M., K. Schooler, A. Wells, H.S. Wiley, and D.A. Lauffenburger. 1999b. Effect of epidermal growth factor receptor internalization on regulation of the phospholipase C-gamma1 signaling pathway. *J Biol Chem*. 274:8958-8965.

Herbst, J.J., L.K. Opresko, B.J. Walsh, D.A. Lauffenburger, and H.S. Wiley. 1994. Regulation of Postendocytic Trafficking of the Epidermal Growth Factor Receptor through Endosomal Retention. *J Biol Chem*. 269:12865-12873.

Hill, T.A., C.P. Gordon, A.B. McGeachie, B. Venn-Brown, L.R. Odell, N. Chau, A. Quan, A. Mariana, J.A. Sakoff, M. Chircop, P.J. Robinson, and A. McCluskey. 2009. Inhibition of dynamin mediated endocytosis by the dynoles--synthesis and functional activity of a family of indoles. *J Med Chem*. 52:3762-3773.

Huang, F., A. Khvorova, W. Marshall, and A. Sorkin. 2004. Analysis of clathrin-mediated endocytosis of epidermal growth factor receptor by RNA interfernce. *J Biol Chem*. 279:16657-16661.

Hyatt, D.C., and B.P. Ceresa. 2008. Cellular localization of the activated EGFR determines its effect on cell growth in MDA-MB-468 cells. *Exp Cell Res*. 314:3415-3425.

Hynes, N.E., and G. MacDonald. 2009. ErbB receptors and signaling pathways in cancer. *Curr Opin Cell Biol*. 21:177-184.

Johanessen, L.E., T. Ringerike, J. Molnes, and I.H. Madshus. 2000. Epidermal growth factor receptor efficiently activates mitogen-activated protein kinase in HeLa cells and HepG2 cells conditionally defective in clathrin-dependent endocytosis. *Exp Cell Res*. 260:136-145.

Jorissen, R.N., F. Walker, N. Pouliot, T.P.J. Garrett, C.W. Ward, and A.W. Burgess. 2003. Epidermal Growth Factor Receptor: Mechanisms of Activation and Signalling. *Exp Cell Res*. 284:31-53.

Kempiak, S.J., S.-C. Yip, J.M. Backer, and J.E. Segall. 2003. Local signaling by the EGF receptor. *J Cell Biol*. 162:781-787.

King, A.C. 1984. Monensin, like methylamine, prevents degradation of 125I-epidermal growth factor, causes intracellular accumulation of receptors and blocks the mitogenic response. *Biochem Biophys Res Commun*. 124:585-591.

Kottke, T.J., A.L. Blajeski, L.M. Martins, P.W. Mesner Jr., N.E. Davidson, W.C. Earnshaw, D.K. Armstrong, and S.H. Kaufmann. 1999. Comparison of Paclitaxel-, 5-Fluoro-2'-deoxyuridine-, and Epidermal Growth Factor (EGF)-induced Apoptosis. *J Biol Chem*. 274:15927-15936.

Larkin, J.M., M.S. Brown, J.L. Goldstein, and R.G. Anderson. 1983. Depletion of intracellular potassium arrests coated pit formation and receptor-mediated endocytosis in fibroblasts. *Cell*. 33:273-285.

Liao, H.J., and G. Carpenter. 2007. Role of the Sec61 translocon in EGF receptor trafficking to the nucleus and gene expression. *Mol Biol Cell*. 18:1064-1072.

Luetteke, N.C., T.H. Qiu, S.E. Fenton, K.L. Troyer, R.F. Riedel, A. Chang, and D.C. Lee. 1999. Targeted inactivation of the EGF and amphiregulin genes reveals distinct roles for

EGF receptor ligands in mouse mammary gland development. *Development*. 126:2739-2750.

Masui, H., L. Castro, and J. Mendelsohn. 1993. Consumption of EGF by A431 cells: evidence for receptor recycling. *J Cell Biol*. 120:85-93.

Matsui, Y., S.A. Halter, J.T. Holt, B.L. Hogan, and R.J. Coffey. 1990. Development of mammary hyperplasia and neoplasia in MMTV-TGF alpha transgenic mice. *Cell*. 61:1147-1155.

McClintock, J.L., and B.P. Ceresa. 2010. Transforming Growth Factor-α (TGF-α) Enhances Corneal Epithelial Cell Migration by Promoting EGFR Recycling. *Inv Opth Vis Sci*. doi:10.1167/iovs.09-4386.

Miettinen, P.J., J.E. Berger, J. Meneses, Y. Phung, R.A. Pedersen, Z. Werb, and R. Derynck. 1995. Epithelial immaturity and multi-organ failure in mice lacking epidermal growth factor receptor. *Nature*. 376:337-341.

Mosesson, Y., G.B. Mills, and Y. Yarden. 2008. Derailed endocytosis: an emerging feature of cancer. *Nat Rev Cancer*. 8:835-850.

Nicholson, R.I., J.M. Gee, and M.E. Harper. 2001. EGFR and cancer prognosis. *Eur J Cancer*. 37 Suppl 4:S9-15.

Offterdinger, M., and P.I. Bastiaens. 2008. Prolonged EGFR signaling by ERBB2-mediated sequestration at the plasma membrane. *Traffic*. 9:147-155.

Presly, J.F., S. Mayor, T.E. McGraw, K.W. Dunn, and F.R. Maxfield. 1997. Bafilomycin A1 treatment retards transferrin receptor recycling more than bulk membrane recycling. *J Biol Chem*. 272:13929-13936.

Ray, E., and A.K. Samanta. 1996. Dansyl Cadaverine regulates ligand induced endocytosis of interleukin-8 receptor in human polymorphonuclear neutrophils. *FEBS Lett*. 378:235-239.

Ringerike, T., E. Stang, L.E. Johanessen, D. Sandnes, F.O. Levy, and I.H. Madshus. 1998. High-affinity binding of epidermal growth factor (EGF) to EGF receptor is disrupted by overexpression of mutant dynamin (K44A). *J Biol Chem*. 273:16639-16642.

Roepstorff, K., M.V. Grandal, L. Henriksen, S.L. Knudsen, M. Lerdrup, L. Grovdal, B.M. Willumsen, and B. van Deurs. 2009. Differential Effects of EGFR Ligands on Endocytic Sorting of the Receptor. *Traffic*.

Rowinsky, E.K. 2004. The erbB Family: Targets for Therapeutic Develpment Against Cancer and Therapeutic strategies Using Monoclonal Antibodies and Tyrosine Kinase Inhibitors *Ann Rev of Med*. 55:433-457.

Rutten, M.J., P.J. Dempsey, C.A. Luttropp, M.A. Hawkey, B.C. Sheppard, R.A. Crass, C.W. Deveney, and R.J. Coffey, Jr. 1996. Identification of an EGF/TGF-alpha receptor in primary cultures of guinea pig gastric mucous epithelial cells. *Am J Physiol*. 270:G604-612.

Sandgren, E.P., N.C. Luetteke, T.H. Qiu, R.D. Palmiter, R.L. Brinster, and D.C. Lee. 1993. Transforming growth factor alpha dramatically enhances oncogene-induced carcinogenesis in transgenic mouse pancreas and liver. *Mol Cell Biol*. 13:320-330.

Sibilia, M., and E.F. Wagner. 1995. Strain-dependent epithelial defects in mice lacking the EGFR. *Science*. 269:234-238.

Stefonek, T.J., and K.S. Masters. 2007. Immobilized gradients of epidermal growth factor promote accelerated and directed keratinocyte migration. *Wound Repair Regen*. 15:847-855.

Stoscheck, C.M., and G. Carpenter. 1984. Down regulation of epidermal growth factor receptors: direct demonstration of receptor degradation in human fibroblasts. *J Cell Biol.* 98:1048-1053.

Threadgill, D.W., A.A. Dlugosz, L.A. Hansen, T. Tennenbaum, U. Lichti, D. Yee, C. LaMantia, T. Mourton, K. Herrup, R.C. Harris, and et al. 1995. Targeted disruption of mouse EGF receptor: effect of genetic background on mutant phenotype. *Science.* 269:230-234.

Tikhomirov, O., and G. Carpenter. 2004. Ligand-induced, p38-dependent Apoptosis in Cells Expressing High Levels of Epidermal Growth Factor Receptor and ErbB-2. *J Biol Chem.* 279:12988-12996.

Tullo, A.B., B. Esmaeli, P.I. Murray, E. Bristow, B.J. Forsythe, and K. Faulkner. 2005. Ocular findings in patients with solid tumour treated with the epidermal growth factor receptor tyrosine kinase inhibitor gefitinib ('Iressa', ZD1839) in Phase I and II clinical trials. *Eye.* 19:729-738.

Uberall, I., Z. Kolar, R. Trojanec, J. Berkovcova, and M. Hajduch. 2008. The status and role of ErbB receptors in human cancer. *Exp Mol Pathol.* 84:79-89.

Vanlandingham, P.A., and B.P. Ceresa. 2009. Rab7 regulates late endocytic trafficking downstream of multivesicular body biogenesis and cargo sequestration. *J Biol Chem.* 284:12110-12124.

Verveer, P.J., F.S. Wouters, A.R. Reynolds, and P.I.H. Bastiaens. 2000. Quantitative Imaging of Lateral ErbB1 Receptor Signal Propagation in the Plasma Membrane. *Science.* 290:1567-1570.

Vieira, A.V., C. Lamaze, and S.L. Schmid. 1996. Control of EGF Receptor Signaling by Clathrin-Mediated Endocytosis. *Science.* 274:2086-2089.

Wang, Y.N., H. Yamaguchi, J.M. Hsu, and M.C. Hung. 2010. Nuclear trafficking of the epidermal growth factor receptor family membrane proteins. *Oncogene.* 29:3997-4006.

Wells, A., J.B. Welsh, C.S. Lazar, H.S. Wiley, G.N. Gill, and M.G. Rosenfeld. 1990. Ligand-Induced Transformation by a Noninternalizing Epidermal Growth Factor Receptor. *Science.* 247:962-964.

Wikstrand, C.J., L.P. Hale, S.K. Batra, M.L. Hill, P.A. Humphrey, S.N. Kurpad, R.E. McLendon, D. Moscatello, C.N. Pegram, C.J. Reist, and et al. 1995. Monoclonal antibodies against EGFRvIII are tumor specific and react with breast and lung carcinomas and malignant gliomas. *Cancer Res.* 55:3140-3148.

Worthylake, R., L.K. Opresko, and H.S. Wiley. 1999. ErbB-2 amplification inhibits down-regulation and induces constitutive activation of both ErbB-2 and epidermal growth factor receptors. *J Biol Chem.* 274:8865-8874.

Zhang, G., S. Basti, and L.M. Jampol. 2007. Acquired trichomegaly and symptomatic external ocular changes in patients receiving epidermal growth factor inhibitors: case reports and a review of literature. *Cornea.* 26:858-860.

9

Roles of SWI/SNF Complex Genes in Breast Cancer

Esra Gunduz[1], Mehmet Gunduz[2],
Bunyamin Isik[3] and Omer Faruk Hatipoglu[4]
[1]*Departments of Medical Genetics, School of Medicine, Fatih University, Ankara,*
[2]*Departments of Medical Genetics and Otolaryngology, School of Medicine, Fatih University, Ankara*
[3]*Department of Family Medicine, School of Medicine, Fatih University, Ankara*
[4]*Department of Molecular Biology and Biochemistry, Graduate School of Medicine, Dentistry and Pharmaceutical Sciences, Okayama*
[1,2,3]*Turkey*
[4]*Japan*

1. Introduction

Cancer is a multifactorial genetic disease which is characterized by uncontrolled proliferation of the cells. Cells undergo mutational changes in a multistep process. Cancer developes from a tumor clone though the firstly mutated cell doesn't present all the features of a cancer cell. Accumulation of the mutations lead cells to display the properties of the cancer. The proliferating cells which have the capacity to survive and invade result in hyperplasia followed by dysplasia and invasion and metastasis at the end [1].
Breast cancer is the most common cancer type and one of the leading cause of cancer mortality in women. Various factors including estrogens and its signaling, EGFR signaling pathway, other oncogenes and tumor suppressor genes including chromatin remodeling factors contribute to development of breast cancer.

At molecular level two major group of genes are responsible for cancer development. These genes, proto- oncogenes and tumor suppressor genes (TSG) control cell growth together in cells at a balance. They are normally required for cell survival and have a direct role in carcinogenesis and cancer progression. When the balance is broken between oncogenes and TSGs due to activation of proto-oncogene or inactivation tumor suppressor genes, cancer develops (**Figure 1, 2**).

In cellular functions proto-oncogenes serve as growth factors, growth factor receptors, transcription factors and signal transduction elements. The mutated proto-oncogenes are named as oncogenes. An oncogene, when mutated or altered, contributes to conversion of a normal cell into a cancer cell. The activation of a proto-oncogene may occur during replication; by a translocation; by gene amplification or by the alterations in mRNA expression. TSGs are also normal cellular genes taking part in regulation of the cell cycle,

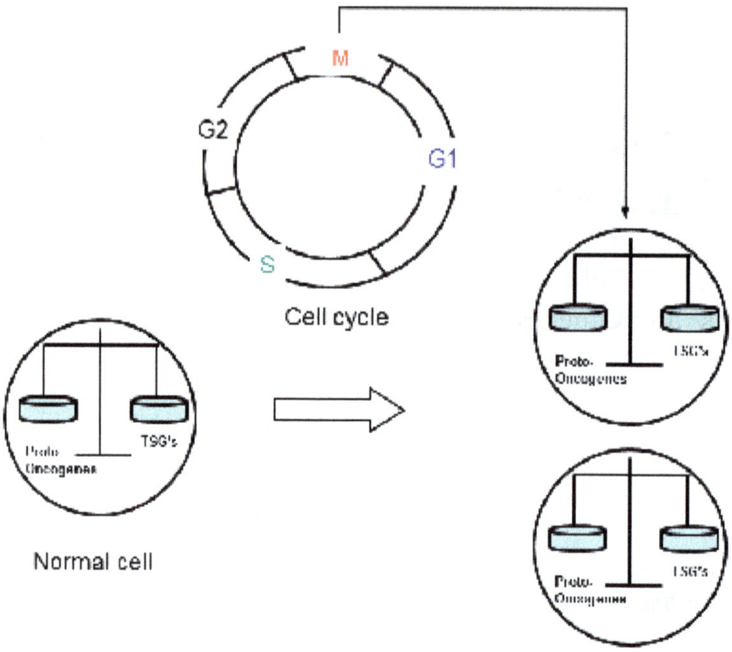

Fig. 1. In human cells proto-oncogenes and tumor suppressor genes are at a balance. There exists a controlled cell division and proliferation.

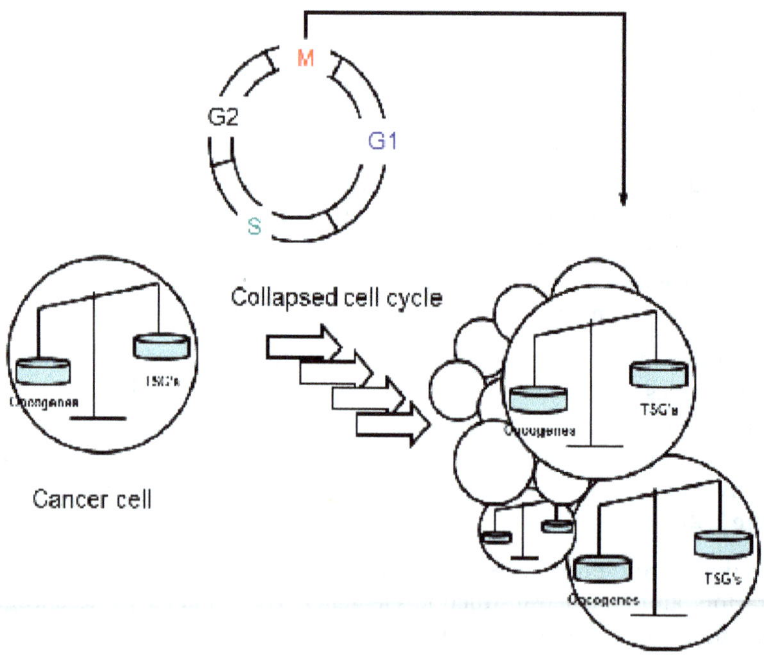

Fig. 2. In a cancer cell, over expression of oncogenes (activation) or low expression of TSGs (inactivation) leads cells to uncontrolled proliferation.

apoptosis, differentiation, surveillance of genomic integrity and repair of DNA errors, chromatin remodeling, signal transduction, and cell adhesion. The activation of the oncogenes and the inactivation of tumor suppressor genes lead cells to proliferate in an uncontrolled manner. Usually one mutation is sufficient for the activation mechanism of oncogenes whereas two hits are necessary for the inactivation of tumor suppressor genes [2,3]. However, a new class of tumor suppressor gene, in which one of the alleles is lost while the rest allele is kept, has recently been defined. Such a tumor suppressor gene is called as haploinsufficient and supposed to be in a cancer-prone state [4-6]. These patients develop cancer when they are exposed to the various carcinogens such as smoking, x-ray and chemicals.

In eukaryotic cells, genetic information encoded by DNA is packaged into chromatin and kept in the nucleus. Thus chromatin is composed of DNA and proteins. The primary proteins of chromatin are histones. A nucleosome, basic unit of chromatin, consists of 146 base-pairs of duplex DNA wrapped around a histone octamer composed of two of each of the conventional histone proteins: H2A, H2B, H3 and H4. Another histon, H1, provides compaction of neighboring nucleosomes by linking them. These compact situation of chromatin reversibly changes in an open and closed situation by various molecules such as histon acetyl transferases (HAT), histon deacetyl transferases (HDAC) and chromatin remodeling molecules, which then influence on transcriptional regulation of gene expression through accesibility of transcription factors by these molecules.

Transcription is an important step to control gene expression from the very early step of life to the end. To maintain transcription every human cell has to deal with the step of an access to DNA either through histone acetylases or chromating remodelling complexes. Many activator proteins of transcription use both of these mechanisms. Histone Acetyl Transferases (HATs) add acetyl groups to the tails of the histones that protrude out of nucleosomes which lead to the binding of the transcription factors. Chromatin remodeling complexes use ATP to open or close the chromatin (**Figure 3**).

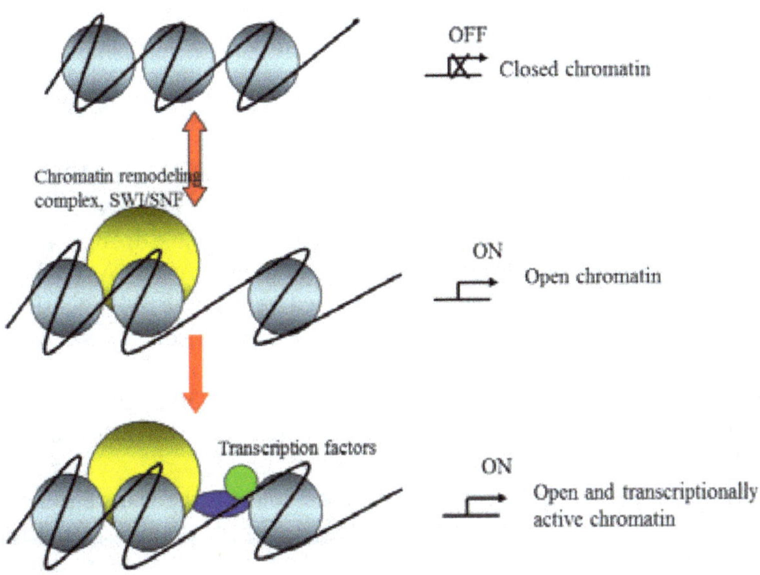

Fig. 3. The binding of chromatin remodeling complex changes conformationally closed chromatin to open chromatin that enables the transcription factors to bind and start transcription.

By cooperation of members of these two classes of complexes, the structure of chromatin is dynamically regulated and thus they play important roles in the control of gene expression. ATP-dependent chromatin remodelers are divided into families according to the subunit composition and biochemical activity such as SWI/SNF, ISWI, INO80, SWR1 and NURD/Mi2/CHD complexes. Of these in particular, some of the members SWI/SNF complexes are emerging tumor suppressors, as genetic and epigenetic inactivation events in several SWI/SNF subunits have been detected in various human cancers [7-10].

2. Function of SWI/SNF family members

Transcription factor action and then the targeted gene expression are mainly regulated by SWI/SNF family of chromatin remodeling complexes. SWI/SNF complexes are large 2-MDa (1.14 MDa in yeast) multi-subunit conglomerates that are involved in either enhancement or suppression of the downstream genes [7-12]. SWI/SNF complex genes were identified through two screens in yeast Saccharomyces cerevisiae. The first identified gene that is required for the expression of SUC2 for sucrose metabolism (sucrose non-fermenting (SNF) mutants), and the second screen showed another gene required for the activation of HO for mating-type switching (switch (SWI) mutants [7, 13-15].

SWI/SNF complex is composed of three groups of subunits; 1) enzymatic (ATPase), 2) core subunits, and 3) accessory subunits [8,11]. Though the exact mechanisms for modification of chromatin structure by SWI/SNF complexes remain incompletely understood, current knowledge suggests that ATPase-dependent disruption of histone-DNA association and resultant nucleosome "sliding" is the main mechanism [8,12]. The mammalian genome encodes 29 different SWI/SNF-like ATPases [12]. Accordingly, each SWI/SNF complex consists of only one of two ATPases, BRM (Brahma) or BRG1 (Brahma-Related Gene 1), which show 74% homology.

SWI/SNF complexes are classified into two major classes as BAF (BRG1 or BRM-Associated Factor; also known as SWI/SNF-A) or PBAF (Polybromo-Associated BAF; also known as SWI/SNF-B) complexes (**Figure 4**). BAF complexes contain either BRG1 (also known as SMARCA4, SNF2b, BAF190) or BRM (also known as SMARCA2, SNF2a) and PBAF complexes include only BRG1 as ATPase subunit. Each ATPase is accompanied with 10 to 12 proteins as core and accessory subunits. The core subunits include BAF155 (also known as SWI3, SRG3, SMARC1), BAF170 (also known as SMARCC2), and SNF5 (also known as SMARCB1, BAF47, INI1). Accessory subunits consist of BAF45 (a,b,c,d; encoded gene names PHF10, DPF1, DPF2, DPF3), BAF53 (a,b; encoded gene names ACTL6A, ACTL6B), BAF57 (encoded gene name SMARCE1), BAF60 (a,b,c; encoded gene name SMARCD1, SMARCD2, SMARCD3), BAF180 (encoded gene name PBRM1), BAF200 (encoded gene name ARID2), BRD7 and BAF250 (a,b; a: also known as ARID1A, SMARCF1, OSA1; b: also known as ARID1B, OSA2) [7,8]. ARID1A (BAF250a) and ARID1B (BAF250b) subunits are mutually exclusive and exist only in BAF complexes. BAF180, BAF200 and BRD7 are exclusively present in PBAF complexes [7,8] [**Figure 4**].

SWI/SNF complexes were found to be based on their roles in the transcription activation. However, studies show that mammalian SWI/SNF complexes have function to both repression and activation of the targeted genes. For development of mammalian T lymphocyte, BRG1 and BAF57 are necessary both for silencing CD4 and activating CD8 expression [7,16,17]. Specific combinations of individual SWI/SNF components were reported to generate sub-complexes with specialized functions that are involved in

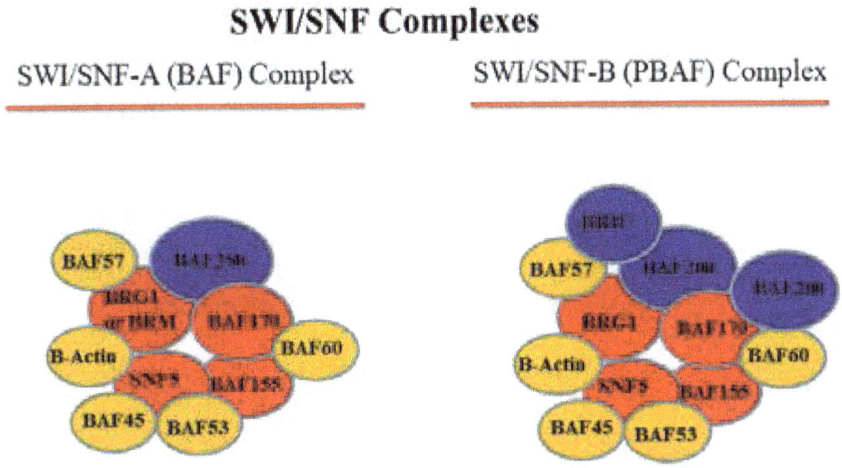

Fig. 4. SWI/SNF complexes are classified into two major classes as BAF (SWI/SNF-A) or PBAF (SWI/SNF-B) complexes. BAF complexes contain either BRG1 or BRM and PBAF complexes include only BRG1 as ATPase subunit. The core subunits include BAF155, BAF170, and SNF5. Accessory subunits consist of BAF45, BAF53, BAF57, BAF60, BAF180, BAF200, BRD7 and BAF250. BAF250a and BAF250b subunits are mutually exclusive and exist only in BAF complexes. BAF180, BAF200 and BRD7 are exclusively present in PBAF complexes.

sequential stages of muscle-gene activation--i.e., initial displacement of the nucleosome followed by the loading of the complete myogenic transcriptosome that promotes gene transcription [18]. Immunoprecipitation analysis of osteocalcin promoter showed that BRM- and BRG1-containing complexes have different roles on it. BRG1 complexes were associated with the promoter induction, while BRM-specific complexes were present only on the repressed promoter and were required for association of the co-repressor HDAC1 [19]. In embryonic stem (ES) cells, BRG1 was reported to act as a repressor to inhibit programmes that are associated with differentiation. On the other hand, it also facilitates the expression of core pluripotency programmes [20,21]. Loss of *Snf5* in murine fibroblasts results in more genes being activated such as E2F targeted genes than repressed [22]. Another example of repression of gene expression is recruitment histone deacetylases (HDACs), which remove activating acetyl marks from histone tails, by SWI/SNF complexes. By this mechanism, SNF5 suppresses cyclin expression in an HDAC1-dependent manner [23]. In conclusion, mammalian SWI/SNF complexes are composed of dynamic units with essential roles in regulating both the activation and the repression of gene expression programmes.

3. Roles of SWI/SNF proteins in cancer

Findings of abnormalities at genetic, epigenetic as well as protein levels of SWI/SNF complexes in various cancers provide a link between chromatin remodelling and tumour suppression. Tumor suppressor role of SWI/SNF complexes was first demonstrated with loss of BRG1 and BRM expression in many cancer cell lines and arrest of growth or slower growth after introduction of BRG1 or hBRM [24]. Brg mutant mice die at early embryonic days due to growth arrest of the inner cell mass and trophoblast [25,26]. Mice with Brg 1 heterozygosity develop mammary adenocarcinomas, suggesting an occurrence of cancer prone state due to haploinsufficiency of Brg1. On the other hand, the mouse with inactivation of BRM by homologous recombination (BRM-/- mice) is born alive and develops normally. Adult mutant mice were approximately 15% heavier than control littermates. This phenomenon was suggested to be caused by increased cell proliferation, because a higher mitotic index was detected in mutant livers and it was further supported by the observation that mutant embryonic fibroblasts were significantly deficient in their ability to arrest in the G0/G1 phase of the cell cycle in response to cell confluency or DNA damage. These studies suggested that BRM plays a role in the regulation of cell proliferation in adult mice and have some defects in control of cellular proliferation [27].

Chromosome transfer studies mapped tumor suppressor gene(s) at 19p13 chromosome locus [28,29]. Studies with microsatellite analysis and functional as well as cancer tissue examination for abnormalities of candidate tumor suppressor gene indicated that chromosome 19p13 locus includes at least two putative tumor suppressor genes namely STK11/LKB1 and BRG1 [30]. STK11 maps about 8.5 Mb distally from BRG1. Loss of heterozygosity of 19p13 was reported in various cancers including thyroid cancer, sex cord stromal tumors, breast cancer, oral carcinoma, prostate cancer, pancreas carcinoma, brain tumors, colorectal carcinoma, gynecological tumors, lung cancers and ovarian carcinoma [31-46]. Some of the studies included genetic analysis of STK11/LKB1 and showed mutation in a subset of tumors especially related with Peutz-Jeugher Syndrome such as breast, colorectal, lung, pancreatic, biliary and ovarian cancer [41-49]. On the other hand, quite a lot of studies reported mutations and/or loss or various alterations of BRG1 in human cancer lines and primary tumors [50-61]. Thus genes at this chromosomal locus may involve in various type cancer exclusively or in cooperation in some cancer types. It should be also noticed that some studies showed only LOH without alteration of either one of these genes. In this situation, each of them can still be involved in carcinogenesis due to haploinsufficiency. At least haploinsufficiency of BRG1 is recognized [25-27,62], while further studies are necessary whether such a role exists for STK11/LKB1 or not. Similar to BRG1, abnormalities of BRM in various cancers have been reported [58-61,63-69].

Though the early studies of cell lines and animal models strongly suggested subunits of SWI/SNF proteins as tumor suppressor, the first definitive evidence that members of these complexes function as tumor suppressive was shown by Versteege and colleagues. They demonstrated occurrence of LOH of BAF47 (SNF5) in almost all cases of pediatric rhabdoid sarcoma, in which the other allele was mutated or silenced by methylation [70]. Inactivation of SNF5 subunit of SWI/SNF is via biallelic mutations, including deletion, nonsense, missense and frameshift mutations was also shown by other studies, supporting SNF5 as a strong tumor suppressor gene at least in this kind of tumors [71-73].

SNF5 alterations have also been shown in other types of tumors though it is much rare as compared to malignant rhabdoid tumors. In a recent study, the effects of Ini1 haploinsufficiency (loss of one allele) on cell growth and immortalization in mouse embryonic fibroblasts were examined. Their results revealed that heterozygosity for Ini1 up-regulated cell growth and immortalization and that exogenous Ini1 down-regulated the growth of primary cells in a Rb-dependent manner. Furthermore, loss of Ini1 was redundant with loss of Rb function in the formation of pituitary tumors in Rb heterozygous mice and gave rise to the formation of large, atypical Rb(+/-) tumor cells lacking adrenocorticotropic hormone expression, confirming in vivo the relationship between Rb and Ini1 in tumor suppression [74]. Mutations and alterations of SNF5 were also reported in familial schwannomatosis and other cancer types [75-84]. Germ line mutations of SNF5 were detected in brain tumors and rhabdoid tumors, suggesting its link with familial cancers [85-88]. In some other tumors, no alteration of SNF was detected [89,90].

Complete loss of Snf5 in genetically engineered mouse leads to early embryonic death. However, heterozygote mice with haploinsufficient Snf5 (snf5+/-) develop tumors similar to malignant rhabdoid tumors in about one third of the animals [91-93]. On the other hand, conditional biallelic inactivation of Snf5 (Snf5-/- mice) resulted in tumors including lymphomas and rhabdoid tumors in 100% of mice [94]. Onset of these tumors occurred in a median period of 11 weeks for a single gene inactivation. When compared to this period with most commonly mutated genes in human cancer i.e. p53 and RB1, p53 loss gave rise to lymphomas and sarcomas at 20 weeks and RB1 heterozygosity together with p53 deficiency resulted in similar tumors and other cancers at 16 weeks [95]. Thus shorter onset time for tumor occurrence in Snf5 inactivation as compared to other well-known tumor suppressors indicates strong tumor suppressor character of this gene. Tumor formation in the absence of SNF5 has been supposed to be due to loss of function of the SWI/SNF complex. However, this view has been challenged by several findings of a recent research. Using both human cell lines and mouse models, Wang et al. [96] showed that cancer formation in the absence of SNF5 does not result from SWI/SNF inactivation but rather that oncogenesis is dependent on continued presence of BRG1 activation than tumor suppressor loss. Thus Snf5 loss would lead to effects more frequently associated with oncogene activation than tumor suppressor loss.

Other than BRG1 and SNF5, alterations of other member of SWI/SNF complexes have been reported in various cancer types. For example mutations of BAF180 (PBRM1) were identified in 41% of renal cell carcinomas, making this gene as the second most frequently mutated gene in these cancers after VHL50 [97]. The ARID1A subunit of SWI/SNF complexes was also recently shown to have mutation or loss of protein in primary human cancers including ovarian clear cell carcinomas, low and high grade endometrioid carcinomas [98-101].ARID1A was also rarely mutated in medulloblastoma, breast and lung cancer [102,103].

4. Alterations and roles of SWI/SNF proteins in breast cancer

Breast cancer is among the most common tumors affecting women. It is characterized by a number of genetic aberrations. Some 5-10% of cases are thought to be inherited. Estrogen plays an important role in normal physiology and malignancy of breast tissue. Biological functions of estrogen are mediated by estrogen receptor (ER). ER controls transcription of ER targeted genes by binding to estrogen responsive elements in their promoters. ATP-dependent chromatin remodeling complexes also influence this signaling pathway by changing the chromatin open/close state. In this respect, heterozygous state of a SWI/SNF subunit, Brg1 in mice leads to mammary carcinomas, indicating roles of SWI/SNF proteins in breast cancer [25]. On the other hand, BRCA1 and BRCA2 genes are already known to have roles both in familial and sporadic breast cancers [104-106]. Breast tumors of patients with germ-line mutations in the BRCA1 and BRCA2 genes have more genetic defects than sporadic breast tumors.

Bochar et al. [107] isolated a predominant form of a multiprotein BRCA1-containing complex from human cells displaying chromatin-remodeling activity using a combination of affinity- and conventional chromatographic techniques. Mass spectrometric sequencing of components of this complex proved that BRCA1 is associated with a SWI/SNF-related complex. They also demonstrated that BRCA1 directly interacts with the BRG1 subunit of the SWI/SNF complex. Furthermore, p53-mediated stimulation of transcription by BRCA1 was completely abrogated by either a dominant-negative mutant of BRG1 or the cancer-causing deletion in exon 11 of BRCA1, revealing that BRCA1 has a direct function in transcriptional control through modulation of chromatin structure [107].

To investigate abnormalities SWI/SNF complex subunits in breast cancer, Decristofaro et al. [108] determined the protein status of the core subunits of BAF170, BAF155, BAF57, BAF53a, and BAF47 in 21 breast cancer cell lines. The authors also determined the protein status of the BRM, BRG1 as well as two other proteins found in human SWI/SNF complexes, BAF180 and BAF250. A breast cancer cell line negative for the BAF57 protein was identified [108].

Deficiency of p270 protein (ARID1A) was shown in a subset of breast cancer. BAF180, a subunit of the PBAP type SWI/SNF chromatin remodeling complex maps to 3p21, in a region where frequent allele loss has been detected in various cancers. A study which used screening for tumor suppressor genes in breast cancer revealed multiple truncating mutations of PB1, which encodes the BAF180 subunit and the mutation was associated with loss of heterozygosity of the wild-type allele [109]. Functional studies showed binding of endogenous wild-type BAF180 to the p21 promoter, which was required for proper p21 expression and G1 arrest after transforming growth factor-beta and gamma-radiation treatment, making BAF180 as a physiologic mediator of p21 expression [109].

In a study, Wang et al. [110] examined the role of BAF57 in breast cancer using the cell line, BT549, which is an invasive human breast carcinoma cell line that lacks expression of BAF57 [111]. They prepared a BT549 stable cell line with expression of the full-length BAF57 protein. The results showed that BT549 clones expressing BAF57 revealed remarkable phenotypic changes, slow growth kinetics, and restoration of contact inhibition. Moreover, microarray analysis showed that BAF57-mediated cell death was associated with up-regulation of proapoptotic genes including the tumor suppressor familial cylindromatosis (CYLD). CYLD was found to be a direct target of BAF57 by chromatin immunoprecipitation analysis. Increased expression of CYLD in BT549 cells induced apoptosis, while its suppression by small interfering RNA inhibited cell death in BAF57 expressing BT549 cells, suggesting the crucial role of BAF57 in cell growth regulation and provided a novel link between hSWI/SNF chromatin remodeling factors and apoptosis [112]. P270 subunit of SWI/SNF complexes was found to be essential for normal cell cycle arrest, providing a direct biological basis to support the implication from tumor tissue screens that deficiency of p270 plays a causative role in carcinogenesis [113]. In a separate study, BAF57 was found to be an ER subtype-selective modulator that specifically regulates ERalpha-mediated transcription, linking ER with SWI/SNF proteins [114].

Harte et al. [115] identified BRD7 as a novel binding partner of BRCA1 with a yeast two-hybrid screen using a BRCA1 bait composed of amino acids 1 to 1142. To determine the functional consequences of the BRCA1-BRD7 interaction, they examined the role of BRD7 in BRCA1-dependent transcription with microarray-based expression profiling. A variety of target genes such as ERalpha was found to be coordinately regulated by BRCA1 and BRD7 complex [115]. In a recent study, two novel mutations were found in one out of 95 breast cancer samples by sequencing BAF57 gene [116].

5. Conclusion and future aspects

Important function of subunits of SWI/SNF complexes arises from their roles in chromatin remodeling and trancription regulation. Mutation and other alterations of these proteins lead to cancer development. Researches on roles of SWI/SNF subunits in development and cancer are increasingly performed yet much work is necessary for clarifying the exact functions of these genes to provide therapy for various human cancers. Promising results are noticed at the moment for usability of some of these genes as a therapeutic and diagnostic target. Thus progress on the knowledge of functions of subunits of SWI/SNF complexes as well as the relationship with other breast cancer-related molecules such as BRCA1-2 and p53 will clarify their roles in human cancer including breast cancer, which will result in their uses in cancer diagnostics as well as therapy in near future.

6. References

Renan MJ. How many mutations are required for tumorigenesis? Implications from human cancer data. Mol Carcinog 7: 139-146, 1993

Hinds PW and Weinberg RA. Tumor suppressor genes. Curr Opin Genet Dev 4: 135-141, 1994

Knudson AG Jr. Mutation and cancer: statistical study of retinoblastoma. Proc Natl Acad Sci USA 68: 820-823, 1971

Mduff FK, Hook CE, Tooze RM, Huntly BJ, Pandolfi PP, Turner SD. Determining the contribution of NPM1 heterozygosity to NPM-ALK-induced lymphomagenesis. Lab Invest. 2011 Jun 27. doi: 10.1038/labinvest.2011.96. [Epub ahead of print]

Zhou XZ, Huang P, Shi R, Lee TH, Lu G, Zhang Z, Bronson R, Lu KP. The telomerase inhibitor PinX1 is a major haploinsufficient tumor suppressor essential for chromosome stability in mice. J Clin Invest 121(4):1266-82, 2011

Bouwman P, Drost R, Klijn C, Pieterse M, van der Gulden H, Song JY, Szuhai K, Jonkers J. Loss of p53 partially rescues embryonic development of Palb2 knockout mice but does not foster haploinsufficiency of Palb2 in tumour suppression. J Pathol 224:10- 21, 2011

Wilson BG, Roberts CW. SWI/SNF nucleosome remodellers and cancer. Nat Rev Cancer 11:481-92, 2011

Weissman B, Knudsen KE. Hijacking the chromatin remodeling machinery: impact of SWI/SNF perturbations in cancer. Cancer Res 69:8223-30, 2009

Hargreaves DC, Crabtree GR. ATP-dependent chromatin remodeling: genetics, genomics and mechanisms. Cell Res 21:396-420, 2011

Reisman D, Glaros S, Thompson EA. The SWI/SNF complex and cancer. Oncogene 28:1653-68, 2009

Wu JI, Lessard J, Crabtree GR. Understanding the words of chromatin regulation. Cell 136:200-6, 2009

Lessard J, Wu JI, Ranish JA, Wan M, Winslow MM, Staahl BT, Wu H, Aebersold R, Graef IA, Crabtree GR. An essential switch in subunit composition of a chromatin remodeling complex during neural development. Neuron 55:201-15, 2007

Neigeborn L, Carlson M. Genes affecting the regulation of SUC2 gene expression by glucose repression in Saccharomyces cerevisiae. Genetics 108:845–858, 1984

Stern M, Jensen R, Herskowitz I. Five SWI genes are required for expression of the HO gene in yeast. J Mol Biol 178:853–868, 1984

Breeden L, Nasmyth K. Cell cycle control of the yeast HO gene: cis- and trans-acting regulators. Cell 48:389–397, 1987

Chi TH, Wan M, Zhao K, Taniuchi I, Chen L, Littman DR, Crabtree GR. Reciprocal regulation of CD4/CD8 expression by SWI/SNF-like BAF complexes. Nature 418:195-9, 2002

Wan M, Zhang J, Lai D, Jani A, Prestone-Hurlburt P, Zhao L, Ramachandran A, Schnitzler GR, Chi T. Molecular basis of CD4 repression by the Swi/Snf-like BAF chromatin remodeling complex. Eur J Immunol 39:580-8, 2009

Albini S, Puri PL. SWI/SNF complexes, chromatin remodeling and skeletal myogenesis: it's time to exchange!. Exp Cell Res 316:3073-80, 2010

Flowers S, Nagl NG Jr, Beck GR Jr, Moran E. Antagonistic roles for BRM and BRG1 SWI/SNF complexes in differentiation. J Biol Chem 284:10067-75, 2009

Ho L, Ronan JL, Wu J, Staahl BT, Chen L, Kuo A, Lessard J, Nesvizhskii AI, Ranish J, Crabtree GR. An embryonic stem cell chromatin remodeling complex, esBAF, is essential for embryonic stem cell self-renewal and pluripotency. Proc Natl Acad Sci U S A 106:5181-6, 2009

Ho L, Jothi R, Ronan JL, Cui K, Zhao K, Crabtree GR. An embryonic stem cell chromatin remodeling complex, esBAF, is an essential component of the core pluripotency transcriptional network. Proc Natl Acad Sci U S A 106:5187-91, 2009

Isakoff MS, Sansam CG, Tamayo P, Subramanian A, Evans JA, Fillmore CM, Wang X, Biegel JA, Pomeroy SL, Mesirov JP, Roberts CW. Inactivation of the Snf5 tumor suppressor stimulates cell cycle progression and cooperates with p53 loss in oncogenic transformation. Proc Natl Acad Sci U S A 102:17745-50, 2005

Zhang ZK, Davies KP, Allen J, Zhu L, Pestell RG, Zagzag D, Kalpana GV. Cell cycle arrest and repression of cyclin D1 transcription by INI1/hSNF5. Mol Cell Biol 22:5975-88, 2002

Dunaief JL, Strober BE, Guha S, Khavari PA, Alin K, Luban J, Begemann M, Crabtree GR, Goff SP. The retinoblastoma protein and BRG1 form a complex and cooperate to induce cell cycle arrest. Cell 79:119-30, 1994

Bultman, S. J. Herschkowitz JI, Godfrey V, Gebuhr TC, Yaniv M, Perou CM, Magnuson T. Characterization of mammary tumors from Brg1 heterozygous mice. Oncogene 27:460–468, 2008

Bultman, S. Gebuhr T, Yee D, La Mantia C, Nicholson J, Gilliam A, Randazzo F, Metzger D, Chambon P, Crabtree G, Magnuson T. A Brg1 null mutation in the mouse reveals functional differences among mammalian SWI/ SNF complexes. Mol Cell 6:1287–1295, 2000

Reyes JC, Barra J, Muchardt C, Camus A, Babinet C, Yaniv M. Altered control of cellular proliferation in the absence of mammalian brahma (SNF2alpha). EMBO J 17:6979-91, 1998

Astbury C, Jackson-Cook CK, Culp SH, Paisley TE, Ware JL. Suppression of tumorigenicity in the human prostate cancer cell line M12 via microcell-mediated restoration of chromosome 19. Genes Chromosomes Cancer 31:143–55, 2011

Gao AC, Lou W, Ichikawa T, Denmeade SR, Barrett JC, Isaacs JT. Suppression of the tumorigenicity of prostatic cancer cells by gene(s) located on human chromosome 19p13.1–13.2. Prostate 38:46–54, 1999

Rodriguez-Nieto S, Sanchez-Cespedes M. BRG1 and LKB1: tales of two tumor suppressor genes on chromosome 19p and lung cancer. Carcinogenesis 30:547-54, 2009

Prazeres HJ, Rodrigues F, Soares P, Naidenov P, Figueiredo P, Campos B, Lacerda M, Martins TC. Loss of heterozygosity at 19p13.2 and 2q21 in tumours from familial clusters of non-medullary thyroid carcinoma. Fam Cancer 7:141-9, 2008

Kato N, Romero M, Catasus L, Prat J. The STK11/LKB1 Peutz-Jegher gene is not involved in the pathogenesis of sporadic sex cord-stromal tumors, although loss of heterozygosity at 19p13.3 indicates other gene alteration in these tumors. Hum Pathol 35:1101-4, 2004 Yang TL, Su YR, Huang CS, Yu JC, Lo YL, Wu PE, Shen CY. High-resolution 19p13.2-13.3 allelotyping of breast carcinomas demonstrates frequent loss of heterozygosity. Genes Chromosomes Cancer 41:250-6, 2004

Dumur CI, Dechsukhum C, Ware JL, Cofield SS, Best AM, Wilkinson DS, Garrett CT, Ferreira-Gonzalez A. Genome-wide detection of LOH in prostate cancer using human SNP microarray technology. Genomics 81:260-9, 2003

Sobottka SB, Haase M, Fitze G, Hahn M, Schackert HK, Schackert G. Frequent loss of heterozygosity at the 19p13.3 locus without LKB1/STK11 mutations in human carcinoma metastases to the brain. J Neurooncol 49:187-95, 2000

Oesterreich S, Allredl DC, Mohsin SK, Zhang Q, Wong H, Lee AV, Osborne CK, O'Connell P. High rates of loss of heterozygosity on chromosome 19p13 in human breast cancer. Br J Cancer 84:493-8, 2001

Connolly DC, Katabuchi H, Cliby WA, Cho KR. Somatic mutations in the STK11/LKB1 gene are uncommon in rare gynecological tumor types associated with Peutz-Jegher's syndrome. Am J Pathol 156:339-45, 2000

Gunduz E, Gunduz M, Ouchida M, Nagatsuka H, Beder L, Tsujigiwa H, Fukushima K, Nishizaki K, Shimizu K, Nagai N. Genetic and epigenetic alterations of BRG1 promote oral cancer development. Int J Oncol 26:201-10, 2005

Sentani K, Oue N, Kondo H, Kuraoka K, Motoshita J, Ito R, Yokozaki H, Yasui W. Increased expression but not genetic alteration of BRG1, a component of the SWI/SNF complex, is associated with the advanced stage of human gastric carcinomas. Pathobiology 69:315-20, 2001

Valdman A, Nordenskjöld A, Fang X, Naito A, Al-Shukri S, Larsson C, Ekman P, Li C. Mutation analysis of the BRG1 gene in prostate cancer clinical samples. Int J Oncol 22:1003-7, 2003

Sato N, Rosty C, Jansen M, Fukushima N, Ueki T, Yeo CJ, Cameron JL, Iacobuzio-Donahue CA, Hruban RH, Goggins M. STK11/LKB1 Peutz-Jeghers gene inactivation in intraductal papillary-mucinous neoplasms of the pancreas. Am J Pathol 159:2017-22, 2001

Trojan J, Brieger A, Raedle J, Esteller M, Zeuzem S. 5'-CpG island methylation of the LKB1/STK11 promoter and allelic loss at chromosome 19p13.3 in sporadic colorectal cancer. Gut 47:272-6, 2000

Nishioka Y, Kobayashi K, Sagae S, Sugimura M, Ishioka S, Nagata M, Terasawa K, Tokino T, Kudo R. Mutational analysis of STK11 gene in ovarian carcinomas. Jpn J Cancer Res 90:629-32, 1999

Wang ZJ, Churchman M, Campbell IG, Xu WH, Yan ZY, McCluggage WG, Foulkes WD, Tomlinson IP. Allele loss and mutation screen at the Peutz-Jeghers (LKB1) locus (19p13.3) in sporadic ovarian tumours. Br J Cancer 80:70-2, 1999

Gill RK, Yang SH, Meerzaman D, et al. Frequent homozygous deletion of the LKB1/STK11 gene in non-small cell lung cancer. Oncogene. 2011 May 2. [Epub ahead of print]

Papp J, Kovacs ME, Solyom S, Kasler M, Børresen-Dale AL, Olah E. High prevalence of germline STK11 mutations in Hungarian Peutz-Jeghers Syndrome patients. BMC Med Genet 11:169, 2010

Su GH, Hruban RH, Bansal RK, Bova GS, Tang DJ, Shekher MC, Westerman AM, Entius MM, Goggins M, Yeo CJ, Kern SE. Germline and somatic mutations of the STK11/LKB1 Peutz-Jeghers gene in pancreatic and biliary cancers. Am J Pathol 154:1835-40, 1999

Nakanishi C, Yamaguchi T, Iijima T, Saji S, Toi M, Mori T, Miyaki M. Germline mutation of the LKB1/STK11 gene with loss of the normal allele in an aggressive breast cancer of Peutz-Jeghers syndrome. Oncology 67:476-9, 2004

McCarthy A, Lord CJ, Savage K, Grigoriadis A, Smith DP, Weigelt B, Reis-Filho JS, Ashworth A. Conditional deletion of the Lkb1 gene in the mouse mammary gland induces tumour formation. J Pathol 219:306-16, 2009

Wong AK, Shanahan F, Chen Y, et al. BRG1, a component of the SWI-SNF complex, is mutated in multiple human tumor cell lines. Cancer Res 60:6171–7, 2000

Rodriguez-Nieto S, Cañada A, Pros E, Pinto AI, Torres-Lanzas J, Lopez-Rios F, Sanchez- Verde L, Pisano DG, Sanchez-Cespedes M. Massive parallel DNA pyrosequencing analysis of the tumor suppressor BRG1/SMARCA4 in lung primary tumors. Hum Mutat 32:E1999-2017, 2011

Schneppenheim R, Frühwald MC, Gesk S, Hasselblatt M, Jeibmann A, Kordes U, Kreuz M, Leuschner I, Martin Subero JI, Obser T, Oyen F, Vater I, Siebert R. Germline nonsense mutation and somatic inactivation of SMARCA4/BRG1 in a family with rhabdoid tumor predisposition syndrome. Am J Hum Genet 86:279-84, 2010

Bartlett C, Orvis TJ, Rosson GS, Weissman BE. BRG1 mutations found in human cancer cell lines inactivate Rb-mediated cell-cycle arrest. J Cell Physiol 226:1989-97, 2011

Medina PP, Romero OA, Kohno T, Montuenga LM, Pio R, Yokota J, Sanchez-Cespedes M. Frequent BRG1/SMARCA4-inactivating mutations in human lung cancer cell lines. Hum Mutat 29:617-22, 2008

Gunduz E, Gunduz M, Nagatsuka H, Beder L, Demircan K, Tamamura R, Hatipoglu OF, Mahmut N, Katase N, Naomoto Y, Nagai N. Epigenetic alterations of BRG1 leads to cancer development through its nuclear-cytoplasmic shuttling abnormalities. Med Hypotheses 67:1313-6, 2006

Medina PP, Carretero J, Fraga MF, Esteller M, Sidransky D, Sanchez-Cespedes M. Genetic and epigenetic screening for gene alterations of the chromatin-remodeling factor, SMARCA4/BRG1, in lung tumors. Genes Chromosomes Cancer 41:170-7, 2004. Erratum in: Genes Chromosomes Cancer. 2005 Feb;42(2):211.

Decristofaro MF, Betz BL, Rorie CJ, Reisman DN, Wang W, Weissman BE. Characterization of SWI/SNF protein expression in human breast cancer cell lines and other malignancies. J Cell Physiol 186:136–45, 2001

Fukuoka J, Fujii T, Shih JH, Dracheva T, Meerzaman D, Player A, Hong K, Settnek S, Gupta A, Buetow K, Hewitt S, Travis WD, Jen J. Chromatin remodeling factors and BRM/BRG1 expression as prognostic indicators in non-small cell lung cancer. Clin Cancer Res 10:4314–24, 2004

Reisman DN, Sciarrotta J, Wang W, Funkhouser WK, Weissman BE. Loss of BRG1/BRM in human lung cancer cell lines and primary lung cancers: correlation with poor prognosis. Cancer Res 63:560–6, 2003

Reisman DN, Strobeck MW, Betz BL, Sciariotta J, Funkhouser W Jr, Murchardt C, Yaniv M, Sherman LS, Knudsen ES, Weissman BE. Concomitant down-regulation of BRM and BRG1 in human tumor cell lines: differential effects on RB-mediated growth arrest vs CD44 expression. Oncogene 21:1196–207, 2002

Bock VL, Lyons JG, Huang XX, Jones AM, McDonald LA, Scolyer RA, Moloney FJ, Barnetson RS, Halliday GM. BRM and BRG1 subunits of the SWI/SNF chromatin remodelling complex are downregulated upon progression of benign skin lesions into invasive tumours. Br J Dermatol 164:1221-7, 2011

Glaros S, Cirrincione GM, Palanca A, Metzger D, Reisman D. Targeted knockout of BRG1 potentiates lung cancer development. Cancer Res 68:3689-96, 2008

Liu G, Gramling S, Munoz D, Cheng D, Azad AK, Mirshams M, Chen Z, Xu W, Roberts H, Shepherd FA, Tsao MS, Reisman D. Two novel BRM insertion promoter sequence variants are associated with loss of BRM expression and lung cancer risk. Oncogene. 2011 Apr 11. [Epub ahead of print]

Glaros S, Cirrincione GM, Muchardt C, Kleer CG, Michael CW, Reisman D. The reversible epigenetic silencing of BRM: implications for clinical targeted therapy. Oncogene 26:7058–66, 2007

Gunduz E, Gunduz M, Ali MA, Beder L, Tamamura R, Katase N, Tominaga S, Yamanaka N, Shimizu K, Nagatsuka H. Loss of heterozygosity at the 9p21-24 region and identification of BRM as a candidate tumor suppressor gene in head and neck squamous cell carcinoma. Cancer Invest 27:661-8, 2009

Shen H, Powers N, Saini N, et al. The SWI/SNF ATPase Brm is a gatekeeper of proliferative control in prostate cancer. Cancer Res 68:10154-62, 2008

Moloney FJ, Lyons JG, Bock VL, Huang XX, Bugeja MJ, Halliday GM. Hotspot mutation of Brahma in non-melanoma skin cancer. J Invest Dermatol 129:1012-5, 2009

Yamamichi N, Inada K, Ichinose M, et al. Frequent loss of Brm expression in gastric cancer correlates with histologic features and differentiation state. Cancer Res 67:10727-35, 2007

Strobeck MW, Reisman DN, Gunawardena RW, Betz BL, Angus SP, Knudsen KE, Kowalik TF, Weissman BE, Knudsen ES. Compensation of BRG-1 function by Brm: insight into the role of the core SWI-SNF subunits in retinoblastoma tumor suppressor signaling. J Biol Chem 277:4782-9, 2002

Versteege I, Sévenet N, Lange J, Rousseau-Merck MF, Ambros P, Handgretinger R, Aurias A, Delattre O. Truncating mutations of hSNF5/INI1 in aggressive paediatric cancer. Nature 394:203-6, 1998

Eaton KW, Tooke LS, Wainwright LM, Judkins AR, Biegel JA. Spectrum of SMARCB1/INI1 mutations in familial and sporadic rhabdoid tumors. Pediatr Blood Cancer. 56:7-15, 2011

Jackson, E. M. Sievert AJ, Gai X, Hakonarson H, Judkins AR, Tooke L, Perin JC, Xie H, Shaikh TH, Biegel JA Genomic analysis using high-density single nucleotide polymorphism-based oligonucleotide arrays and multiplex ligation-dependent probe amplification provides a comprehensive analysis of INI1/SMARCB1 in malignant rhabdoid tumors. Clin Cancer Res 15:1923–1930, 2009

Biegel, J. A. Zhou JY, Rorke LB, Stenstrom C, Wainwright LM, Fogelgren B. Germ-line and acquired mutations of INI1 in atypical teratoid and rhabdoid tumors. Cancer Res 59:74–79, 1999

Guidi CJ, Mudhasani R, Hoover K, Koff A, Leav I, Imbalzano AN, Jones SN. Functional interaction of the retinoblastoma and Ini1/Snf5 tumor suppressors in cell growth and pituitary tumorigenesis. Cancer Res 66:8076-82, 2006

Sevenet N, Lellouch-Tubiana A, Schofield D, Hoang-Xuan K, Gessler M, Birnbaum D, Jeanpierre C, Jouvet A, Delattre O. Constitutional mutations of the hSNF5/INI1 gene predispose to a variety of cancers. Am J Hum Genet 65:1342–1348, 1999

Trobaugh-Lotrario AD, Tomlinson GE, Finegold MJ, Gore L, Feusner JH. Small cell undifferentiated variant of hepatoblastoma: adverse clinical and molecular features similar to rhabdoid tumors. Pediatr Blood Cancer 52:328–334, 2009

Kohashi K, Izumi T, Oda Y, Yamamoto H, Tamiya S, Taguchi T, Iwamoto Y, Hasegawa T, Tsuneyoshi M. Infrequent SMARCB1/INI1 gene alteration in epithelioid sarcoma: a useful tool in distinguishing epithelioid sarcoma from malignant rhabdoid tumor. Hum Pathol 40:349-55, 2009

Kohashi, K. Oda Y, Yamamoto H, Tamiya S, Oshiro Y, Izumi T, Taguchi T, Tsuneyoshi M. SMARCB1/INI1 protein expression in round cell soft tissue sarcomas associated with chromosomal translocations involving EWS: a special reference to SMARCB1/INI1 negative variant extraskeletal myxoid chondrosarcoma. Am J Surg Pathol 32:1168–1174, 2008

Kreiger PA, Judkins AR, Russo PA, Biegel JA, Lestini BJ, Assanasen C, Pawel BR. Loss of INI1 expression defines a unique subset of pediatric undifferentiated soft tissue sarcomas. Mod Pathol 22:142–150, 2009

Modena P, Lualdi E, Facchinetti F, Galli L, Teixeira MR, Pilotti S, Sozzi G. SMARCB1/INI1 tumor suppressor gene is frequently inactivated in epithelioid sarcomas. Cancer Res. 65:4012–4019, 2005

Schmitz U, Mueller W, Weber M, Sévenet N, Delattre O, von Deimling A. INI1 mutations in meningiomas at a potential hotspot in exon 9. Br J Cancer 84:199-201, 2001

Lin H, Wong RP, Martinka M, Li G. Loss of SNF5 expression correlates with poor patient survival in melanoma. Clin Cancer Res 15:6404-11, 2009

Mobley BC, McKenney JK, Bangs CD, Callahan K, Yeom KW, Schneppenheim R, Hayden MG, Cherry AM, Gokden M, Edwards MS, Fisher PG, Vogel H. Loss of SMARCB1/INI1 expression in poorly differentiated chordomas. Acta Neuropathol 120:745–753, 2010

Gessi M, Giangaspero F, Pietsch T. Atypical teratoid/rhabdoid tumors and choroid plexus tumors: when genetics "surprise" pathology. Brain Pathol 13:409-1, 2003

Hulsebos TJ, Plomp AS, Wolterman RA, Robanus-Maandag EC, Baas F, Wesseling P. Germline mutation of INI1/ SMARCB1 in familial schwannomatosis. Am J Hum Genet 80:805–810, 2007

Christiaans I, Kenter SB, Brink HC, van Os TA, Baas F, van den Munckhof P, Kidd AM, Hulsebos TJ. Germline SMARCB1 mutation and somatic NF2 mutations in familial multiple meningiomas. J Med Genet 48:93-7, 2011

Bourdeaut F, Lequin D, Brugières L, et al. Frequent hSNF5/INI1 germline mutations in patients with rhabdoid tumor. Clin Cancer Res 17:31-8, 2011

Rousseau G, Noguchi T, Bourdon V, Sobol H, Olschwang S. SMARCB1/INI1 germline mutations contribute to 10% of sporadic schwannomatosis. BMC Neurol 11:9, 2011

Yamamoto H, Kohashi K, Tsuneyoshi M, Oda Y. Heterozygosity Loss at 22q and Lack of INI1 Gene Mutation in Gastrointestinal Stromal Tumor. Pathobiology 78:132-9, 2011

Mori N, Inoue K, Okada M, Motoji T. Absence of Mutations on the SNF5 Gene in Hematological Neoplasms with Chromosome 22 Abnormalities. Acta Haematol 126:69-75, 2011

Roberts CW, Galusha SA, McMenamin ME, Fletcher CD, Orkin SH. Haploinsufficiency of Snf5 (integrase interactor 1) predisposes to malignant rhabdoid tumors in mice. Proc Natl Acad Sci USA 97:13796–13800, 2000

Klochendler-Yeivin, A. Fiette L, Barra J, Muchardt C, Babinet C, Yaniv M. The murine SNF5/INI1 chromatin remodeling factor is essential for embryonic development and tumor suppression. EMBO Rep 1:500–506, 2000

Guidi, C. J. Sands AT, Zambrowicz BP, Turner TK, Demers DA, Webster W, Smith TW, Imbalzano AN, Jones SN. Disruption of Ini1 leads to peri-implantation lethality and tumorigenesis in mice. Mol Cell Biol 21:3598–3603, 2001

Roberts CW, Leroux MM, Fleming MD, Orkin SH. Highly penetrant, rapid tumorigenesis through conditional inversion of the tumor suppressor gene Snf5. Cancer Cell 2:415–425, 2002

Williams BO, Remington L, Albert DM, Mukai S, Bronson RT, Jacks T. Cooperative tumorigenic effects of germline mutations in Rb and p53. Nat Genet 7:480-4, 1994

Wang X, Sansam CG, Thom CS, Metzger D, Evans JA, Nguyen PT, Roberts CW. Oncogenesis caused by loss of the SNF5 tumor suppressor is dependent on activity of BRG1, the ATPase of the SWI/SNF chromatin remodeling complex. Cancer Res 69:8094-101, 2009

Varela I, Tarpey P, Raine K, et al. Exome sequencing identifies frequent mutation of the SWI/SNF complex gene PBRM1 in renal carcinoma. Nature 469:539-42, 2011

Wiegand KC, Lee AF, Al-Agha OM, Chow C, Kalloger SE, Scott DW, Steidl C, Wiseman SM, Gascoyne RD, Gilks B, Huntsman DG. Loss of BAF250a (ARID1A) is frequent in high-grade endometrial carcinomas. J Pathol 224:328-33, 2011

Guan B, Mao TL, Panuganti PK, Kuhn E, Kurman RJ, Maeda D, Chen E, Jeng YM, Wang TL, Shih IeM. Mutation and loss of expression of ARID1A in uterine low- grade endometrioid carcinoma. Am J Surg Pathol 35:625-32, 2011

Wiegand KC, Shah SP, Al-Agha OM et al. ARID1A mutations in endometriosis-associated ovarian carcinomas. N Engl J Med 363:1532–1543, 2010

Jones, S. Wang TL, Shih IeM, et al. Frequent mutations of chromatin remodeling gene ARID1A in ovarian clear carcinoma. Science 330:228–231, 2010

Parsons, D. W. Li M, Zhang X, et al. The Genetic Landscape of the Childhood Cancer Medulloblastoma. Science 331:435–439, 2011

Huang J, Zhao YL, Li Y, Fletcher JA, Xiao S. Genomic and functional evidence for an ARID1A tumor suppressor role. Genes Chromosom Cancer 46:745–750, 2007

Wang F, Fang Q, Ge Z, Yu N, Xu S, Fan X. Common BRCA1 and BRCA2 mutations in breast cancer families: a meta-analysis from systematic review. Mol Biol Rep. 2011 Jun 4. [Epub ahead of print]

Nanda R. Targeting" triple-negative breast cancer: the lessons learned from BRCA1-associated breast cancers. Semin Oncol 38:254-62, 2011

Milne RL, Antoniou AC. Genetic modifiers of cancer risk for BRCA1 and BRCA2 mutation carriers. Ann Oncol Suppl 1:i11-7, 2011

Bochar DA, Wang L, Beniya H, Kinev A, Xue Y, Lane WS, Wang W, Kashanchi F, Shiekhattar R. BRCA1 is associated with a human SWI/SNF-related complex: linking chromatin remodeling to breast cancer. Cell 102:257-65, 2000

Decristofaro MF, Betz BL, Rorie CJ, Reisman DN, Wang W, Weissman BE. Characterization of SWI/SNF protein expression in human breast cancer cell lines and other malignancies. J Cell Physiol 186:136-45, 2001

Wang X, Nagl NG Jr, Flowers S, Zweitzig D, Dallas PB, Moran E. Expression of p270 (ARID1A), a component of human SWI/SNF complexes, in human tumors. Int J Cancer 112:636, 2004

Xia W, Nagase S, Montia AG, Kalachikov SM, Keniry M, Su T, Memeo L, Hibshoosh H, Parsons R. BAF180 is a critical regulator of p21 induction and a tumor suppressor mutated in breast cancer. Cancer Res 68:1667-74, 2008

Kiskinis E, García-Pedrero JM, Villaronga MA, Parker MG, Belandia B. Identification of BAF57 mutations in human breast cancer cell lines. Breast Cancer Res Treat 98:191-8, 2006

Wang L, Baiocchi RA, Pal S, Mosialos G, Caligiuri M, Sif S. The BRG1- and hBRM-associated factor BAF57 induces apoptosis by stimulating expression of the cylindromatosis tumor suppressor gene. Mol Cell Biol 25:7953-65, 2005

Nagl NG Jr, Patsialou A, Haines DS, Dallas PB, Beck GR Jr, Moran E. The p270 (ARID1A/SMARCF1) subunit of mammalian SWI/SNF-related complexes is essential for normal cell cycle arrest. Cancer Res 65:9236-44, 2005

García-Pedrero JM, Kiskinis E, Parker MG, Belandia B. The SWI/SNF chromatin remodeling subunit BAF57 is a critical regulator of estrogen receptor function in breast cancer cells. J Biol Chem 281:22656-64, 2006

Harte MT, O'Brien GJ, Ryan NM, Gorski JJ, Savage KI, Crawford NT, Mullan PB, Harkin DP. BRD7, a subunit of SWI/SNF complexes, binds directly to BRCA1 and regulates BRCA1-dependent transcription. Cancer Res 70:2538-47, 2010

Villaronga MA, López-Mateo I, Markert L, Espinosa E, Fresno Vara JA, Belandia B. Identification and characterization of novel potentially oncogenic mutations in the human BAF57 gene in a breast cancer patient.Breast Cancer Res Treat. 2011 Apr 5. [Epub ahead of print]

10

Estrogen-Related Receptors and Breast Cancer

Christina T. Teng[1] and Peggy R. Teng[2]
[1]*Division of National Toxicology Program, National Institute of Environmental Health Sciences, National Institutes of Health, Durham*
[2]*Department of Experimental Pathology and Laboratory Medicine, Anderson School of Management, UCLA Alumnus, Los Angeles*
United States of America

1. Introduction

The estrogen-related receptors (ERRs) α, β and γ comprise the NR3B orphan subgroup within the nuclear receptor superfamily. Although the ERRs were identified based on their sequence homology to estrogen receptor alpha (ERα), they do not bind estrogen or any other natural hormones. Recent studies have defined the roles of ERRs in the regulation of target genes at the transcriptional level as well as their participation in a broad range of physiological functions such as energy metabolism and growth progression. The expression of ERRs has been shown to be up-regulated in advanced breast cancer cells and is considered to be a negative prognostic marker for the diagnosis of the disease. This review will cover what is currently known in regards to the gene structure of ERRs in addition to their regulation, function and relationship to breast cancer.

Breast cancer is a complicated disease with 200,000 women diagnosed in the United States each year. There are many factors that influence breast cancer development and progression with hormone and nuclear receptors playing critical roles. Several reviews have been written on the emerging roles of estrogen and nuclear receptors in breast cancer (reviews (Conzen 2008; Hayashi, Niwa et al. 2009; Riggins, Mazzotta et al. 2010)). In this review we will focus on the estrogen-related receptor alpha, beta and gamma (ERRα, β and γ). ERRα and ERRβ were the first orphan nuclear receptors to be cloned in the late 1980's (Giguere, Yang et al. 1988) with ERRγ following 10 years later (Eudy, Yao et al. 1998; Hong, Yang et al. 1999; Heard, Norby et al. 2000). Although these receptors were cloned many years ago based on their sequence homology at the DNA binding domain to estrogen receptor alpha (ERα), their biological relevance (s) has only recently been uncovered (Giguere 2008; Villena and Kralli 2008) along with potential roles in cancer, and more specifically breast cancer.

1.1 Background of nuclear receptor family

ERRs belong to the orphan nuclear receptor NR3B subfamily which do not bind to any known natural ligands and are constitutively active in transcription (Benoit, Cooney et al. 2006). Crystal structure analyses of the ERRs revealed that the AF-2 containing helix 12, essential for coactivator interaction (Nettles and Greene 2005), is in an active conformation while the ligand-binding pocket (LBP) remains empty (Greschik, Wurtz et al. 2002; Kallen, Schlaeppi et al. 2004). ERRs bind to TCAA/GGTCA elements called SFRE/ERRE and continually transactivate the target gene (Yang, Shigeta et al. 1996; Sladek, Beatty et al. 1997). While there are three members in this subfamily, both ERRβ (Zhou, Liu et al. 2006; Bombail, Collins et al. 2010) and ERRγ (Heard, Norby et al. 2000) have multiple variants that are expressed in a tissue-specific manner whereas there are no reports on variants of ERRα.

Although ERRs have high amino acid sequence homology, they are located on different chromosomes and cover a wide range of genomic space. The ESRRA gene is located at chromosome 11q13.1 (Shi, Shigeta et al. 1997) with a processed pseudogene present at 13q12.1 (Sladek, Beatty et al. 1997). It contains 7 exons and spans approximately 11 kbp genomic-space. The ESRRB gene is located at chromosome 14q24.3, has 12 exons and at least 5 variants from alternative splicing. It covers 130 kbp genomic-space ((Zhou, Liu et al. 2006; Collin, Kalay et al. 2008); Ensembl genome browser 61). The ESRRG gene spans 635 kbp genomic space, is located at chromosome 1q41 with 9 exons and 5 variants ((Eudy, Yao et al. 1998; Hong, Yang et al. 1999; Heard, Norby et al. 2000); Ensembl genome browser). A diagrammatic presentation of the relationship between ERRs and the ERs protein demonstrated that the highly conserved DNA binding domain (DBD) among the ERRs is closely related to the ERs DBD (Fig. 1). As indicated above, the ERR genes are located on different chromosomes which suggests that the gene and/or genome duplication event occurred over a long period of evolutionary time. Additionally, some of the coding exons are separated by large introns while others are clustered together.

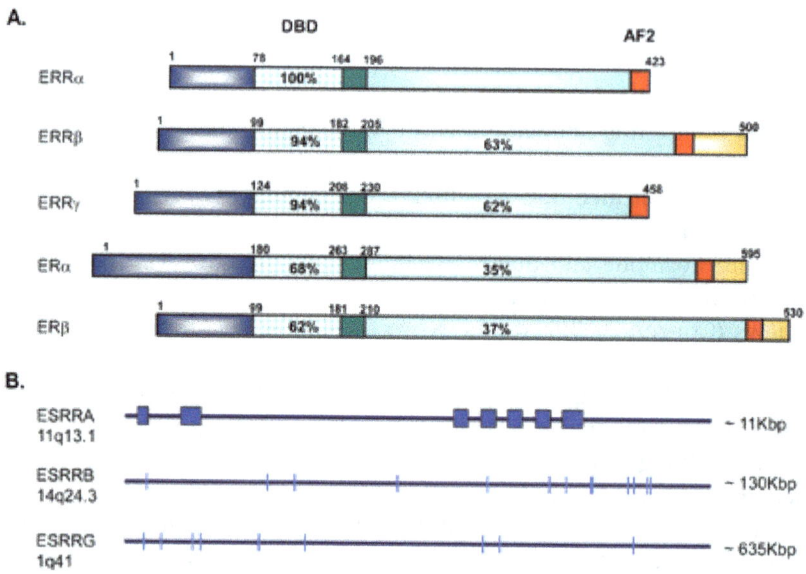

Fig. 1. A. Protein structures of the ERRs and ERs. DBD, DNA binding domain; AF2, activation function 2. Number on top indicates the amino acid position of the modular domains for the nuclear receptor. % in the box indicates the amino acid sequence homology to ERRα within the same domain. B: Gene structures of the ERRs. The size of the gene and the locations of the exons (vertical bar or box) are in approximation. Chromosome locations and the approximate gene sizes are indicated.

1.2 Expression of ERRs

Surveying the expression of all 49 nuclear receptors from 39 mouse tissues uncovered the coordination of several nuclear receptor groups with the transcriptional programs necessary to affect distinct physiologic pathways (Bookout, Jeong et al. 2006). Indeed expression of some of the nuclear receptors including the ERRs is linked to the circadian clock in key metabolic tissues suggesting their role in regulation of nutrient and energy metabolism (Horard, Castet et al. 2004; Yang, Downes et al. 2006; Giguere 2008; Villena and Kralli 2008). These studies underscore the importance of regulation and expression of nuclear receptors in normal and abnormal physiological conditions. ERRα is ubiquitously expressed in all tissues examined and is especially abundant in those with high metabolic needs such as heart, skeletal muscle and kidney (Giguere 2008). In addition, ERRα is expressed in both human and mouse embryonic stem cells (Xie, Jeong et al. 2009), during adipocyte differentiation (Fu, Sun et al. 2005) and bone morphogenesis (Bonnelye and Aubin 2002; Bonnelye, Kung et al. 2002) suggesting its roles in differentiation and development. Although expression of ERRγ is more restricted and not detectable in every tissue examined with levels that are lower than ERRα, it is still highly expressed in metabolically active tissues such as brain, skeletal muscle, heart and kidney (Zhang and Teng 2007; Giguere 2008). It was thought that ERRβ was mainly expressed in embryo (Giguere, Yang et al. 1988; Luo, Sladek et al. 1997), however as detection methods improved, ERRβ expression was found to be present in eye, brain, thyroid, kidney and the heart of adult tissues (Bookout, Jeong et al. 2006). Although ERRβ is present at lower levels as compared to ERRα and ERRγ, it also exhibited a distinct diurnal rhythmic expression much like the other two in white fat (WAT), brown fat (BAT), liver and skeletal muscle. This suggests a potential role in the coordination of oxidative metabolism in these tissues (Yang, Downes et al. 2006). The expression of ERRs in these metabolically active tissues under circadian rhythm hints to potential overlapping functions in energy metabolism.

As stated earlier, the expression level of the receptors could be closely linked to their biological function in a cell-type specific manner. This is particularly relevant for a constitutive activator since they are not regulated by the addition of ligands. Therefore the function of ERRs could be controlled by their expression level; however information regarding the mechanisms and signals that regulate their expression is limited.

1.3 Regulation of ERRs

1.3.1 Estrogen regulation of ERRs

ERRα was demonstrated to be the target gene for estrogen in the mouse uterus (Shigeta, Zuo et al. 1997) 15 years ago. Later, a combinatorial estrogen response element which can bind several nuclear receptors termed multiple hormone response element (MHRE) was identified in the human ERRα gene promoter (Liu, Zhang et al. 2003). Under the influence of estrogen, the estrogen receptor alpha (ERα), (but not the estrogen receptor beta (ERβ)) was recruited to the chromatin of the human ERRα promoter which interacted with the MHRE in an indirect tethering manner and transactivated the promoter (Liu, Zhang et al. 2003; Hu, Kinyamu et al. 2008). Surprisingly, in a similar experiment conducted with ER negative SKBR3 cells, estrogen treatment also induced chromatin modification around the MHRE region and recruited the coregulators and RNA polymerase II to the ERRα promoter (Li, Birnbaumer et al. 2010). This suggests that the ERRα gene can be regulated by estrogen in a non-ER dependent manner. Indeed, the MHRE (a 57 bp region in human and a 34 bp region) in mouse of the ERRα gene is a pleiopropic response element for multiple nuclear receptors

(Liu, Zhang et al. 2005) and also serves as the binding site for ERRα and ERRγ (Laganiere, Tremblay et al. 2004; Mootha, Handschin et al. 2004; Liu, Zhang et al. 2005). ERRγ was recently found to be responsive to estrogen, its expression able to be stimulated in a dose dependent manner. Furthermore, this response can be blocked by the pure estrogen antagonist ICI 182,780 (Ijichi, Shigekawa et al. 2011). By using chromatin immunoprecipitation (ChIP)-on chip analysis with MCF-cells, a number of potential EREs in the second intron of the human ERRγ gene were previously identified (Carroll, Meyer et al. 2006). These studies demonstrated a functional cross-talk between ERs and ERRs in the estrogen signaling pathway.

1.3.2 PCG-1α regulation of ERRα

While nuclear receptor binding to its target gene is important for transcriptional activation, it requires specific interactions with coregulatory proteins (Glass, Rose et al. 1997; McKenna, Lanz et al. 1999). One of the key regulators in energy metabolism is peroxisome proliferator-activated receptor γ coactivator -1α (PGC-1α). PGC-1α not only interacts with and stimulates ERRα transcriptional activity, it also enhances its expression in an autoregulatory loop mechanism (Schreiber, Knutti et al. 2003; Laganiere, Tremblay et al. 2004; Mootha, Handschin et al. 2004; Zhang and Teng 2007; Wang, Li et al. 2008). By combining PGC-1α induced genome-wide transcriptional profiles with a computational strategy to detect cis-regulatory motifs approach, ERRα was discovered to be a key transcription factor that is involved in cross-talk with PGC-1α in regulating the oxidative phosphorylation pathway (Mootha, Handschin et al. 2004). PGC-1α is capable of co-activating nearly all known nuclear receptors and many other transcription factors (Puigserver and Spiegelman 2003), yet it possesses a unique protein interaction surface that is dedicated specifically to the ERRs (see review and references therein (Villena and Kralli 2008)). With this unique relationship, ERRα expression is co-regulated with PGC-1α under various physiological stimuli such as during fasting (Ichida, Nemoto et al. 2002), under cold exposure (Schreiber, Knutti et al. 2003) and exercise (Cartoni, Leger et al. 2005). Therefore, induction of PGC-1α expression by physiological stimuli also induces ERRα expression in a positive feed-forward mechanism. The expression level of ERRα is also affected by ERRγ (Liu, Zhang et al. 2005; Zhang and Teng 2007) and cAMP (Liu, Benlhabib et al. 2009). These studies showed that multiple mechanisms are involved in the regulation of ERRs expression and function.

1.4 Function of the ERRs

1.4.1 ERRs interactions with ERs and other nuclear receptors

Understanding the role of ERRs in ER-mediated function starts with their cloning. ERRα and ERRβ were identified based on a search for genes with sequence homology at the DNA binding domain to ERα (Giguere, Yang et al. 1988). Eight years later, ERRα was re-cloned as a specific binding protein to an extended hormone response element (HRE) half-site, the TCAAGGTCATC region of the human lactoferrin gene promoter (Yang, Shigeta et al. 1996). This finding revealed that ERRα binds to the steroidogenic factor 1 (SF-1) binding element termed SFRE and later renamed this element to ERRE as estrogen-related receptor response element whenever addressing the ERRs binding (Sladek, Bader et al. 1997). It was demonstrated that binding of ERRα to this ERRE enhances the ER-mediated estrogen response of the lactoferrin gene (Yang, Shigeta et al. 1996). ERRα was later shown to bind a variety of EREs as a monomer or homodimer (Johnston, Liu et al. 1997; Vanacker, Pettersson et al. 1999; Zhang and Teng 2000; Zhang and Teng 2001) and genes possessing such ERE or

ERRE or both were subject to ERRα regulation (Sladek, Beatty et al. 1997; Vega and Kelly 1997; Vanacker, Bonnelye et al. 1998; Vanacker, Delmarre et al. 1998; Sumi and Ignarro 2003). Other than the binding elements, ERRs and ERs recognize similar co-activators and co-repressors (Xie, Hong et al. 1999; Zhang and Teng 2000). Therefore, an extensive cross-talk between the ERRα and ERα occurs at the multiple steps of the transcriptional process ((Giguere 2002) and references therein). Depending on the EREs and the surrounding elements, ERRα could either enhance or inhibit the estrogen responsiveness of the target genes (Yang, Shigeta et al. 1996; Kraus, Ariazi et al. 2002; Zhang, Chen et al. 2006).
ERRβ represses glucocorticoid receptor (GR) activity (Trapp and Holsboer 1996) and inhibits the function of NF-E2 Related Factor 2 (Nrf2) on antioxidant response element mediated gene expression (Zhou, Lo et al. 2007) in a cell-specific manner. Recently, variant isoforms (Long and Short) of ERRβ were found in the human endometrium. Increasing the expression of the Long form enhanced the ERα-mediated stimulation of c-myc expression and cell proliferation in Ishikawa cells whereas the Short form had no effect (Bombail, Collins et al. 2010). Interestingly, ERRγ (but not ERRα or ERRβ) was shown to activate the orphan nuclear receptor small heterodimer partner (SHP; NR0B2) (Sanyal, Kim et al. 2002) and the dosage-sensitive sex reversal (DAX-1) promoter (Park, Ahn et al. 2005). ERRs could bind to the promoter of other nuclear receptors such as thyroid hormone receptor (TR) (Vanacker, Bonnelye et al. 1998; Castet, Herledan et al. 2006), PPARα (Huss, Torra et al. 2004), RXRα and RXRβ (Sonoda, Laganiere et al. 2007) thus potentially regulating their expression. These nuclear receptors are also involved in a wide range of physiological functions. Therefore, the cross-talk of ERRs with other nuclear receptors expands their functional roles and points to the importance of their expression in normal and diseased conditions.

1.4.2 The role of ERRs in homeostasis

A major advance in understanding the role of ERRα in energy homeostasis comes from the observation that the medium-chain acyl-coenzyme A dehydrogenase (MCAD) is an ERRα target (Sladek, Bader et al. 1997; Vega and Kelly 1997). The MCAD is an enzyme that mediates the first step in the mitochondrial β-oxidation of fatty acids (Schulz 1991). This was followed by the discovery of a close relationship between ERRα and PGC-1α in transcriptional regulation (Huss, Kopp et al. 2002; Ichida, Nemoto et al. 2002; Schreiber, Knutti et al. 2003). Evidence indicates that PGC-1α serves as a key regulator of mitochondrial biogenesis in mammals. This includes the activation of the transcription of mitochondrial uncoupling protein -1 (UCP-1) and the induction of the expression of NRF-1, NRF-2 and Tfam, all critical factors for mitochondrial function and maintenance. Furthermore, PGC-1α up-regulates the expression of genes involved in mitochondrial fatty acid oxidation and triggers mitochondrial proliferation (see review (Kelly and Scarpulla 2004)). The regulatory roles of PGC-1α in these key metabolic processes were mediated by ERRα (see review and references therein (Giguere 2008; Villena and Kralli 2008)). In microarray studies, over expression of PGC-1α in culture cells induced hundred of genes encoding mitochondrial proteins involved in fatty acid oxidation (FAO), the tricarboxylic acid cycle (TCA), oxidative phosphorylation (OXPHOS), mitochondrial membrane and carbohydrate metabolism. Interestingly, these PGC-1α effects can be blocked by siRNA against ERRα or be induced by over expression of constitutively active ERRα (Mootha, Handschin et al. 2004; Schreiber, Emter et al. 2004). Taken together, ERRα plays a major role in the regulation of sets of genes involved in a wide range of energy balance activities such as lipid transport, fatty acid oxidation, TCA cycle, oxidative phosphorylation, and mitochondrial biogenesis to name a few.

2. ERRs in breast cancer

Searching for therapeutic targets in cancer biology is an important endeavor and the nuclear receptor has been shown to be one such target. Recently, the expression profile of 48 nuclear receptors in 51 human cancer cell lines derived from nine different tissues from the NC160 collection was investigated (Holbeck, Chang et al. 2010). The results uncovered a number of potential receptor-drug interactions and demonstrated that the individual receptor levels may predict a response to therapeutic intervention. Like all cancers, breast cancer is a complicated disease and many factors, estrogen in particular, contributes to its development and progression (Kelsey and Bernstein 1996). Although estrogen action is mediated through two receptors (ERα (Greene, Gilna et al. 1986) and ERβ (Kuiper, Enmark et al. 1996)), 70% of breast cancers express ERα which serves as the mediator for estrogen action (Russo, Hu et al. 2000; Conzen 2008; Hayashi, Niwa et al. 2009). In view of the structural similarity and functional cross-talk of the ERs and ERRs, it is possible that ERRs are also involved in breast cancer biology (review and references therein (Ariazi and Jordan 2006; Riggins, Mazzotta et al. 2010)).

2.1 ERRs as potential biomarkers

Using qPCR to measure the mRNA levels of ERs, epidermal growth factor receptor, ErbB family members, and ERR mRNA levels in 38 unselected primary breast tumors and 9 normal mammary gland epithelial cells from breast reduction surgery revealed that ERRα is highly expressed in a subset of tumors with elevated levels of ErbB2, an indicator of aggressive tumor behavior and nonfunctional ERα. Unlike ERRα, expression of ERRγ in breast tumors correlates with ER-positive status and ErbB4 expression which is a preferred clinical marker. These studies suggest that ERRα can be used as an unfavorable whereas ERRγ can serve as a favorable marker for diagnosis of clinical outcome. The mRNA level of ERRβ in the above mentioned breast tumor samples is very low and the potential as a biomarker unclear (Ariazi, Clark et al. 2002). Despite the proposed use of ERRγ as a favorable marker, over expression of ERRγ contributed to the development of tamoxifen (TAM)- resistance in cell lines derived from invasive lobular carcinoma (Riggins, Lan et al. 2008). Additional studies using an immunohistochemistry approach combined with RT-PCR supports the earlier findings that ERRα expression in breast carcinoma is associated with an increased risk of recurrence and an adverse clinical outcome (Suzuki, Miki et al. 2004).

2.2 ERRα and breast cancer cell growth

ERRα has been extensively studied in the context of breast cancer (Ariazi, Clark et al. 2002; Suzuki, Miki et al. 2004; Barry and Giguere 2005; Ariazi and Jordan 2006; Ariazi, Kraus et al. 2007; Stein, Chang et al. 2008; Chisamore, Wilkinson et al. 2009; Deblois, Hall et al. 2009; Stein, Gaillard et al. 2009; Dwyer, Joseph et al. 2010). Correlation between the expression of ERRs and disease outcome presents a first glimpse of the potential role of ERRs in breast cancer. Further studies using an unbiased microarray approach to understand the cross-talk between ERs and ERRs in MCF-7 cells yielded unexpected results (Stein, Chang et al. 2008). Despite the functional cross-talk between ERs and ERRs presented earlier, ERRα was found to regulate a smaller set of genes that overlapped with ERα despite regulating many more genes not involved in estrogen signaling. Analysis of the microarray data from ER-regulated and ERR-regulated genes in MCF-7 cells by gene ontology (GO) showed that the majority of genes regulated by ERRα are involved in energy metabolism, oxidative stress and detoxification as expected. Interestingly, ERRα also induces vascular endothelial growth factor (VEGF), a highly angiogenic factor. Importantly, knockdown ERRα expression in MDA-MB-231 cells reduced tumor cell migration *in vitro* and tumor growth as xenografts *in vivo* (Stein, Chang et al. 2008). Further studies demonstrated that ERRα-dependent activation of VEGF mRNA expression occurs in several different breast cancer cell lines (Stein, Gaillard et al. 2009). This suggests that ERRα promotes tumor cell growth by stimulating VEGF expression. These studies together with the finding that ERRα also induces the pro-migratory factor, WNT11 (Dwyer, Joseph et al. 2010) provides a basis for highly expressed ERRα to be considered an overall negative phenotype of breast cancers.

2.3 ERRα and aromatase

As indicated above, there is much evidence that points to potential mechanisms of how ERRα influences breast cancer biology. ERRα plays a role in the local production of estrogen in breast cancer cells with levels in tumor tissue being several-fold higher than in normal circulating estrogen (Thorsen, Tangen et al. 1982; van Landeghem, Poortman et al. 1985) and aromatase, a key enzyme in converting androgens to estrogens, is also up-regulated in tumor cells (Miller and O'Neill 1987; Sasano and Harada 1998; Chen, Zhou et al. 1999). The presence of aromatase mRNA in the intra-tumoral location of 19 breast carcinoma tissues was detected using laser capture microdissection (LCM) and quantitative reverse transcription-PCR (q-PCR) while aromatase protein was verified by immunohistochemistry (Miki, Suzuki et al. 2007). Furthermore, microarray expression profiling of aromatase and ERRα mRNA in isolated carcinoma cells demonstrated a significant positive correlation (Miki, Suzuki et al. 2007). Although regulation of aromatase expression is tissue- and promoter-specific, its activity in breast carcinoma is higher than in normal tissue of the same patients (Silva, Rowlands et al. 1989; Miller, Anderson et al. 1990; Lipton, Santen et al. 1992). This suggests that the regulation of aromatase expression in breast cancer cells of the patient has been changed. Indeed, promoter switching in breast cancer tissue has been reported (Chen, Zhou et al. 1999; Chen, Reierstad et al. 2009) and ERRα plays a positive role (Yang, Zhou et al. 1998; Miao, Shi et al. 2010). Taken together, ERRα functions as a key modulator of intratumoral estrogen production in human breast carcinoma by stimulating the expression of the androgen-estrogen key converting enzyme, aromatase via tumor specific promoter usage.

2.4 ERRα and EGFR

ERRα has a close relationship with the ErbB2/epidermal growth factor receptor (EGFR) signaling pathway. ErbB2 is a receptor tyrosine kinase and in combination with EGFR, activates a complex array of downstream signaling pathways which leads to phosphorylation of multiple transcription factors including ERRα. Phosphorylation of these transcription factors promotes growth and proliferation (reviewed in ref. (Yarden and Sliwkowski 2001)). Upon EGF treatment, ERRα in MCF-7 cells was phosphorylated and preferentially recruited to the pS2 promoter. Furthermore, phosphorylated ERRα showed enhanced DNA binding capability in an *in vitro* study (Barry and Giguere 2005). Additionally, mitogen-activated protein kinases (MAPK) and Akts (components of the

ErbB2 pathway) are involved in ERRα phorphorylation and transactivation since inhibitors to MAPK and Akt also block ERRα target gene activation (Ariazi, Kraus et al. 2007). These observations suggest that ERRα phosphorylation provides a mechanism of enhanced transactivation function in breast cancer cells. Recently, using a mouse model of ErbB2-initiated mammary tumorigenesis found that ablation of ERRα significantly delays ErbB2-induced tumor development, lowers the levels of ErbB2 and co-amplifies transcripts within the 17q12-21 chromosomal region (the ErbB2 amplicon) (Deblois, Chahrour et al. 2010). The minimal 17q12 amplicon houses not only the ErbB2 gene; it also includes those involved in signal transduction, transcription, cell migration and invasion, inhibition of apotosis, genomic instability and tamoxifen resistance. ERRα binds to those genes and directs the recruitment of co-activators PGC-1β and RNA polymerase II to their promoters (Deblois, Chahrour et al. 2010). Furthermore, ERRα antagonists repress the effect of ERα on the ErbB2 promoter which leads to the development of tamoxifen resistance in breast cancer cells.

2.5 ERRα and AIB1

Comparing the co-activators along with the expression of various nuclear receptors in 48 primary breast tumor samples, a positive correlation between ERRα and AIB1 (amplified in breast cancer-1) (Anzick, Kononen et al. 1997) was found. AIB1 is an oncogenic co-activator of ERα that is frequently amplified and over expressed in human breast carcinomas (Anzick, Kononen et al. 1997; Liao, Kuang et al. 2002). In addition, these two proteins were abundant in the tumor samples and a direct interaction of the receptor and co-activator was demonstrated by fluorescence-resonance energy transfer, mammalian two-hybrid, and coimmunoprecipitation assay with endogenous proteins. On the other hand, the levels of PGC-1α (a well characterized ERRα co-activator) in primary breast carcinoma was low and no detectable association with ERRα was found (Heck, Rom et al. 2009). The enhanced association of ERRα with AIB1 underscores the functional significance of ERRα/AIB1 rather than the ERRα/PGC-1α interaction for breast tumor development and progression.

2.6 ERRγ and PGC-1β

Although direct evidence between cellular metabolism and breast cancer development is lacking, switching from aerobic oxidative phosphorylation to glycolytic metabolism is a typical feature of cancer cells (Warburg 1956). Recent reports demonstrated that the expression of miR-378, an ErbB2-regulated microRNA, correlates with the progression of human breast cancer by inducing the metabolic shift from an oxidative to a glycolytic pathway (Eichner, Perry et al. 2010). The miR-378 is embedded within PGC-1β and when expressed, inhibits the expression of ERRγ and GABPA (PGC-1β partners), a function that is opposite to the PGC-1 family of co-activators. In view of the close relationship of ERRs and PGC-1 coactivator family in the context of energy metabolism (Giguere 2008; Villena and Kralli 2008), the finding that miR-378 targets ERRγ but not ERRα demonstrated again that the isoforms of ERR possess differential functions as well as overlapping activities either in regulating energy or in breast cancer biology.

3. The potential agonist and antagonist of ERRs

As mentioned earlier, the ERR-coactivator or corepressor interaction determines the receptor's functional activity. Any factor that interrupts this interaction has the ability to modulate ERR function (Huss, Kopp et al. 2002; Kamei, Ohizumi et al. 2003; Schreiber, Knutti et al. 2003;

Debevec, Christian et al. 2007), therefore could be a potential therapeutic target site. Small-molecule agonists for ERRβ and ERRγ have been identified and characterized. However, identifying an agonist for ERRα has proved to be difficult (Yu and Forman 2005; Hyatt, Lockamy et al. 2007). Nonetheless, novel synthetic antagonists of ERRs, especially for ERRα, are emerging (Yang and Chen 1999; Coward, Lee et al. 2001; Tremblay, Bergeron et al. 2001; Tremblay, Kunath et al. 2001; Busch, Stevens et al. 2004; Willy, Murray et al. 2004; Chisamore, Cunningham et al. 2009). By disrupting the constitutive ERR/co-activator interaction or by inducing proteosome-dependent protein degradation of the receptor, these small molecules inhibit the function of ERRs and thus tumor growth and progression (Ariazi and Jordan 2006; Stein, Chang et al. 2008; Chisamore, Wilkinson et al. 2009; Heck, Rom et al. 2009; Wu, Wang et al. 2009). Recently, a series of diaryl ether-based ligands for ERRα were developed and demonstrated in animal models to be antidiabetic agents (Patch, Searle et al. 2011). Taken together, these studies provide a basis for the further development of therapeutics to treat breast cancers based on suppressing ERRα expression and activity. Recently, environmental estrogenic compounds were found to modulate ERRα (Suetsugi, Su et al. 2003) and ERRγ (Matsushima, Kakuta et al. 2007; Takashima-Sasaki, Mori et al. 2007; Wang, Fang et al. 2009; Hirvonen, Rajalin et al. 2011) activities in either a positive or negative manner. The impact of environmental factors on breast cancer via ERRs is currently unclear.

4. ERRs in other cancers

Since the over expression of ERRα in breast cancer was discovered (Ariazi, Clark et al. 2002; Suzuki, Miki et al. 2004), additional studies have found an association between the abnormal expression of ERRs and a variety of tumors and cancers such as prostate (Cheung, Yu et al. 2005; Yu, Wang et al. 2007; Yu, Wong et al. 2008), ovarian (Sun, Sehouli et al. 2005), colon-rectal (Cavallini, Notarnicola et al. 2005) and endometrium (Gao, Sun et al. 2006). In neoplastic prostatic tissues, ERRβ and ERRγ show levels that are either reduced or undetectable as compared to normal prostatic epithelial cells (Cheung, Yu et al. 2005). This suggests a down-regulation of these two receptors in prostate cancer. In a series of experiments, the forced induction of ERRβ or ERRγ in androgen sensitive (LNCaP) and androgen-insensitive (DU145) prostate cancer cells demonstrated that over expression of these two receptors suppresses cell proliferation and tumorigenicity of the cancer cells. The inhibition of prostate cancer cell proliferation was due to cell cycle arrest as demonstrated by the induction of cyclin-dependent kinase inhibitor p21 by ERRβ and p21/p27 by ERRγ. Moreover, ERRβ and ERRγ-mediated growth inhibition could be potentiated by their specific agonist DY131 and reduced by siRNA (Yu, Wang et al. 2007; Yu, Wong et al. 2008). The expression of ERRβ and ERRγ in prostate cancer is in contrast to ERRα in breast cancer cells, colorectal tumor, and malignant colon cells (Cavallini, Notarnicola et al. 2005). ERRα expression in endometrial adenocarcinoma is positively correlated with myometrial invasion while a negative correlation was observed between the expression of ERRγ mRNA and nodal metastasis (Gao, Sun et al. 2006). Therefore, the expression levels of the subtype ERRs in cancer cells provides a potential prognostic strategy for the therapeutic treatment of the cancer.

5. Conclusion

The studies cited in this review demonstrate that ERRs are differentially expressed in normal and cancer cells. While many factors influence their expression, ERRs in turn, regulate many sets of genes involved in a wide variety of signaling pathways. As of today, the majority of studies are on ERRα and its relationship with breast cancer development and progression. How ERRα is involved in breast cancer biology is summarized in Figure 2.

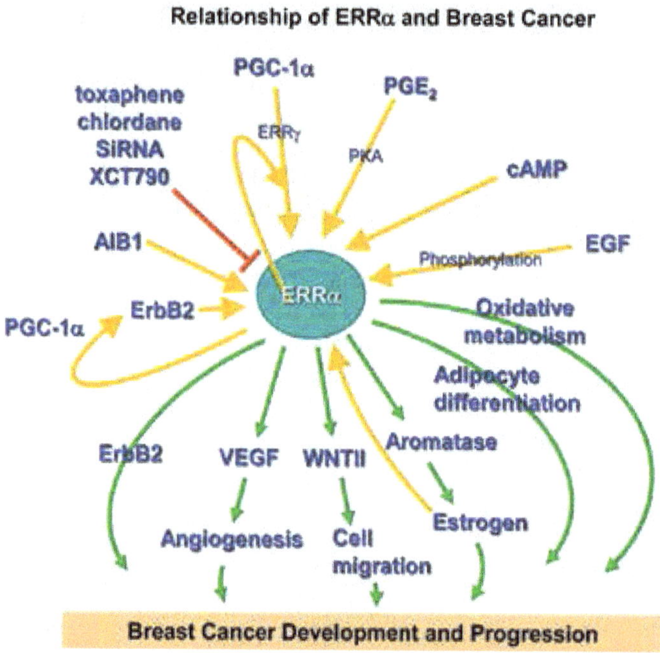

Fig. 2. Potential pathways that regulate ERRα expression and influences breast cancer development and progression. Yellow arrow, upregulates ERRα expression; red arrow, downregulates ERRα activity; green arrow, potential mechanisms of ERRα action on breast cancer.

The roles of ERRγ in breast cancer have yet to be established. While ERRγ targets the same metabolic gene network as ERRα, it may perform distinct physiological functions such as participation in the metabolic shift pathway in breast cancer cells. ERRγ was recently demonstrated as a target for endocrine disruptors, the estrogen-mimic of the environmental chemicals which may be involved in breast cancer development or progression. Compared to ERRα and ERRγ, the number of functional studies on ERRβ has been relatively slim. Nonetheless, the report on the repressive function of ERRβ in prostate cancer cells will certainly garner additional attention to this orphan receptor. Collectively, the role of these ERRs in this disease state is emerging and they could prove to be a viable therapeutic target in the treatment of breast cancer.

6. References

Anzick, S. L., J. Kononen, et al. (1997). "AIB1, a steroid receptor coactivator amplified in breast and ovarian cancer." *Science* 277(5328): 965-968.

Ariazi, E. A., G. M. Clark, et al. (2002). "Estrogen-related receptor alpha and estrogen-related receptor gamma associate with unfavorable and favorable biomarkers, respectively, in human breast cancer." *Cancer Res* 62(22): 6510-6518.

Ariazi, E. A. and V. C. Jordan (2006). "Estrogen-related receptors as emerging targets in cancer and metabolic disorders." *Curr Top Med Chem* 6(3): 203-215.

Ariazi, E. A., R. J. Kraus, et al. (2007). "Estrogen-related receptor alpha1 transcriptional activities are regulated in part via the ErbB2/HER2 signaling pathway." *Mol Cancer Res* 5(1): 71-85.

Barry, J. B. and V. Giguere (2005). "Epidermal growth factor-induced signaling in breast cancer cells results in selective target gene activation by orphan nuclear receptor estrogen-related receptor alpha." *Cancer Res* 65(14): 6120-6129.

Benoit, G., A. Cooney, et al. (2006). "International Union of Pharmacology. LXVI. Orphan nuclear receptors." *Pharmacological reviews* 58(4): 798-836.

Bombail, V., F. Collins, et al. (2010). "Modulation of ER alpha transcriptional activity by the orphan nuclear receptor ERR beta and evidence for differential effects of long- and short-form splice variants." *Molecular and cellular endocrinology* 314(1): 53-61.

Bonnelye, E. and J. E. Aubin (2002). "Differential expression of estrogen receptor-related receptor alpha and estrogen receptors alpha and beta in osteoblasts in vivo and in vitro." *J Bone Miner Res* 17(8): 1392-1400.

Bonnelye, E., V. Kung, et al. (2002). "Estrogen receptor-related receptor alpha impinges on the estrogen axis in bone: potential function in osteoporosis." *Endocrinology* 143(9): 3658-3670.

Bookout, A. L., Y. Jeong, et al. (2006). "Anatomical profiling of nuclear receptor expression reveals a hierarchical transcriptional network." *Cell* 126(4): 789-799.

Busch, B. B., W. C. Stevens, Jr., et al. (2004). "Identification of a selective inverse agonist for the orphan nuclear receptor estrogen-related receptor alpha." *J Med Chem* 47(23): 5593-5596.

Carroll, J. S., C. A. Meyer, et al. (2006). "Genome-wide analysis of estrogen receptor binding sites." *Nat Genet* 38(11): 1289-1297.

Cartoni, R., B. Leger, et al. (2005). "Mitofusins 1/2 and ERR{alpha} expression are increased in human skeletal muscle after physical exercise." *J Physiol.*

Castet, A., A. Herledan, et al. (2006). "Receptor-interacting protein 140 differentially regulates estrogen receptor-related receptor transactivation depending on target genes." *Molecular Endocrinology* 20(5): 1035-1047.

Cavallini, A., M. Notarnicola, et al. (2005). "Oestrogen receptor-related receptor alpha (ERRalpha) and oestrogen receptors (ERalpha and ERbeta) exhibit different gene expression in human colorectal tumour progression." *Eur J Cancer* 41(10): 1487-1494.

Chen, D., S. Reierstad, et al. (2009). "Regulation of breast cancer-associated aromatase promoters." *Cancer Lett* 273(1): 15-27.

Chen, S., D. Zhou, et al. (1999). "Breast tumor aromatase: functional role and transcriptional regulation." *Endocr Relat Cancer* 6(2): 149-156.

Cheung, C. P., S. Yu, et al. (2005). "Expression and functional study of estrogen receptor-related receptors in human prostatic cells and tissues." *J Clin Endocrinol Metab* 90(3): 1830-1844.

Chisamore, M. J., M. E. Cunningham, et al. (2009). "Characterization of a novel small molecule subtype specific estrogen-related receptor alpha antagonist in MCF-7 breast cancer cells." *PLoS One* 4(5): e5624.

Chisamore, M. J., H. A. Wilkinson, et al. (2009). "Estrogen-related receptor-alpha antagonist inhibits both estrogen receptor-positive and estrogen receptor-negative breast tumor growth in mouse xenografts." *Mol Cancer Ther* 8(3): 672-681.

Collin, R. W., E. Kalay, et al. (2008). "Mutations of ESRRB encoding estrogen-related receptor beta cause autosomal-recessive nonsyndromic hearing impairment DFNB35." *American journal of human genetics* 82(1): 125-138.

Conzen, S. D. (2008). "Minireview: nuclear receptors and breast cancer." *Mol Endocrinol* 22(10): 2215-2228.

Coward, P., D. Lee, et al. (2001). "4-Hydroxytamoxifen binds to and deactivates the estrogen-related receptor gamma." *Proc Natl Acad Sci U S A* 98(15): 8880-8884.

Debevec, D., M. Christian, et al. (2007). "Receptor interacting protein 140 regulates expression of uncoupling protein 1 in adipocytes through specific peroxisome proliferator activated receptor isoforms and estrogen-related receptor alpha." *Mol Endocrinol* 21(7): 1581-1592.

Deblois, G., G. Chahrour, et al. (2010). "Transcriptional control of the ERBB2 amplicon by ERRalpha and PGC-1beta promotes mammary gland tumorigenesis." *Cancer Res* 70(24): 10277-10287.

Deblois, G., J. A. Hall, et al. (2009). "Genome-wide identification of direct target genes implicates estrogen-related receptor alpha as a determinant of breast cancer heterogeneity." *Cancer Res* 69(15): 6149-6157.

Dwyer, M. A., J. D. Joseph, et al. (2010). "WNT11 expression is induced by estrogen-related receptor alpha and beta-catenin and acts in an autocrine manner to increase cancer cell migration." *Cancer Res* 70(22): 9298-9308.

Eichner, L. J., M. C. Perry, et al. (2010). "miR-378(*) mediates metabolic shift in breast cancer cells via the PGC-1beta/ERRgamma transcriptional pathway." *Cell Metab* 12(4): 352-361.

Eudy, J. D., S. Yao, et al. (1998). "Isolation of a gene encoding a novel member of the nuclear receptor superfamily from the critical region of Usher syndrome type IIa at 1q41." *Genomics* 50(3): 382-384.

Fu, M., T. Sun, et al. (2005). "A Nuclear Receptor Atlas: 3T3-L1 adipogenesis." *Molecular Endocrinology* 19(10): 2437-2450.

Gao, M., P. Sun, et al. (2006). "Expression of estrogen receptor-related receptor isoforms and clinical significance in endometrial adenocarcinoma." *Int J Gynecol Cancer* 16(2): 827-833.

Giguere, V. (2002). "To ERR in the estrogen pathway." *Trends Endocrinol Metab* 13(5): 220-225.

Giguere, V. (2008). "Transcriptional control of energy homeostasis by the estrogen-related receptors." *Endocr Rev* 29(6): 677-696.

Giguere, V., N. Yang, et al. (1988). "Identification of a new class of steroid hormone receptors." *Nature* 331: 91-94.

Glass, C. K., D. W. Rose, et al. (1997). "Nuclear receptor coactivators." *Current opinion in cell biology* 9(2): 222-232.

Greene, G. L., P. Gilna, et al. (1986). "Sequence and expression of human estrogen receptor complementary DNA." *Science* 231(4742): 1150-1154.

Greschik, H., J. M. Wurtz, et al. (2002). "Structural and functional evidence for ligand-independent transcriptional activation by the estrogen-related receptor 3." *Mol Cell* 9(2): 303-313.

Hayashi, S., T. Niwa, et al. (2009). "Estrogen signaling pathway and its imaging in human breast cancer." *Cancer Sci* 100(10): 1773-1778.

Heard, D. J., P. L. Norby, et al. (2000). "Human ERR gamma, a third member of the estrogen receptor- related receptor (ERR) subfamily of orphan nuclear receptors: Tissue-specific isoforms are expressed during development and in the adult." *Molecular Endocrinology* 14(3): 382-392.

Heck, S., J. Rom, et al. (2009). "Estrogen-related receptor alpha expression and function is associated with the transcriptional coregulator AIB1 in breast carcinoma." *Cancer Res* 69(12): 5186-5193.

Hirvonen, J., A.-M. Rajalin, et al. (2011). "Transcriptional activity of estrogen-related receptor [gamma] (ERR[gamma]) is stimulated by the phytoestrogen equol." *The Journal of Steroid Biochemistry and Molecular Biology* 123(1-2): 46-57.

Holbeck, S., J. Chang, et al. (2010). "Expression profiling of nuclear receptors in the NCI60 cancer cell panel reveals receptor-drug and receptor-gene interactions." *Mol Endocrinol* 24(6): 1287-1296.

Hong, H., L. Yang, et al. (1999). "Hormone-independent transcriptional activation and coactivator binding by novel orphan nuclear receptor ERR3." *J Biol Chem* 274(32): 22618-22626.

Horard, B., A. Castet, et al. (2004). "Dimerization is required for transactivation by estrogen-receptor-related (ERR) orphan receptors: evidence from amphioxus ERR." *J Mol Endocrinol* 33(2): 493-509.

Hu, P., H. K. Kinyamu, et al. (2008). "Estrogen induces estrogen-related receptor alpha gene expression and chromatin structural changes in estrogen receptor (ER)-positive and ER-negative breast cancer cells." *J Biol Chem* 283(11): 6752-6763.

Huss, J. M., R. P. Kopp, et al. (2002). "Peroxisome proliferator-activated receptor coactivator-1alpha (PGC-1alpha) coactivates the cardiac-enriched nuclear receptors estrogen-related receptor-alpha and -gamma. Identification of novel leucine-rich interaction motif within PGC-1alpha." *J Biol Chem* 277(43): 40265-40274.

Huss, J. M., I. P. Torra, et al. (2004). "Estrogen-related receptor alpha directs peroxisome proliferator-activated receptor alpha signaling in the transcriptional control of energy metabolism in cardiac and skeletal muscle." *Mol Cell Biol* 24(20): 9079-9091.

Hyatt, S. M., E. L. Lockamy, et al. (2007). "On the intractability of estrogen-related receptor alpha as a target for activation by small molecules." *J Med Chem* 50(26): 6722-6724.

Ichida, M., S. Nemoto, et al. (2002). "Identification of a specific molecular repressor of the peroxisome proliferator-activated receptor gamma Coactivator-1 alpha (PGC-1alpha)." *J Biol Chem* 277(52): 50991-50995.

Ijichi, N., T. Shigekawa, et al. (2011). "Estrogen-related receptor gamma modulates cell proliferation and estrogen signaling in breast cancer." *J Steroid Biochem Mol Biol* 123(1-2): 1-7.

Johnston, S. D., X. Liu, et al. (1997). "Estrogen-related receptor alpha 1 functionally binds as a monomer to extended half-site sequences including ones contained within estrogen- response elements." *Mol Endocrinol* 11(3): 342-352.

Kallen, J., J. M. Schlaeppi, et al. (2004). "Evidence for Ligand-independent Transcriptional Activation of the Human Estrogen-related Receptor {alpha} (ERR{alpha}): CRYSTAL STRUCTURE OF ERR{alpha} LIGAND BINDING DOMAIN IN

COMPLEX WITH PEROXISOME PROLIFERATOR-ACTIVATED RECEPTOR COACTIVATOR-1{alpha}." *J Biol Chem* 279(47): 49330-49337.

Kamei, Y., H. Ohizumi, et al. (2003). "PPARgamma coactivator 1beta/ERR ligand 1 is an ERR protein ligand, whose expression induces a high-energy expenditure and antagonizes obesity." *Proc Natl Acad Sci U S A* 100(21): 12378-12383.

Kelly, D. P. and R. C. Scarpulla (2004). "Transcriptional regulatory circuits controlling mitochondrial biogenesis and function." *Genes & development* 18(4): 357-368.

Kelsey, J. L. and L. Bernstein (1996). "Epidemiology and prevention of breast cancer." *Annu Rev Public Health* 17: 47-67.

Kraus, R. J., E. A. Ariazi, et al. (2002). "Estrogen-related receptor alpha 1 actively antagonizes estrogen receptor-regulated transcription in MCF-7 mammary cells." *J Biol Chem* 277(27): 24826-24834.

Kuiper, G. G., E. Enmark, et al. (1996). "Cloning of a novel receptor expressed in rat prostate and ovary." *Proc Natl Acad Sci U S A* 93(12): 5925-5930.

Laganiere, J., G. B. Tremblay, et al. (2004). "A Polymorphic Autoregulatory Hormone Response Element in the Human Estrogen-related Receptor {alpha} (ERR{alpha}) Promoter Dictates Peroxisome Proliferator-activated Receptor {gamma} Coactivator-1{alpha} Control of ERR{alpha} Expression." *J Biol Chem* 279(18): 18504-18510.

Li, Y., L. Birnbaumer, et al. (2010). "Regulation of ERRalpha gene expression by estrogen receptor agonists and antagonists in SKBR3 breast cancer cells: differential molecular mechanisms mediated by g protein-coupled receptor GPR30/GPER-1." *Molecular Endocrinology* 24(5): 969-980.

Liao, L., S. Q. Kuang, et al. (2002). "Molecular structure and biological function of the cancer-amplified nuclear receptor coactivator SRC-3/AIB1." *J Steroid Biochem Mol Biol* 83(1-5): 3-14.

Lipton, A., R. J. Santen, et al. (1992). "Prognostic value of breast cancer aromatase." *Cancer* 70(7): 1951-1955.

Liu, D., H. Benlhabib, et al. (2009). "cAMP Enhances estrogen-related receptor {alpha} (ERR{alpha}) transcriptional activity at the SP-A promoter by increasing its interaction with protein kinase A and steroid receptor coactivator 2 (SRC-2)." *Mol Endocrinol* 23(6): 772-783.

Liu, D., Z. Zhang, et al. (2003). "Estrogen Stimulates Estrogen-Related Receptor {alpha} Gene Expression Through Conserved Hormone Response Elements." *Endocrinology* 144(11): 4894-4904.

Liu, D., Z. Zhang, et al. (2005). "Estrogen-related receptor-gamma and peroxisome proliferator-activated receptor-gamma coactivator-1alpha regulate estrogen-related receptor-alpha gene expression via a conserved multi-hormone response element." *J Mol Endocrinol* 34(2): 473-487.

Luo, J., R. Sladek, et al. (1997). "Placental abnormalities in mouse embryos lacking the orphan nuclear receptor ERR-beta." *Nature* 388(6644): 778-782.

Matsushima, A., Y. Kakuta, et al. (2007). "Structural evidence for endocrine disruptor bisphenol A binding to human nuclear receptor ERR gamma." *J Biochem* 142(4): 517-524.

McKenna, N. J., R. B. Lanz, et al. (1999). "Nuclear receptor coregulators: cellular and molecular biology." *Endocrine reviews* 20(3): 321-344.

Miao, L., J. Shi, et al. (2010). "Estrogen receptor-related receptor alpha mediates up-regulation of aromatase expression by prostaglandin E2 in prostate stromal cells." *Mol Endocrinol* 24(6): 1175-1186.

Miki, Y., T. Suzuki, et al. (2007). "Aromatase localization in human breast cancer tissues: possible interactions between intratumoral stromal and parenchymal cells." *Cancer Res* 67(8): 3945-3954.

Miller, W. R., T. J. Anderson, et al. (1990). "Relationship between tumour aromatase activity, tumour characteristics and response to therapy." *J Steroid Biochem Mol Biol* 37(6): 1055-1059.

Miller, W. R. and J. O'Neill (1987). "The importance of local synthesis of estrogen within the breast." *Steroids* 50(4-6): 537-548.

Mootha, V. K., C. Handschin, et al. (2004). "Err{alpha} and Gabpa/b specify PGC-1{alpha}-dependent oxidative phosphorylation gene expression that is altered in diabetic muscle." *Proc Natl Acad Sci U S A.*

Nettles, K. W. and G. L. Greene (2005). "Ligand control of coregulator recruitment to nuclear receptors." *Annual review of physiology* 67: 309-333.

Park, Y. Y., S. W. Ahn, et al. (2005). "An autoregulatory loop controlling orphan nuclear receptor DAX-1 gene expression by orphan nuclear receptor ERRgamma." *Nucleic acids research* 33(21): 6756-6768.

Patch, R. J., L. L. Searle, et al. (2011). "Identification of Diaryl Ether-Based Ligands for Estrogen-Related Receptor alpha as Potential Antidiabetic Agents." *J Med Chem.*

Puigserver, P. and B. M. Spiegelman (2003). "Peroxisome proliferator-activated receptor-gamma coactivator 1 alpha (PGC-1 alpha): transcriptional coactivator and metabolic regulator." *Endocr Rev* 24(1): 78-90.

Riggins, R. B., J. P. Lan, et al. (2008). "ERR{gamma} Mediates Tamoxifen Resistance in Novel Models of Invasive Lobular Breast Cancer." *Cancer Res* 68(21): 8908-8917.

Riggins, R. B., M. M. Mazzotta, et al. (2010). "Orphan nuclear receptors in breast cancer pathogenesis and therapeutic response." *Endocr Relat Cancer* 17(3): R213-231.

Russo, J., Y. F. Hu, et al. (2000). "Developmental, cellular, and molecular basis of human breast cancer." *J Natl Cancer Inst Monogr*(27): 17-37.

Sanyal, S., J. Y. Kim, et al. (2002). "Differential regulation of the orphan nuclear receptor small heterodimer partner (SHP) gene promoter by orphan nuclear receptor ERR isoforms." *The Journal of biological chemistry* 277(3): 1739-1748.

Sasano, H. and N. Harada (1998). "Intratumoral aromatase in human breast, endometrial, and ovarian malignancies." *Endocr Rev* 19(5): 593-607.

Schreiber, S. N., R. Emter, et al. (2004). "The estrogen-related receptor {alpha} (ERR{alpha}) functions in PPAR{gamma} coactivator 1{alpha} (PGC-1{alpha})-induced mitochondrial biogenesis." *Proc Natl Acad Sci U S A.*

Schreiber, S. N., D. Knutti, et al. (2003). "The transcriptional coactivator PGC-1 regulates the expression and activity of the orphan nuclear receptor ERRalpha." *J Biol Chem.*

Schulz, H. (1991). "Beta oxidation of fatty acids." *Biochimica et biophysica acta* 1081(2): 109-120.

Shi, H., H. Shigeta, et al. (1997). "Human estrogen receptor-like 1 (ESRL1) gene: genomic organization, chromosomal localization, and promoter characterization." *Genomics* 44(1): 52-60.

Shigeta, H., W. Zuo, et al. (1997). "The mouse estrogen receptor-related orphan receptor alpha 1: molecular cloning and estrogen responsiveness." *J Mol Endocrinol* 19(3): 299-309.

Silva, M. C., M. G. Rowlands, et al. (1989). "Intratumoral aromatase as a prognostic factor in human breast carcinoma." *Cancer Res* 49(10): 2588-2591.

Sladek, R., J. A. Bader, et al. (1997). "The orphan nuclear receptor estrogen-related receptor alpha is a transcriptional regulator of the human medium-chain acyl coenzyme A dehydrogenase gene." *Mol Cell Biol* 17(9): 5400-5409.

Sladek, R., B. Beatty, et al. (1997). "Chromosomal mapping of the human and murine orphan receptors ERR alpha (ESRRA) and ERR beta (ESRRB) and identification of a novel human ERR alpha-related pseudogene." *Genomics* 45(2): 320-326.

Sonoda, J., J. Laganiere, et al. (2007). "Nuclear receptor ERR alpha and coactivator PGC-1 beta are effectors of IFN-gamma-induced host defense." *Genes & development* 21(15): 1909-1920.

Stein, R. A., C. Y. Chang, et al. (2008). "Estrogen-Related Receptor {alpha} Is Critical for the Growth of Estrogen Receptor-Negative Breast Cancer." *Cancer Res* 68(21): 8805-8812.

Stein, R. A., S. Gaillard, et al. (2009). "Estrogen-related receptor alpha induces the expression of vascular endothelial growth factor in breast cancer cells." *J Steroid Biochem Mol Biol* 114(1-2): 106-112.

Suetsugi, M., L. Su, et al. (2003). "Flavone and isoflavone phytoestrogens are agonists of estrogen-related receptors." *Mol Cancer Res* 1(13): 981-991.

Sumi, D. and L. J. Ignarro (2003). "Estrogen-related receptor {alpha}1 up-regulates endothelial nitric oxide synthase expression." *Proc Natl Acad Sci U S A* 100(24): 14451-14456.

Sun, P., J. Sehouli, et al. (2005). "Expression of estrogen receptor-related receptors, a subfamily of orphan nuclear receptors, as new tumor biomarkers in ovarian cancer cells." *J Mol Med* 83(6): 457-467.

Suzuki, T., Y. Miki, et al. (2004). "Estrogen-related receptor alpha in human breast carcinoma as a potent prognostic factor." *Cancer Res* 64(13): 4670-4676.

Takashima-Sasaki, K., C. Mori, et al. (2007). "Exposure of juvenile female mice to isoflavone causes lowered expression of estrogen-related receptor gamma gene in vagina." *Reprod Toxicol* 23(4): 507-512.

Thorsen, T., M. Tangen, et al. (1982). "Concentration of endogenous oestradiol as related to oestradiol receptor sites in breast tumor cytosol." *Eur J Cancer Clin Oncol* 18(4): 333-337.

Trapp, T. and F. Holsboer (1996). "Nuclear orphan receptor as a repressor of glucocorticoid receptor transcriptional activity." *The Journal of biological chemistry* 271(17): 9879-9882.

Tremblay, G. B., D. Bergeron, et al. (2001). "4-Hydroxytamoxifen is an isoform-specific inhibitor of orphan estrogen-receptor-related (ERR) nuclear receptors beta and gamma." *Endocrinology* 142(10): 4572-4575.

Tremblay, G. B., T. Kunath, et al. (2001). "Diethylstilbestrol regulates trophoblast stem cell differentiation as a ligand of orphan nuclear receptor ERR beta." *Genes Dev* 15(7): 833-838.

van Landeghem, A. A., J. Poortman, et al. (1985). "Endogenous concentration and subcellular distribution of estrogens in normal and malignant human breast tissue." *Cancer Res* 45(6): 2900-2906.

Vanacker, J. M., E. Bonnelye, et al. (1998). "Activation of the thyroid hormone receptor alpha gene promoter by the orphan nuclear receptor ERR alpha." *Oncogene* 17(19): 2429-2435.

Vanacker, J. M., C. Delmarre, et al. (1998). "Activation of the osteopontin promoter by the orphan nuclear receptor estrogen receptor related alpha." *Cell Growth Differ* 9(12): 1007-1014.

Vanacker, J. M., K. Pettersson, et al. (1999). "Transcriptional targets shared by estrogen receptor- related receptors (ERRs) and estrogen receptor (ER) alpha, but not by ERbeta." *Embo J* 18(15): 4270-4279.

Vega, R. B. and D. P. Kelly (1997). "A role for estrogen-related receptor alpha in the control of mitochondrial fatty acid beta-oxidation during brown adipocyte differentiation." *J Biol Chem* 272(50): 31693-31699.

Villena, J. A. and A. Kralli (2008). "ERRalpha: a metabolic function for the oldest orphan." *Trends Endocrinol Metab* 19(8): 269-276.

Wang, J., F. Fang, et al. (2009). "Kaempferol is an estrogen-related receptor alpha and gamma inverse agonist." *FEBS Lett* 583(4): 643-647.

Wang, L., Y. Li, et al. (2008). "PGC-1 alpha induces dynamic protein interactions on the ERR alpha gene multi-hormone response element nucleosome in kidney cells." *Biochem J* 416: 407-419.

Warburg, O. (1956). "On respiratory impairment in cancer cells." *Science* 124(3215): 269-270.

Willy, P. J., I. R. Murray, et al. (2004). "Regulation of PPARgamma coactivator 1alpha (PGC-1alpha) signaling by an estrogen-related receptor alpha (ERRalpha) ligand." *Proc Natl Acad Sci U S A* 101(24): 8912-8917.

Wu, F., J. Wang, et al. (2009). "Estrogen-related receptor alpha (ERRalpha) inverse agonist XCT-790 induces cell death in chemotherapeutic resistant cancer cells." *Chem Biol Interact* 181(2): 236-242.

Xie, C. Q., Y. Jeong, et al. (2009). "Expression profiling of nuclear receptors in human and mouse embryonic stem cells." *Molecular Endocrinology* 23(5): 724-733.

Xie, W., H. Hong, et al. (1999). "Constitutive activation of transcription and binding of coactivator by estrogen-related receptors 1 and 2." *Mol Endocrinol* 13(12): 2151-2162.

Yang, C. and S. Chen (1999). "Two organochlorine pesticides, toxaphene and chlordane, are antagonists for estrogen-related receptor alpha-1 orphan receptor." *Cancer Res* 59(18): 4519-4524.

Yang, C., D. Zhou, et al. (1998). "Modulation of aromatase expression in the breast tissue by ERR alpha-1 orphan receptor." *Cancer Res* 58(24): 5695-5700.

Yang, N., H. Shigeta, et al. (1996). "Estrogen-related receptor, hERR1, modulates estrogen receptor-mediated response of human lactoferrin gene promoter." *J Biol Chem* 271(10): 5795-5804.

Yang, X., M. Downes, et al. (2006). "Nuclear receptor expression links the circadian clock to metabolism." *Cell* 126(4): 801-810.

Yarden, Y. and M. X. Sliwkowski (2001). "Untangling the ErbB signalling network." *Nat Rev Mol Cell Biol* 2(2): 127-137.

Yu, D. D. and B. M. Forman (2005). "Identification of an agonist ligand for estrogen-related receptors ERRbeta/gamma." *Bioorg Med Chem Lett* 15(5): 1311-1313.

Yu, S., X. Wang, et al. (2007). "ERRgamma suppresses cell proliferation and tumor growth of androgen-sensitive and androgen-insensitive prostate cancer cells and its implication as a therapeutic target for prostate cancer." *Cancer Res* 67(10): 4904-4914.

Yu, S., Y. C. Wong, et al. (2008). "Orphan nuclear receptor estrogen-related receptor-beta suppresses in vitro and in vivo growth of prostate cancer cells via p21(WAF1/CIP1) induction and as a potential therapeutic target in prostate cancer." *Oncogene* 27(23): 3313-3328.

Zhang, Z., K. Chen, et al. (2006). "Estrogen-related receptors-stimulated monoamine oxidase B promoter activity is down-regulated by estrogen receptors." *Mol Endocrinol* 20(7): 1547-1561.

Zhang, Z. and C. T. Teng (2000). "Estrogen receptor-related receptor alpha 1 interacts with coactivator and constitutively activates the estrogen response elements of the human lactoferrin gene." *J Biol Chem* 275(27): 20837-20846.

Zhang, Z. and C. T. Teng (2001). "Estrogen receptor alpha and estrogen receptor-related receptor alpha1 compete for binding and coactivator." *Mol Cell Endocrinol* 172(1-2): 223-233.

Zhang, Z. and C. T. Teng (2007). "Interplay between estrogen-related receptor alpha (ERRalpha) and gamma (ERRgamma) on the regulation of ERRalpha gene expression." *Mol Cell Endocrinol* 264(1-2): 128-141.

Zhou, W., Z. Liu, et al. (2006). "Identification and characterization of two novel splicing isoforms of human estrogen-related receptor beta." *The Journal of clinical endocrinology and metabolism* 91(2): 569-579.

Zhou, W., S. C. Lo, et al. (2007). "ERRbeta: a potent inhibitor of Nrf2 transcriptional activity." *Molecular and cellular endocrinology* 278(1-2): 52-62.

11

p53, p63 and p73 Network in Breast Cancers

Chee-Onn Leong
International Medical University,
Malaysia

1. Introduction

Inactivation of the tumor suppressor p53 is the single most common genetic defect in all human cancers. The p53 tumor suppressor is critically important in regulation of cell cycle progression, senescence, differentiation, DNA repair and apoptosis. The discovery of two closely related homologues, p63 and p73, in 1997 generated instant excitement and quick expectations about their tumor suppressor functions. However, despite a remarkable structural and partial functional similarity among p53, initial p63 and p73 mouse knockout studies revealed an unexpected functional diversity among them. p63 and p73 knockouts exhibit severe developmental abnormalities but no increased cancer susceptibility. While p53 is frequently mutated during tumorigenesis (in over 50% of human tumors), p63 and p73 are rarely mutated. Instead, the p63 locus is amplified in squamous cell carcinomas (Bjorkqvist et al., 1998; Massion et al., 2003) and p73 is overexpressed in many tumor types including breast cancers (Moll and Slade, 2004; Zaika and El-Rifai, 2006; Zaika et al., 1999). Although p63 and p73 can activate apoptosis *in vitro*, it is clear that they are not classic Knudson-like tumor suppressors like p53.

Throughout the years, impressive number of evidences has been uncovered, suggesting that the p53-family play an important role in breast cancers. The emerging picture is that of an interconnected pathway, in which all p53-family proteins are involved in the response to oncogenic stress and physiological inputs. The p53/p63/p73 family members are capable of interacting in many ways that involve direct or indirect protein interactions, regulation of same target gene promoter and regulation of each other's promoters. As such, fluctuations in the levels of selected p53 family members (or their isoforms) might change the relative availability of shared protein partners, as multiple p53-family proteins compete for interaction. Also, differential expression of selected interactors - linked with genetic variation - may distinguish the response of the p53 pathway to the same potentially oncogenic stimuli in diverse individuals.

Despite the recent advances in understanding the unique roles of p53 family protein in breast cancers, there are many outstanding questions. What are the unique functions of the TA and ΔN isoforms of p63 and p73? How is individual p53 family member mediates gene expression regulated by the interaction with mutant p53 and other family member and their splicing variants in the cell? What are the patterns of p53 family isoform expression during normal development and tumorigenesis? What are the upstream signaling pathways that regulate individual p53 family member? What are the p53, p63 and p73 target genes? Do p53, p63 and p73 regulate distinct and/or overlapping sets of genes? Understanding the complexity of these interactions allow us to delineate the function of p53 family in human tumorigenesis and enable the development of new cancer therapeutics.

2. The origins and gene architecture of the p53 family proteins

The tumor suppressor gene, p53, was discovered in 1979 (Lane and Crawford, 1979; Linzer and Levine, 1979). Until recently, *p53* was thought to be a unique gene with no genetic paralogues. In 1997, however, Caput and coworkers serendiptiously identified a human homolog of p53 which they called p73 (Irwin and Kaelin, 2001; Kaelin, 1999; Kaghad et al., 1997). Shortly thereafter, several groups identified a third member of the family variably called Ket, p40, p51, p73L and p63 (Irwin and Kaelin, 2001; Kaelin, 1999; Osada et al., 1998; Schmale and Bamberger, 1997; Senoo et al., 1998; Trink et al., 1998; Yang et al., 1998). While p53 was discovered first, evolutionary conservation of DNA sequence suggests that p63 arose first during evolution, then p73 and finally p53 (Johnson et al., 2005).

Like many transcription factors, p53 are modular proteins with a conserved N-terminal transcriptional activation domain (TA), central DNA-binding domain (DBD) and a C-terminal oligomerization domain (OD) (Fig. 1) (Arrowsmith, 1999). The DBD has the highest degree of homology, where p63 and p73 share 65% amino-acid identity with p53, and even higher identity with each other. All three genes express many spliced isoforms – a feature that was thought to be unique for p63 and p73 but has recently found to be true for p53.

The existence of an internal promoter within the p53 family was first discovered in *p63* (Yang et al., 1998). The human and mouse *p63* genes express at least three alternatively spliced C-terminal isoforms (α, β, γ), and can be transcribed from an alternative promoter located in the intron 3 (Fig. 1). The transactivating isoforms (TAp63) are generated using the promoter upstream of exon 1 while the alternative promoter in intron 3 leads to the expression of N-terminal truncated isoforms (ΔNp63) lacking the transactivation domain. Altogether, the *p63* gene expresses at least six mRNA variants which encode for six different p63 protein isoforms (TAp63α, TAp63β, TAp63γ, ΔNp63α, ΔNp63β, and ΔNp63γ) (Murray-Zmijewski et al., 2006).

The p73 gene expresses at least seven alternatively spliced C-terminal isoforms (α, β, γ, δ, ε, ζ and η) and at least four alternatively spliced N-terminal isoforms (Melino et al., 2003; Moll and Slade, 2004; Stiewe et al., 2002b). Like p63, the p73 gene can be transcribed from an alternative promoter located in the intron 3 (Fig. 1). The transactivating isoforms are generated by the activity of the promoter upstream of exon 1 while the alternative promoter in intron 3 leads to the expression of the N-terminal truncated isoforms (ΔNp73) lacking the transactivation domain. Altogether, the p73 gene expresses at least 35 mRNA variants, which can encode theoretically 29 different p73 protein isoforms (Fig. 1). So far, 14 different p73 protein isoforms have been described. In contrast to p63, p73 isoforms can be initiated from different ATG and contain different part of the N-terminal domain, suggesting that they can have distinct protein interactions and specific activities (Murray-Zmijewski et al., 2006).

3. Developmental phenotypes of p53, p63 and p73 knockout mice

Since p53 is a powerful tumor suppressor gene, its loss in mice predisposes the animals to cancers of various organs (involving tissues such as blood, muscle and bone) with no visible developmental defects. Similarly, human patients with Li Fraumeni syndrome, the disease

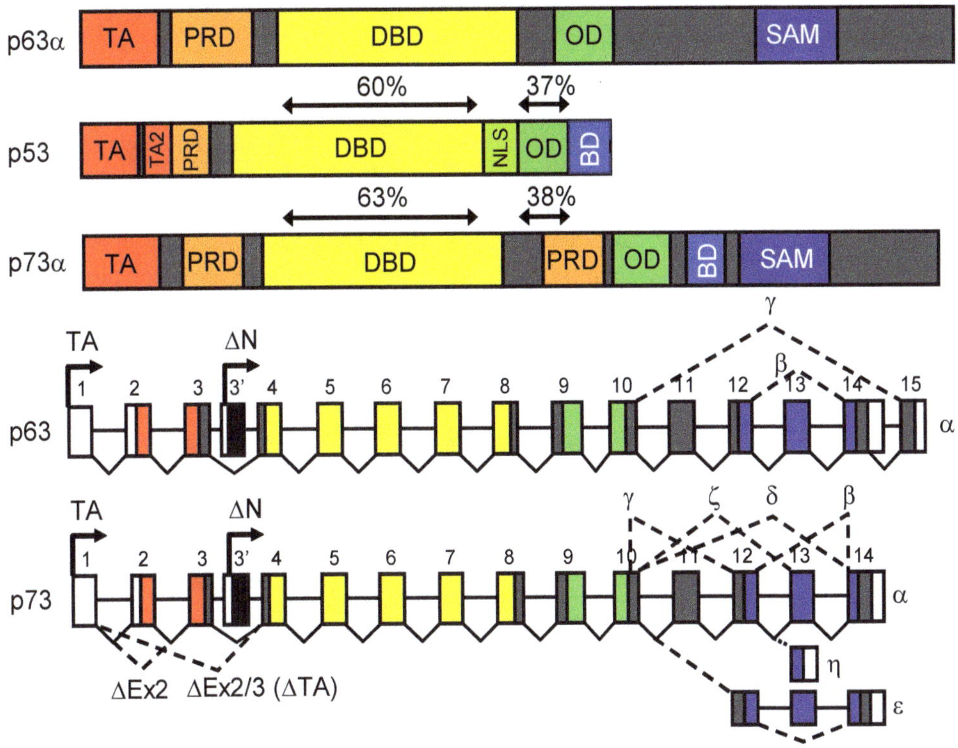

Fig. 1. **Gene architecture of the p53 family.** The p53 family includes the three genes p53, p63, and p73. Each of them has a modular structure consisting of the transactivation domain (TA), the DNA binding domain (DBD), and the oligomerization domain (OD). In addition to the 3 common domains, p63 and p73 also harbor a C-terminal sterile alpha-motif (SAM) domain in the α isoform. All p53 family genes are expressed as two major types: the full-length proteins containing the TA domain and ΔN proteins missing the TA domain. The P1 promoter in the 5′-untranslated region produces TA proteins that are transcriptionally active, whereas the P2 promoter produces ΔN proteins with dominant-negative functions toward themselves and toward wild-type p53. In addition, both p63 and p73 also undergo extensive C-terminal alternative splicing generating a myriad of isoforms with different transcriptional activity and specificity.

caused by germ line mutation of human p53, also predisposes to various cancer especially breast cancers (Johnson et al., 2005). While p53 seems to play little role in embryonic development, the p63 and p73 deficient mice have severe developmental abnormalities (Westfall and Pietenpol, 2004).

3.1 p63 in development: Role in epithelial differentiation and proliferation

p63-deficient mice are born alive but the limbs are absent or truncated owing to a malfunction of the apical ectodermal ridge (Mills et al., 1999; Yang et al., 1999). They fail to develop a stratified epidermis and most epithelial tissues (for example, hair follicles, teeth, prostate, lacrimal and salivary glands, and mammary glands), and eventually die from dehydration within hours of birth (Stiewe, 2007). Reminiscent of the knockout phenotype in mice, heterozygous germ line point mutations of p63 in humans also cause striking autosomal dominant developmental disorders including ectrodactyly-ectodermal dysplasia (EEC) (Celli et al., 1999), ankyloblepharon-ectodermal dysplasia clefting (Hay-Wells Syndrome) (Fomenkov et al., 2003), acro-dermato-ungual-lacrimal-tooth (ADULT) syndrome (Duijf et al., 2002), limb-mammary syndrome (LMF) (van Bokhoven et al., 2001), Rapp-Hodgkin syndrome (Chan et al., 2005), and split hand-split foot malformation syndrome (Brunner et al., 2002; Johnson et al., 2005; van Bokhoven et al., 2001).

Although the p63-deficient mice and human cases showed prominent phenotypes, the actual function of p63 in developmental processes remain controversial. The two groups that generated the p63-deficient mice reported identical phenotypes, the conclusions drawn from examination of the murine tissues differed (Westfall and Pietenpol, 2004). In one case clumps of differentiated cells were detected in the epidermis (Yang et al., 1999), whereas in the other, uncommitted ectodermal cells covered the body surface (Mills et al., 1999). This lead to two divergent points of view emerged from these analyses: one group attributed the p63-null phenotype to an absence of lineage commitment and an early block in epithelial differentiation (Mills et al., 1999); the other postulated that the phenotype was secondary to a defect in epithelial stem-cell renewal (Yang et al., 1999). It thus remained uncertain whether the primary function of p63 was in control of differentiation or self-renewal, or both (Blanpain and Fuchs, 2007).

Subsequent studies on p63 attempted to clarify this issue, but were further complicated with the discovery that the two principal isoforms of p63, ΔNp63 and TAp63, each of which have distinct roles in epithelial development. When transgenic mice expressing either TAp63 and/or ΔNp63 were bred on the p63-null background, mice expressing ΔNp63, but not TAp63, partially rescued basal epidermal gene expression, whereas only mice coexpressing both isoforms presented a significant improvement in expression of terminal differentiation marker. This data is consistent with the notion that ΔNp63 governs basal-epidermal gene expression, whereas TAp63 (possibly together with ΔNp63) promote terminal differentiation. Taken together, these studies supported a role for p63 in differentiation and not self-renewal. However, a later study by Senoo et al. (2007) demonstrated that p63 is not required for lineage commitment and differentiation of epithelial cells, as these cells present the typical markers for epithelial development and, in the case of the thymic epithelia, are fully competent to support the maturation of developing T cells in the thymus (Senoo et al., 2007). The study provides compelling evidence that p63 functions specifically to maintain the extraordinary proliferative capacity of the epithelial stem cells of the thymus and epidermis, suggesting a general function of the p63 transcription factor in maintaining the stem cells of a broad array of stratified epithelia. Thus, the question whether p63 functions in control of differentiation, self-renewal, or both remain debatable.

3.2 p73 in development: Role in neuronal and pheromonal pathways

The p73 knock-out mice have profound developmental defects including hippocampal dysgenesis, hydrocephalus, chronic infections and inflammation (Abraham and Meyer, 2003). They also exhibit abnormal reproductive and social behavior due to defects in pheromone detection, attributed to a dysfunctional nasal organ that normally expresses high levels of p73 (Johnson et al., 2005). The tissue specificity of the p73 deficient phenotype (concentrated to the brain and related structures) may be associated with variable patterns of isoforms expressed in brain vs. other tissues (Hu et al., 2000; Johnson et al., 2005).

ΔNp73 is the predominant isoform in the developing mouse brain and might act as a transcriptional repressor (Pozniak et al., 2000; Yang et al., 1998). *In situ* hybridization reveals strong ΔNp73 expression in E12.5 fetal mouse brain in the preplate layer, bed nucleus of stria terminalis, choroid plexus, vomeronasal area, and preoptic area (Yang et al., 2000). Moreover, ΔNp73 is the only form of p73 found in mouse brain and the sympathetic superior cervical ganglia in P10 neonatal mice (Pozniak et al., 2000). Functional studies and knockout mice showed ΔNp73 is required to counteract p53-mediated neuronal death during the normal development of the mouse neuronal system (Pozniak et al., 2000). Withdrawal of nerve growth factor, an obligate survival factor for mouse sympathetic neurons, leads to p53 induction and p53-dependent cell death. In pull-down assays, mixed protein complexes of p53/ΔNp73 were demonstrated, suggesting one biochemical basis for transdominance in addition to possible promoter competition. Together, these data demonstrated that ΔNp73 is downstream of nerve growth factor in the nerve growth factor survival pathway and explains why p73-deficient mice, missing all forms of p73 including protective ΔNp73, undergo accelerated neuronal death in postnatal superior cervical ganglia (Moll and Slade, 2004; Pozniak et al., 2000).

To date, there are no human developmental syndromes associated with germ line p73 mutations (Johnson et al., 2005). Unlike p53-decifiency, p73 knock-out mice show no increased susceptibility to spontaneous tumorigenesis (Stiewe and Putzer, 2002; Yang et al., 2000).

4. Role of p53 family in breast malignancy: Tumor suppressor or oncogene?

p53 is a powerful tumor suppressor, as proven by a wealth of in vivo models and dramatically confirmed by frequent mutation in human cancers. However, the role of p63 and p73 in tumor suppression is less obvious, because they are rarely deleted or mutated in cancer and the respective homozygous knockout mice die tumor-free from developmental defects in the initial studies.

4.1 p63 and cancer

p63, mainly its ΔN isoform, is highly expressed in embryonic epidermis and act as a molecular switch for initiation of an epithelial stratification program (Koster et al., 2004). In postnatal epidermis, ΔNp63 expression is restricted to the nuclei of basal cells of normal epithelia (skin, esophagus, tonsil, prostate, urothelium, ectocervix, and vagina) and to certain populations of basal cells in glandular structures of prostate, breast, and bronchi (Di Como et al., 2002; Yang et al., 1998). Specifically, p63 is expressed in myoepithelial cells of the breast that play an important role in differentiation and carcinogenesis of the breast (Davis et al., 2002; Garraway et al., 2003; Moll and Slade, 2004; Reis-Filho et al., 2003a; Ribeiro-Silva et al., 2003). p63 expression was not detected in mesenchymal, neural, endothelial, smooth muscle or adipose cells consistent with restricted p63 expression in squamous and basal epithelial tissues (Reis-Filho et al., 2003b; Westfall and Pietenpol, 2004). The initial findings showed that ΔNp63α can act antagonistically toward p53 (Yang et al., 1998). Subsequent studies found dysregulated expression of p63, sometimes in conjunction with amplification of its genomic region at 3q27-28 in a many human epithelial cancers (Crook et al., 2000; Hibi et al., 2000; Massion et al., 2003; Park et al., 2000; Yamaguchi et al., 2000). Amplification of the p63 gene frequently leads to overexpression of the ΔNp63α variant (Hibi et al., 2000). Regardless, ΔNp63α have been reported to be frequently overexpressed in bladder, breast, cervix, head and neck, lung, prostate and nasopharyngeal carcinoma (Crook et al., 2000; Moll and Slade, 2004; Westfall and Pietenpol, 2004). Overexpression of the ΔNp63 variant in Rat 1a cells have also been shown to increase growth of these cells in soft agar and as xenograft tumors (Hibi et al., 2000). Thus, the maintenance of the ΔNp63 isoforms in squamous cancers may contribute to keeping the cells in a stem cell-like phenotype, thereby promoting tumor growth. Of note, analysis of p63 sequence isolated from various human tumors and numerous human cancer cell lines showed that p63 rarely, if ever, mutated (Hagiwara et al., 1999; Osada et al., 1998). Collectively these data suggest that p63 does not function as a tumor suppressor but rather as an oncogene (Westfall and Pietenpol, 2004).

Nevertheless, studies on the TA isoform of p63 suggest an opposite view. Transient transfection of TAp63 has been shown to induce cell cycle arrest and apoptosis (Osada et al., 1998; Westfall and Pietenpol, 2004; Yang et al., 1998). The TAp63 isoforms are able to bind to DNA through p53 response element (p53RE) and activate transcription of a subset of p53 target genes (Murray-Zmijewski et al., 2006). Interestingly, TAp63γ had the greatest transactivation activity and TAp63α had the minimal activity (Westfall and Pietenpol, 2004). The ΔNp63 isoforms can also bind DNA through p53RE and can exert dominant-negative effects over p53, p73 and p63 activities by either competing for DNA binding sites or by direct protein interaction (Benard et al., 2003). Moreover, ΔNp63 isoforms were also shown to directly activate specific gene targets not induced by TA isoforms (Dohn et al., 2001; Wu et al., 2003). Thus, p63 has the ability to regulate a number of genes with diverse roles and possesses opposing regulatory effect by expressing different amount of TAp63 and ΔNp63 isoforms. Thus, an abnormal alteration in expression of these isoforms is likely to play an important role in tumorigenesis.

4.2 p73 and cancer

Like p63, p73 is rarely, if ever mutated in cancers. Unlike p63 which is frequently amplified in epithelial cancers, p73 frequently undergoes loss of heterozygosity in breast and colon cancer, neuroblastoma, oligodendroglioma, and melanoma. This fact, in conjunction with the functional similarity to p53, originally led to the proposal that p73 is a tumor suppressor gene (Kaghad et al., 1997). Genetic data on most cancer types, however, exclude p73 as a classic Knudson-type tumor suppressor, which by definition is targeted to undergo loss of expression or function during tumorigenesis. To date, loss of function mutations in p73 are vanishingly rare (0.6%). Moreover, imprinting of the p73 locus, initially thought to be an epigenetic explanation to satisfy the two-hit hypothesis, is rather uncommon and, if present, varies from tissue to tissue and person to person and does not correlate with p73 expression levels (Kovalev et al., 1998; Moll and Slade, 2004; Nomoto et al., 1998; Tsao et al., 1999; Zaika et al., 1999).

In fact, TAp73 overexpression has been found in different tumor types including tumors of breast (Leong et al., 2007; Zaika et al., 1999), neuroblastoma (Kovalev et al., 1998), lung (Mai et al., 1998; Tokuchi et al., 1999), esophagus (Cai et al., 2000), stomach (Kang et al., 2000), colon (Sunahara et al., 1998), bladder (Chi et al., 1999; Yokomizo et al., 1999), ovarian cancer (Chen et al., 2000; Ng et al., 2000; Zwahlen et al., 2000), liver cancer (Tannapfel et al., 1999b), cholangiocellular carcinoma (Tannapfel et al., 1999a), colon carcinoma (Sun, 2002), and head and neck squamous carcinoma (Choi et al., 2002; Rocco et al., 2006; Weber et al., 2002). Of note, primary tumors and tumor cell lines with p73 overexpression tend to simultaneously overexpress a complex profile of shorter C-terminal splice variants (p73γ, p73δ, p73δ, and p73ϕ), whereas the normal tissue of origin is limited to the expression of p73α and p73β (Zaika et al., 1999). Importantly, patients with high global p73 protein expression had a worse survival than patients with undetectable levels (Moll and Slade, 2004; Sun, 2002; Tannapfel et al., 1999b).

Little is known about which genes are regulated specifically by p73 under physiological conditions. When overexpressed p73 also binds to p53 DNA target sites, transactivates p53-responsive genes and is capable of inducing cell cycle arrest and apoptosis in mammalian cells in a p53-like manner (Jost et al., 1997; Kaghad et al., 1997; Stiewe and Putzer, 2002). For example, p73 can activate the promoters of several p53-responsive genes, including *p21, BAX, PUMA, MDM2, GADD45, 14-3-3σ, cyclin G, IGFBP3,* and *p53R2* (Irwin and Kaelin, 2001; Jost et al., 1997; Kaghad et al., 1997; Lee and La Thangue, 1999; Nakano et al., 2000; Ueda et al., 1999; Vikhanskaya et al., 2001; Yang et al., 1998; Yu et al., 1999; Zhu et al., 1998). Nonetheless, there is evidence that p73 can activate many other genes which are not p53 target genes. For example, aquaporin 3 (AQP3), a glycerol and water transporter, has been shown to be a specific p73-responsive gene. It is speculated, that in p73-deficient mice lack of AQP3 induction accounts for the defects in production or reabsorption of cerebrospinal fluid, resulting in hydrocephalus (Stiewe and Putzer, 2002; Zheng and Chen, 2001).

Numerous reports also indicating a quantitative difference in the transcriptional activity of the various p73 splice variants. For example, the TAp73β is a more potent transcriptional activator than TAp73α (De Laurenzi et al., 1998; Lee and La Thangue, 1999; Yu et al., 1999; Zhu et al., 1998). Likewise TAp73β is more potent than TAp73α as an inducer of apoptosis, suggesting that TAp73α contains an 'inhibitory' region not included in the β-isoform. Consistently, a C-terminal deletion mutant of TAp73α lacking the putative inhibitory region showed a significantly higher level of transcriptional activity than wild-type TAp73α (Ozaki et al., 1999; Ueda et al., 2001). Moreover, the transcriptional activity of TAp73β was reduced *in trans* by co-expression with either TAp73α or p73ε, which bears an identical C-terminal structure as TAp73α (Ueda et al., 2001). This suppression effect is most likely mediated by inter-variant associations as it depends on the presence of the oligomerization domain. These observations indicate that p73-mediated gene expression is regulated by the interaction of all p73 isoforms present in the cell. The current data therefore indicate the existence of transciptional specificity among the p53-family members with pronounced differences between p53 and p73 on the one hand and between the various p73 isoforms on the other hand (Stiewe and Putzer, 2002).

5. Regulation of p53 family functions

The p53 family proteins are entangled in a regulatory network with positive or negative modulators. Many regulatory pathways may be shared by multiple p53-family proteins, with similar or different effects (Fig. 2).

5.1 Upstream regulation of p53 family members

One of the clear differences that discriminate p53 family members is the fact that they response to viral oncoproteins differently. Adenovirus E1B55, human papilloma virus E6 protein, and SV40 T antigen bind to and inactivate p53 during viral transformation (Fig. 2)

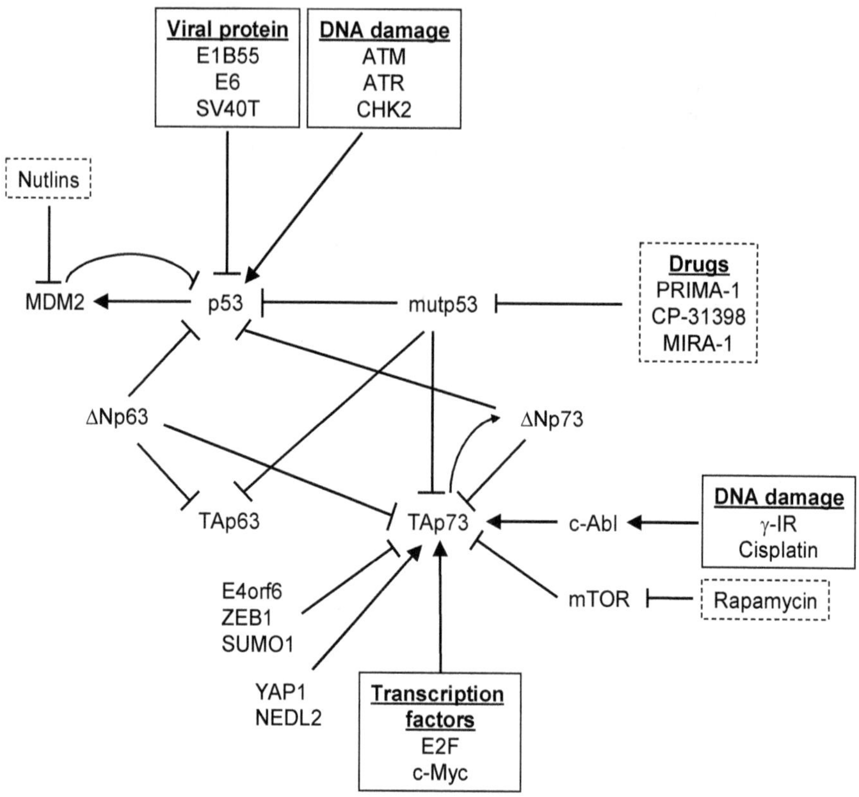

Fig. 2. The p53 family network and its regulation.

(Lechner et al., 1992; Linzer and Levine, 1979; Sarnow et al., 1982; Yew and Berk, 1992). These three proteins, however, do not bind to p73 (Dobbelstein and Roth, 1998; Marin et al., 1998; Roth et al., 1998; Steegenga et al., 1999). In fact, p73β can induce growth inhibition and apoptosis in cancer cells that produce E6 (Prabhu et al., 1998). Likewise, E6 and SV40 T antigen do not interact with p63 (Roth and Dobbelstein, 1999). The adenoviral protein E4orf6 also binds to and antagonizes p53, but there have been conflicting reports as to whether it interacts with p73. Roth *et al.* (1998) reported that E4orf6 does not affect p73 stability or the ability of p73 to activate transcription (Roth et al., 1998). Two other groups reported that E4orf6 binds to the C-terminus of p73 and blocks transcriptional activation and colony suppression by p73 (Higashino et al., 1998; Steegenga et al., 1999). Thus, certain viral oncoproteins preferentially inactivate p53 while sparing p63 and p73, despite the high degree of similarity between these three proteins (Fig. 2).

Several reports have shown that the cellular oncogenes E2F1 and c-Myc can induce and activate the endogenous TAp73α and TAp73β proteins for target gene transactivation, apoptosis, and growth suppression in p53-deficient human tumor cells (Irwin et al., 2000; Lissy et al., 2000; Stiewe and Putzer, 2000; Zaika et al., 2001). E2F1 is a specific and direct transcriptional activator of TAp73 but not p63 (Fig. 2) (Irwin et al., 2000; Stiewe and Putzer, 2000). Because oncogene deregulation of E2F1 and c-Myc are one of the most common genetic alterations in human tumors, these findings might provide a physiologic mechanism for TAp73 overexpression in tumors.

In a recent study, we showed that TAp73 is selective upregulated in BRCA1-associated ovarian tumors. Interestingly, we found that BRCA1-deficient ovarian carcinoma cells exhibit hypermethylation within a p73 regulatory region, which includes the binding site for the transcriptional repressor ZEB1. This hypermethylation leads to the abrogation of ZEB1 binding and hence increased expression of TAp73. Similarly, ZEB1 binding site methylation and TAp73 expression correlated with BRCA1 status in primary ovarian carcinomas and with clinical response to cisplatin (Fig. 2) (Ibrahim et al., 2010). Together, these data establish another important link between p73 and human cancer.

5.2 Regulation of p53 family protein stability

p53 is a short-lived protein, and its stability is very tightly regulated by ubiquitination under physiological condition (Haupt et al., 1997; Honda et al., 1997; Kubbutat et al., 1997). Polyubiquitination of p53 is carried out by the ubiquitin ligase MDM2. The polyubiquitination and degradation of p53 is influenced by a variety of factors including regulated changes in the subcellular localization of p53 and MDM2. Moreover, *MDM2* itself is a p53-inducible gene, and thus activation of p53 establishes a negative feedback loop wherein MDM2 limits p53 accumulation (Fig. 2) (Barak et al., 1993; Irwin and Kaelin, 2001).

In addition to its role in p53 degradation, MDM2 also binds to a sequence in the transactivation domain of p53 (amino acid residues 17–27) and thereby inhibits p53-dependent transactivation (Momand et al., 1992). The MDM2 binding site in p53 is well conserved in both p63 and p73. Several groups have shown that MDM2 bind to p73 and prevent it from binding to the transcriptional coactivators p300 and CBP (Balint et al., 1999; Ongkeko et al., 1999; Zeng et al., 1999; Zeng et al., 2000). This leads to impaired p73-dependent transcriptional activation and diminished apoptosis. Of note, like p53, p73 can activate the *MDM2* promoter (Wang et al., 2001b; Zeng et al., 1999; Zhu et al., 1998). Although MDM2 does not target p73 for polyubiquitination, p73 stability is indirectly dependent upon the activity of the proteasome. Specifically, many proteosome inhibitors have been shown to increase p73 levels (Balint et al., 1999; Irwin and Kaelin, 2001; Ongkeko et al., 1999). Thus, it is possible that p73 is polyubiquitinated in cells by a yet unknown E3 ligase.

Unlike p73 and p53, p63 does not bind to either MDM2 (Wang et al., 2001a). Although there are no data implicating ubiquitination pathways in p63 degradation, Ratovitski *et al.* (2001) showed that p63 abundance could be regulated by caspase-dependent proteolysis due to the presence of a caspase recognition site, YVED, in the amino acid sequence (Irwin and Kaelin, 2001; Ratovitski et al., 2001).

Besides MDM2, the degradation and protein stability of p53 family proteins might be regulated by small ubiquitin-related modifier-1 (SUMO-1) (Minty et al., 2000; Moll and Slade, 2004). Conjugation to SUMO-1 has been shown to affect p53 transcriptional activity but does not appear to influence p53 stability (Fig. 2) (Gostissa et al., 1999; Irwin and Kaelin, 2001; Rodriguez et al., 2001). Nevertheless, modification of p73α by SUMO-1 has been reported to alter p73 subcellular localization and increased the rate of p73 degradation. On the other hand, the novel Hect domain containing NEDD4-like E3 ubiquitin ligase, NEDL2, binds to p73 via its PY motif in the C-terminal region (Miyazaki et al., 2003). p53, which lacks the PY motif, does not bind to NEDL2. Overexpression of NEDL2 results in the ubiquitination of p73. However, rather than mediating degradation, ubiquitination by NEDL2 enhances the stability of p73 and its ability to transactivate p53/p73-responsive promoters (Fig. 2). The differential binding of NEDL2 to p53 family members is thus another factor that might contribute to their functional divergence. Likewise, the NAD(P)H:quinone oxidoreductase-1 (NQO1) stabilizes p73α (as well as p53) but not p73β by binding to the SAM domain of p73α and protect p73α from 20S proteasomal degradation.. This NQO1-mediated stabilization of p73α and p53 might explan why NQO1 knockout mice and human with inactive NQO1 polymorphisms are susceptible to cancer (Asher et al., 2002; Moll and Slade, 2004).

5.3 Regulation of p53 family protein transcriptional activity

The ankyrin-rich, Src holomogy 3 domain, proline-rich proteins, ASPP1 and ASPP2, stimulate the apoptotic function of p53, p63, and p73 (Bergamaschi et al., 2004; Samuels-Lev et al., 2001). By binding to the DBD of p53, p63, and p73, ASPP1 and ASPP2 stimulate the transactivation function of all three proteins on the promoters of *BAX*, *PIG3*, and *PUMA* but not *MDM2* or $p21^{WAF\text{-}1/CIP1}$. Hence, ASPP1 and ASPP2 are the first two identified common activators of all p53 family members.

The transcriptional coactivator Yes-associated protein (YAP) has also been shown to potentiate TAp73-mediated transactivation of BAX after DNA damage. Conversely, Akt phosphorylates YAP, which induces interaction with 14-3-3, relocation of YAP to the cytoplasm, and attenuation of p73-mediated apoptosis (Basu et al., 2003; Moll and Slade, 2004).

5.4 DNA damage response and postranslational modification

p53 stabilization and activation by genotoxic stress is associated with multiple post-translational modifications at the N- and C-termini of p53. Under genotoxic stress, activation of stress kinases such ATM, ATR, and Chk2 lead to phosphorylation of p53 at multiple residues at Ser15, Ser20, Ser33, Ser37, Ser46, Thr18, Thr81, Ser315 and Ser392 to stabilize the protein by interfering with MDM2 binding (Fig. 2). In addition, acetylation at Lys320, Lys373, and Lys382, and sumoylation at Lys386 have also been reported to activate the transcriptional activity of p53 (Appella, 2001).

p73 is also activated for apoptosis in response to various genotoxix agents including cisplatin, taxol, and γ-irradiation. The activation of p73 is highly dependent on the non-receptor tyrosine kinase c-abl (Agami et al., 1999; Gong et al., 1999; Moll and Slade, 2004; Yuan et al., 1999). In response to γ-irradiation and cisplatin, TAp73 undergoes phosphorylation at Tyr99 by c-abl (Fig. 2). This, in turn, lead to the stabilization of the protein and dissociation of TAp73 from the TAp73/ΔNp63 inhibitory complex followed by apoptosis (Agami et al., 1999; Leong et al., 2007; Tsai and Yuan, 2003; Yuan et al., 1999).

The activation and phosphorylation of p73 is mainly through the direct interaction between the PXXP motifs of p73 and the Src homology 3 domain of c-abl (Moll and Slade, 2004). Because c-abl is itself phosphorylated and activated by the ATM, ATM may also be involved in the pathway leading to c-abl-dependent p73 activation (Shaul, 2000). These findings suggest that p73 might participate in a mismatch-repair signaling pathway. Recent microarray gene expression profiles further support a role for p73 in response to and repair of DNA damage (Vikhanskaya et al., 2001). In addition to cisplatin, Taxol also increases p73 accumulation, but UV irradiation, actinomycin D, and methylmethane sulfonate do not (Irwin and Kaelin, 2001; Levrero et al., 1999). As p63 does not have the PXXP motifs, it is unlikely that c-abl will phosphorylate p63 (Moll and Slade, 2004).

In addition to c-abl, p73 proteins may also be regulated by cyclin-CDK complexes and play a role in the regulation of cell cycle. p73 physically interacts with various cyclins and certain cyclin-CDK complexes including cyclin A-CDK1/2, cyclin B-CDK1/ 2, and cyclin E-CDK2, which can phosphorylate various p73 isoforms in vitro at Thr86. This cell cycle-dependent phosphorylation inhibits p73 to induce endogenous p21 expression (Gaiddon et al., 2003). p73 is a physiologic target of the cyclin B-CDK1 mitotic kinase complex in vivo, which results in a decreased ability of p73 to bind DNA and activate transcription in mitotic cells. Thus, both p73α and p73β isoforms have been shown to be hyperphosphorylated in normal mitotic cells (Fulco et al., 2003).

DNA damage also induces acetylation of p73 at Lys321, Lys327, and Lys331 by the acetyltransferase p300/cAMP-responsive element binding protein. Non-acetylated p73 is defective in inducing proapoptotic genes such as p53AIP1 but retains the ability to activate other target genes such as p21. This indicates that DNA damage-dependent p73 acetylation, like in p53, potentiates the apoptotic function of p73 by selectively increasing its ability to induce the transcription of proapoptotic target genes (Costanzo et al., 2002; Moll and Slade, 2004).

Finally, the mammalian target of rapamycin (mTOR) was recently identified as a negative regulator of p73 (Fig. 2). Notably, pharmacologic inhibition of mTOR in primary human mammary epithelial cells resulted in differential regulation of p53 family members (Rosenbluth et al., 2008). Cells exhibited selective up-regulation of TAp73, whereas ΔNp63 and p53 levels were both decreased. Interestingly, inhibition of mTOR by rapamycin synergizes cisplatin sensitivity in breast cancer cells through upregulation of TAp73 (Wong et al., 2010). Since mTOR is a master regulator of energy homeostasis and cell growth, and is often active in tumors (Guertin and Sabatini, 2007), this suggests that mTOR may inhibit TAp73 in tumors. In general, cancer cells may use upstream kinases or cofactors to inhibit p53 family members in different cellular contexts, ultimately maintaining proliferation and survival (Rosenbluth and Pietenpol, 2008).

6. The p53 pathway as a network

The significance interplay between p53 family and their isoforms in tumor is demonstrated by the fact that p53 cannot induce apoptosis in response to DNA damage, without the presence of p63 and p73 (Flores et al., 2002). Various mechanisms by which p53/p63/p73 proteins and their isoforms determine the cell fate through formation of transdominant heterocomplex, promoter competition and autoregulatory feedback loop have been proposed. These mechanisms are likely to play an important role in the transition between normal cell cycling and the onset of tumor formation.

6.1 Homotypic and heterotypic interactions among p53 family members

Physical interaction between oncogenic and antioncogenic p53 family members have been demonstrated to interfere with the tumor suppressor functions of wild-type p53 and TAp73 (Nakagawa et al., 2002; Stiewe et al., 2003; Stiewe et al., 2002a; Zaika et al., 2002). Mixed protein complexes were found between endogenous ΔNp73α or ΔNp73β on the one hand and either wild-type p53, TAp73α, or TAp73β on the other hand in primary human tumors, cultured human tumor cells, and mouse neurons (Moll and Slade, 2004). In human head and neck suqamous cell carcinoma and triple-negative breast cancer, endogenous ΔNp63 was shown to physically interact with TAp73 and suppresses TAp73 tumor suppressor activities (Fig. 2) (Leong et al., 2007; Rocco et al., 2006).

In addition, physical interactions between certain human p53 mutants and TAp73 or TAp63 proteins have been reported in coimmunoprecipitation assays, and these interactions correlate with functional transdominance. In contrast, complexes between wild-type p53 and p73 are not observed in mammalian cells (Di Como et al., 1999; Marin et al., 2000; Pozniak et al., 2000; Vikhanskaya et al., 2000). Unexpectedly, protein contact occurs between the DBD of mutant p53 and the DBD and oligomerization domain of p73 rather than between the respective oligomerization domains (Davison et al., 1999; Gaiddon et al., 2001; Strano et al., 2000; Vikhanskaya et al., 2000). In cotransfection experiments, mixed heterocomplexes were shown between p53 mutants p53Ala143, p53Leu173, p53His175, p53Cys220, p53Trp248, or p53Gly281 and TAp73α, TAp73γ, TAp73δ and TAp63 (Di Como et al., 1999; Gaiddon et al., 2001; Marin et al., 2000; Strano et al., 2000). Physiologic complexes were found in five tumor cell lines between endogenous mutant p53 and p73 (Marin et al., 2000; Strano et al., 2000). Functionally, formation of such stable complexes leads to a loss of p73- and p63-mediated transactivation and proapoptotic abilities. Moreover, E2F1-induced p73 transactivation, apoptosis, and colony suppression was inhibited by coexpressed p53His175 (Stiewe and Putzer, 2000). Interestingly, the Arg/Pro polymorphism at codon 72 of mutant p53 is a biological determinant for binding and inactivation of p73, with 72R mutants of p53 being inhibitory, whereas 72P mutants are not (Fig. 2) (Bergamaschi et al., 2003; Marin et al., 2000; Moll and Slade, 2004).

This functional inhibition of TAp73 or TAp63 by some p53 mutants mirrors the ability of many transdominant missense p53 mutants to abrogate wild-type p53 function (Kern et al., 1992; Unger et al., 1992). It suggests that in tumors that express both TAp73 and mutant p53 (typically at very high levels due to deficient MDM2-mediated degradation), the function of TAp73 and TAp63 might be inactivated. If this occurs in primary human tumors, it might have far-reaching consequences because (a) it argues for a transdominant inhibition of the tumor suppressor function of TAp73 isoforms during tumor development, (b) it could be the underlying mechanism for the gain-of-function activity of certain p53 mutants, and (c) it might further increase chemoresistance in cancer therapy of established tumors.

p53 is exceptional among tumor suppressors in that it selects for the overexpression of missense mutants rather than for loss of expression as most other suppressor genes do. This gain-of function increased tumorigenicity compared with p53-null parental cells, increased resistance to cancer agents, and increased genomic instability due to abrogation of the mitotic spindle checkpoint (Dittmer et al., 1993; Halevy et al., 1990; Shaulsky et al., 1991). Conceivably, p63 might also participates in this network. A recent study shown that mutant p53His273 is required for survival of breast cancer cells as knock-down of endogenous mutant p53His273 in breast cancer cells induces massive apoptosis. Surprisingly, the survival effects of p53His273 is independent of TAp73 or TAp63 function as depletion of both isoforms did not rescue the cells from apoptosis following p53His273 knock-down (Lim et al., 2009). Therefore, it is important to note that not all p53 mutants have transdominant effects against TAp73 or TAp63. Some p53 mutants are clearly recessive toward TAp73 (e.g., p53His283, p53Tyr277 and p53His273) and do not interfere with its action (Gaiddon et al., 2001; Lim et al., 2009; Moll and Slade, 2004).

6.2 Promoter competition

Promoter competition by ΔNp73 and ΔNp63 at TAp73/p53 response elements has been reported previously (Kartasheva et al., 2002; Rocco et al., 2006; Stiewe et al., 2002a). It is conceivable that ΔNp73 or ΔNp63 homo-oligomers might have a stronger affinity to certain target gene promoters than wild-type p53 or TAp73. In those cases, p53 or TAp73 inhibition could occur due to competition at the level of target gene access. In the wild-type p53-containing ovarian carcinoma cell line A2780, coexpression of increasing amounts of either TAp73α, TAp73β, TAp73γ, or TAp73ε inhibits specific DNA binding and transcriptional activity of p53 in the absence of hetero-oligomer formation (Moll and Slade, 2004; Ueda et al., 1999; Vikhanskaya et al., 2000). These results suggest that promoter competition could be another mechanism for transdominance between p53 family proteins.

6.3 Autoregulatory feedback loop among p53, TAp73, and ΔNp73

p53 and TAp73 regulate ΔNp73 but not ΔNp63 levels by binding to the p73 P2 promoter and inducing its transcription (Fig. 2). A p73-specific responsive element was mapped within the P2 region (Nakagawa et al., 2002). This generates a negative feedback loop analogous negatively regulates the activity of p53 and p73 (Grob et al., 2001; Kartasheva et al., 2002; Nakagawa et al., 2002; Vossio et al., 2002). As mentioned earlier, ΔNp73 blocks p53 and TAp73 activity through heterocomplex formation (Nakagawa et al., 2002; Stiewe et al., 2002a; Zaika et al., 2002) or through promoter competition (Kartasheva et al., 2002; Stiewe et al., 2002a) and thus contributes to the termination of the p53/p73 response in cells. In contrast to ΔNp73, ΔNp63 expression is transcriptionally repressed by p53 (Moll and Slade, 2004; Waltermann et al., 2003).

7. Targeting the p53 family for treatment of breast cancers

As described above, activation of wild-type TAp73 (or TAp63) lead to cell death in cancer cells. This hypothesis is intriguing given the fact that p73 and p63 are rarely mutated in cancer. Instead, overexpression of TAp73 has been reported in many tumor types including breast cancers and head and neck squamous carcinoma (Leong et al., 2007; Rocco et al., 2006). As such, selective activaton of TAp73 (or TAp63) might induce tumor specific cell death. In principle, activation of the p53 family tumor suppressive pathways might be achieved in several ways (Kaelin, 1999).

First, induction and activation of TAp73 have been reported in response to wide variety of chemotherapeutic agents including Adriamycin, cisplatin, taxol, and etoposide in different tumor cell lines (Bergamaschi et al., 2003; Irwin et al., 2003; Moll and Slade, 2004). In particular, cisplatin treatment has been shown to induce c-abl dependent phosphorylation of TAp73 and lead to its dissociation from the TAp73/ΔNp63 inhibitory complex in head and neck squamous cell carcinoma and breast cancer cells (Fig. 2) (Leong et al., 2007; Rocco et al., 2006). Similarly, a recent clinical study also shown that cells that co-overexpressed TAp73 and ΔNp63 is more likely to response to cisplatin compare to tumors that have no TAp73 expression. These results suggest that certain chemotherapeutic agents can activate TAp73 even in the presence of high level of ΔN isoforms.

Second, a more detailed understanding of the upstream signals that impinge upon p73 and p63 might allow for the design of drugs that would activate the transcription of these genes or stabilize their protein products. For example, the mammalian target of rapamycin (mTOR) was recently identified as a negative regulator of p73 (Rosenbluth et al., 2008). Inhibition of mTOR in primary human mammary epithelial cells selectively up-regulate TAp73 (Rosenbluth et al., 2008; Rosenbluth and Pietenpol, 2008). Combination of cisplatin and mTOR inhibitor, rapamycin, has also been shown to synergizes cisplatin sensitivity in basal-like breast cancer cells through up-regulation of TAp73 recently (Fig. 2) (Wong et al.,

2010). Of note, a phase II neo-adjuvant clinical trial of cisplatin and mTOR inhibitor, everolimus, in patients with triple-negative breast cancer has recently opened for recruitment (ClinicalTrials.gov Identifier: NCT00930930) and will be able to directly address whether targeting these pathways will increase the sensitivity of tumors towards cisplatin chemotherapy.

Finally, it might be possible to design or discover drugs that block the interaction of mutant p53 with p73 or intreraction of MDM2 with p73 which has been shown to inhibit p73 transcription activity (Kaelin, 1999). In theory, molecules already in development that block the interaction of MDM2 with p53 or molecules that restore mutant p53 function might also function in this setting. For example, PRIMA-1, CP-31398 and MIRA-1 are molecules that have been shown to restore wild-type conformation and transcriptional transactivation to mutant p53 (Fig. 2) (Wiman, 2006). Similarly, MDM2 inhibitor such as Nutlins, might interfere MDM2-p73 binding and hence restore the tumor suppressor function of p73 (Ambrosini et al., 2007; Shangary and Wang, 2008). Whether these molecules will selectively activate TAp73 remain to be investigated.

8. Concluding remarks

In concludion, studies of the newly identified p53 family members, p63 and p73, have revealed several structural and functional similarities. The p53 transactivation, DNA binding, and oligomerization domains are highly conserved among all family members. Like p53, p63 and p73 can form oligomers, bind DNA, and transactivate the promoters of a subset of p53 target genes and induce apoptosis. In addition, certain cellular and viral proteins known to bind and regulate p53 activity likewise can bind to p63 and p73.

Despite the fact that p63 and p73 mimic many p53 activities, more recent studies highlight significant differences between the family members. In contrast to *p53*, *p63* and *p73* give rise to multiple functionally distinct protein isoforms due to alternative promoter utilization and alternative mRNA splicing. The ΔN isoforms, which lack the N-terminal transactivation domain, can function as "dominant-negative" proteins, blocking certain activities of the corresponding full-length proteins.

Differences in the upstream signaling pathways involved in activation of each of the family members are also becoming apparent. Only a subset of the DNA-damaging agents that induce p53 also induce p73. Many cellular and viral oncoproteins also discriminate between p53 and the newer family members. Finally, it is becoming apparent that *p63* and *p73* are not classical Knudson-type tumor suppressor genes. In particular, these genes are not frequently mutated in tumors, and germ-line mutations in these genes do not cause tumors in mice. Instead, mice with deletions in *p63* and *p73* have significant developmental abnormalities.

Despite the significant advances in understanding the unique roles of p53, p63 and p73, there are still several outstanding questions. Understanding the complexity of p53 family members interactions may allow us to to delineate the function of the p53 family network in human tumorigenesis and facilitate the development of anticancer therapeutics that seek to induce the activation of "p53-responsive" genes in cells lacking wild-type p53.

9. References

Abraham, H., and Meyer, G. (2003). Reelin-expressing neurons in the postnatal and adult human hippocampal formation. Hippocampus *13*, 715-727.

Agami, R., Blandino, G., Oren, M., and Shaul, Y. (1999). Interaction of c-Abl and p73alpha and their collaboration to induce apoptosis. Nature *399*, 809-813.

Ambrosini, G., Sambol, E. B., Carvajal, D., Vassilev, L. T., Singer, S., and Schwartz, G. K. (2007). Mouse double minute antagonist Nutlin-3a enhances chemotherapy-induced apoptosis in cancer cells with mutant p53 by activating E2F1. Oncogene *26*, 3473-3481.

Appella, E. (2001). Modulation of p53 function in cellular regulation. Eur J Biochem *268*, 2763.

Arrowsmith, C. H. (1999). Structure and function in the p53 family. Cell Death Differ *6*, 1169-1173.

Asher, G., Lotem, J., Sachs, L., Kahana, C., and Shaul, Y. (2002). Mdm-2 and ubiquitin-independent p53 proteasomal degradation regulated by NQO1. Proc Natl Acad Sci U S A *99*, 13125-13130.

Balint, E., Bates, S., and Vousden, K. H. (1999). Mdm2 binds p73 alpha without targeting degradation. Oncogene *18*, 3923-3929.

Barak, Y., Juven, T., Haffner, R., and Oren, M. (1993). mdm2 expression is induced by wild type p53 activity. EMBO J *12*, 461-468.

Basu, S., Totty, N. F., Irwin, M. S., Sudol, M., and Downward, J. (2003). Akt phosphorylates the Yes-associated protein, YAP, to induce interaction with 14-3-3 and attenuation of p73-mediated apoptosis. Mol Cell *11*, 11-23.

Benard, J., Douc-Rasy, S., and Ahomadegbe, J. C. (2003). TP53 family members and human cancers. Hum Mutat *21*, 182-191.

Bergamaschi, D., Gasco, M., Hiller, L., Sullivan, A., Syed, N., Trigiante, G., Yulug, I., Merlano, M., Numico, G., Comino, A., *et al.* (2003). p53 polymorphism influences response in cancer chemotherapy via modulation of p73-dependent apoptosis. Cancer Cell *3*, 387-402.

Bergamaschi, D., Samuels, Y., Jin, B., Duraisingham, S., Crook, T., and Lu, X. (2004). ASPP1 and ASPP2: common activators of p53 family members. Mol Cell Biol *24*, 1341-1350.

Bjorkqvist, A. M., Husgafvel-Pursiainen, K., Anttila, S., Karjalainen, A., Tammilehto, L., Mattson, K., Vainio, H., and Knuutila, S. (1998). DNA gains in 3q occur frequently in squamous cell carcinoma of the lung, but not in adenocarcinoma. Genes Chromosomes Cancer *22*, 79-82.

Blanpain, C., and Fuchs, E. (2007). p63: revving up epithelial stem-cell potential. Nat Cell Biol *9*, 731-733.

Brunner, H. G., Hamel, B. C., and Bokhoven Hv, H. (2002). P63 gene mutations and human developmental syndromes. Am J Med Genet *112*, 284-290.

Cai, Y. C., Yang, G. Y., Nie, Y., Wang, L. D., Zhao, X., Song, Y. L., Seril, D. N., Liao, J., Xing, E. P., and Yang, C. S. (2000). Molecular alterations of p73 in human esophageal squamous cell carcinomas: loss of heterozygosity occurs frequently; loss of imprinting and elevation of p73 expression may be related to defective p53. Carcinogenesis *21*, 683-689.

Celli, J., Duijf, P., Hamel, B. C., Bamshad, M., Kramer, B., Smits, A. P., Newbury-Ecob, R., Hennekam, R. C., Van Buggenhout, G., van Haeringen, A., *et al.* (1999). Heterozygous germline mutations in the p53 homolog p63 are the cause of EEC syndrome. Cell *99*, 143-153.

Chan, I., McGrath, J. A., and Kivirikko, S. (2005). Rapp-Hodgkin syndrome and the tail of p63. Clin Exp Dermatol *30*, 183-186.

Chen, C. L., Ip, S. M., Cheng, D., Wong, L. C., and Ngan, H. Y. (2000). P73 gene expression in ovarian cancer tissues and cell lines. Clin Cancer Res *6*, 3910-3915.

Chi, S. G., Chang, S. G., Lee, S. J., Lee, C. H., Kim, J. I., and Park, J. H. (1999). Elevated and biallelic expression of p73 is associated withprogression of human bladder cancer. Cancer Res *59*, 2791-2793.

Choi, H. R., Batsakis, J. G., Zhan, F., Sturgis, E., Luna, M. A., and El-Naggar, A. K. (2002). Differential expression of p53 gene family members p63 and p73 in head and neck squamous tumorigenesis. Hum Pathol *33*, 158-164.

Costanzo, A., Merlo, P., Pediconi, N., Fulco, M., Sartorelli, V., Cole, P. A., Fontemaggi, G., Fanciulli, M., Schiltz, L., Blandino, G., *et al.* (2002). DNA damage-dependent acetylation of p73 dictates the selective activation of apoptotic target genes. Mol Cell *9*, 175-186.

Crook, T., Nicholls, J. M., Brooks, L., O'Nions, J., and Allday, M. J. (2000). High level expression of deltaN-p63: a mechanism for the inactivation of p53 in undifferentiated nasopharyngeal carcinoma (NPC)? Oncogene *19*, 3439-3444.

Davis, L. D., Zhang, W., Merseburger, A., Young, D., Xu, L., Rhim, J. S., Moul, J. W., Srivastava, S., and Sesterhenn, I. A. (2002). p63 expression profile in normal and malignant prostate epithelial cells. Anticancer Res *22*, 3819-3825.

Davison, T. S., Vagner, C., Kaghad, M., Ayed, A., Caput, D., and Arrowsmith, C. H. (1999). p73 and p63 are homotetramers capable of weak heterotypic interactions with each other but not with p53. J Biol Chem *274*, 18709-18714.

De Laurenzi, V., Costanzo, A., Barcaroli, D., Terrinoni, A., Falco, M., Annicchiarico-Petruzzelli, M., Levrero, M., and Melino, G. (1998). Two new p73 splice variants, gamma and delta, with different transcriptional activity. J Exp Med *188*, 1763-1768.

Di Como, C. J., Gaiddon, C., and Prives, C. (1999). p73 function is inhibited by tumor-derived p53 mutants in mammalian cells. Mol Cell Biol *19*, 1438-1449.

Di Como, C. J., Urist, M. J., Babayan, I., Drobnjak, M., Hedvat, C. V., Teruya-Feldstein, J., Pohar, K., Hoos, A., and Cordon-Cardo, C. (2002). p63 expression profiles in human normal and tumor tissues. Clin Cancer Res *8*, 494-501.

Dittmer, D., Pati, S., Zambetti, G., Chu, S., Teresky, A. K., Moore, M., Finlay, C., and Levine, A. J. (1993). Gain of function mutations in p53. Nat Genet *4*, 42-46.

Dobbelstein, M., and Roth, J. (1998). The large T antigen of simian virus 40 binds and inactivates p53 but not p73. J Gen Virol *79 (Pt 12)*, 3079-3083.

Dohn, M., Zhang, S., and Chen, X. (2001). p63alpha and DeltaNp63alpha can induce cell cycle arrest and apoptosis and differentially regulate p53 target genes. Oncogene *20*, 3193-3205.

Duijf, P. H., Vanmolkot, K. R., Propping, P., Friedl, W., Krieger, E., McKeon, F., Dotsch, V., Brunner, H. G., and van Bokhoven, H. (2002). Gain-of-function mutation in ADULT syndrome reveals the presence of a second transactivation domain in p63. Hum Mol Genet *11*, 799-804.

Flores, E. R., Tsai, K. Y., Crowley, D., Sengupta, S., Yang, A., McKeon, F., and Jacks, T. (2002). p63 and p73 are required for p53-dependent apoptosis in response to DNA damage. Nature *416*, 560-564.

Fomenkov, A., Huang, Y. P., Topaloglu, O., Brechman, A., Osada, M., Fomenkova, T., Yuriditsky, E., Trink, B., Sidransky, D., and Ratovitski, E. (2003). P63 alpha mutations lead to aberrant splicing of keratinocyte growth factor receptor in the Hay-Wells syndrome. J Biol Chem *278*, 23906-23914.

Fulco, M., Costanzo, A., Merlo, P., Mangiacasale, R., Strano, S., Blandino, G., Balsano, C., Lavia, P., and Levrero, M. (2003). p73 is regulated by phosphorylation at the G2/M transition. J Biol Chem *278*, 49196-49202.

Gaiddon, C., Lokshin, M., Ahn, J., Zhang, T., and Prives, C. (2001). A subset of tumor-derived mutant forms of p53 down-regulate p63 and p73 through a direct interaction with the p53 core domain. Mol Cell Biol *21*, 1874-1887.

Gaiddon, C., Lokshin, M., Gross, I., Levasseur, D., Taya, Y., Loeffler, J. P., and Prives, C. (2003). Cyclin-dependent kinases phosphorylate p73 at threonine 86 in a cell cycle-dependent manner and negatively regulate p73. J Biol Chem *278*, 27421-27431.

Garraway, L. A., Lin, D., Signoretti, S., Waltregny, D., Dilks, J., Bhattacharya, N., and Loda, M. (2003). Intermediate basal cells of the prostate: in vitro and in vivo characterization. Prostate *55*, 206-218.

Gong, J. G., Costanzo, A., Yang, H. Q., Melino, G., Kaelin, W. G., Jr., Levrero, M., and Wang, J. Y. (1999). The tyrosine kinase c-Abl regulates p73 in apoptotic response to cisplatin-induced DNA damage. Nature *399*, 806-809.

Gostissa, M., Hengstermann, A., Fogal, V., Sandy, P., Schwarz, S. E., Scheffner, M., and Del Sal, G. (1999). Activation of p53 by conjugation to the ubiquitin-like protein SUMO-1. EMBO J *18*, 6462-6471.

Grob, T. J., Novak, U., Maisse, C., Barcaroli, D., Luthi, A. U., Pirnia, F., Hugli, B., Graber, H. U., De Laurenzi, V., Fey, M. F., *et al.* (2001). Human delta Np73 regulates a dominant negative feedback loop for TAp73 and p53. Cell Death Differ *8*, 1213-1223.

Guertin, D. A., and Sabatini, D. M. (2007). Defining the role of mTOR in cancer. Cancer Cell *12*, 9-22.

Hagiwara, K., McMenamin, M. G., Miura, K., and Harris, C. C. (1999). Mutational analysis of the p63/p73L/p51/p40/CUSP/KET gene in human cancer cell lines using intronic primers. Cancer Res *59*, 4165-4169.

Halevy, O., Michalovitz, D., and Oren, M. (1990). Different tumor-derived p53 mutants exhibit distinct biological activities. Science *250*, 113-116.

Haupt, Y., Maya, R., Kazaz, A., and Oren, M. (1997). Mdm2 promotes the rapid degradation of p53. Nature *387*, 296-299.

Hibi, K., Trink, B., Patturajan, M., Westra, W. H., Caballero, O. L., Hill, D. E., Ratovitski, E. A., Jen, J., and Sidransky, D. (2000). AIS is an oncogene amplified in squamous cell carcinoma. Proc Natl Acad Sci U S A *97*, 5462-5467.

Higashino, F., Pipas, J. M., and Shenk, T. (1998). Adenovirus E4orf6 oncoprotein modulates the function of the p53-related protein, p73. Proc Natl Acad Sci U S A *95*, 15683-15687.

Honda, R., Tanaka, H., and Yasuda, H. (1997). Oncoprotein MDM2 is a ubiquitin ligase E3 for tumor suppressor p53. FEBS Lett *420*, 25-27.

Hu, J. F., Ulaner, G. A., Oruganti, H., Ivaturi, R. D., Balagura, K. A., Pham, J., Vu, T. H., and Hoffman, A. R. (2000). Allelic expression of the putative tumor suppressor gene p73 in human fetal tissues and tumor specimens. Biochim Biophys Acta *1491*, 49-56.

Ibrahim, N., He, L., Leong, C. O., Xing, D., Karlan, B. Y., Swisher, E. M., Rueda, B. R., Orsulic, S., and Ellisen, L. W. (2010). BRCA1-associated epigenetic regulation of p73 mediates an effector pathway for chemosensitivity in ovarian carcinoma. Cancer Res *70*, 7155-7165.

Irwin, M., Marin, M. C., Phillips, A. C., Seelan, R. S., Smith, D. I., Liu, W., Flores, E. R., Tsai, K. Y., Jacks, T., Vousden, K. H., and Kaelin, W. G., Jr. (2000). Role for the p53 homologue p73 in E2F-1-induced apoptosis. Nature *407*, 645-648.

Irwin, M. S., and Kaelin, W. G. (2001). p53 family update: p73 and p63 develop their own identities. Cell Growth Differ *12*, 337-349.

Irwin, M. S., Kondo, K., Marin, M. C., Cheng, L. S., Hahn, W. C., and Kaelin, W. G., Jr. (2003). Chemosensitivity linked to p73 function. Cancer Cell *3*, 403-410.

Johnson, J., Lagowski, J., Sundberg, A., and Kulesz-Martin, M. (2005). P53 family activities in development and cancer: relationship to melanocyte and keratinocyte carcinogenesis. J Invest Dermatol *125*, 857-864.

Jost, C. A., Marin, M. C., and Kaelin, W. G., Jr. (1997). p73 is a simian [correction of human] p53-related protein that can induce apoptosis. Nature *389*, 191-194.

Kaelin, W. G., Jr. (1999). The p53 gene family. Oncogene *18*, 7701-7705.

Kaghad, M., Bonnet, H., Yang, A., Creancier, L., Biscan, J. C., Valent, A., Minty, A., Chalon, P., Lelias, J. M., Dumont, X., *et al.* (1997). Monoallelically expressed gene related to p53 at 1p36, a region frequently deleted in neuroblastoma and other human cancers. Cell *90*, 809-819.

Kang, M. J., Park, B. J., Byun, D. S., Park, J. I., Kim, H. J., Park, J. H., and Chi, S. G. (2000). Loss of imprinting and elevated expression of wild-type p73 in human gastric adenocarcinoma. Clin Cancer Res *6*, 1767-1771.

Kartasheva, N. N., Contente, A., Lenz-Stoppler, C., Roth, J., and Dobbelstein, M. (2002). p53 induces the expression of its antagonist p73 Delta N, establishing an autoregulatory feedback loop. Oncogene *21*, 4715-4727.

Kern, S. E., Pietenpol, J. A., Thiagalingam, S., Seymour, A., Kinzler, K. W., and Vogelstein, B. (1992). Oncogenic forms of p53 inhibit p53-regulated gene expression. Science *256*, 827-830.

Koster, M. I., Kim, S., Mills, A. A., DeMayo, F. J., and Roop, D. R. (2004). p63 is the molecular switch for initiation of an epithelial stratification program. Genes Dev *18*, 126-131.

Kovalev, S., Marchenko, N., Swendeman, S., LaQuaglia, M., and Moll, U. M. (1998). Expression level, allelic origin, and mutation analysis of the p73 gene in neuroblastoma tumors and cell lines. Cell Growth Differ *9*, 897-903.

Kubbutat, M. H., Jones, S. N., and Vousden, K. H. (1997). Regulation of p53 stability by Mdm2. Nature *387*, 299-303.

Lane, D. P., and Crawford, L. V. (1979). T antigen is bound to a host protein in SV40-transformed cells. Nature *278*, 261-263.

Lechner, M. S., Mack, D. H., Finicle, A. B., Crook, T., Vousden, K. H., and Laimins, L. A. (1992). Human papillomavirus E6 proteins bind p53 in vivo and abrogate p53-mediated repression of transcription. EMBO J *11*, 3045-3052.

Lee, C. W., and La Thangue, N. B. (1999). Promoter specificity and stability control of the p53-related protein p73. Oncogene *18*, 4171-4181.

Leong, C. O., Vidnovic, N., DeYoung, M. P., Sgroi, D., and Ellisen, L. W. (2007). The p63/p73 network mediates chemosensitivity to cisplatin in a biologically defined subset of primary breast cancers. J Clin Invest *117*, 1370-1380.

Levrero, M., De Laurenzi, V., Costanzo, A., Gong, J., Melino, G., and Wang, J. Y. (1999). Structure, function and regulation of p63 and p73. Cell Death Differ *6*, 1146-1153.

Lim, L. Y., Vidnovic, N., Ellisen, L. W., and Leong, C. O. (2009). Mutant p53 mediates survival of breast cancer cells. Br J Cancer *101*, 1606-1612.

Linzer, D. I., and Levine, A. J. (1979). Characterization of a 54K dalton cellular SV40 tumor antigen present in SV40-transformed cells and uninfected embryonal carcinoma cells. Cell *17*, 43-52.

Lissy, N. A., Davis, P. K., Irwin, M., Kaelin, W. G., and Dowdy, S. F. (2000). A common E2F-1 and p73 pathway mediates cell death induced by TCR activation. Nature *407*, 642-645.

Mai, M., Yokomizo, A., Qian, C., Yang, P., Tindall, D. J., Smith, D. I., and Liu, W. (1998). Activation of p73 silent allele in lung cancer. Cancer Res *58*, 2347-2349.

Marin, M. C., Jost, C. A., Brooks, L. A., Irwin, M. S., O'Nions, J., Tidy, J. A., James, N., McGregor, J. M., Harwood, C. A., Yulug, I. G., *et al.* (2000). A common polymorphism acts as an intragenic modifier of mutant p53 behaviour. Nat Genet *25*, 47-54.

Marin, M. C., Jost, C. A., Irwin, M. S., DeCaprio, J. A., Caput, D., and Kaelin, W. G., Jr. (1998). Viral oncoproteins discriminate between p53 and the p53 homolog p73. Mol Cell Biol *18*, 6316-6324.

Massion, P. P., Taflan, P. M., Jamshedur Rahman, S. M., Yildiz, P., Shyr, Y., Edgerton, M. E., Westfall, M. D., Roberts, J. R., Pietenpol, J. A., Carbone, D. P., and Gonzalez, A. L. (2003). Significance of p63 amplification and overexpression in lung cancer development and prognosis. Cancer Res *63*, 7113-7121.

Melino, G., Lu, X., Gasco, M., Crook, T., and Knight, R. A. (2003). Functional regulation of p73 and p63: development and cancer. Trends Biochem Sci *28*, 663-670.

Mills, A. A., Zheng, B., Wang, X. J., Vogel, H., Roop, D. R., and Bradley, A. (1999). p63 is a p53 homologue required for limb and epidermal morphogenesis. Nature *398*, 708-713.

Minty, A., Dumont, X., Kaghad, M., and Caput, D. (2000). Covalent modification of p73alpha by SUMO-1. Two-hybrid screening with p73 identifies novel SUMO-1-interacting proteins and a SUMO-1 interaction motif. J Biol Chem *275*, 36316-36323.

Miyazaki, K., Ozaki, T., Kato, C., Hanamoto, T., Fujita, T., Irino, S., Watanabe, K., Nakagawa, T., and Nakagawara, A. (2003). A novel HECT-type E3 ubiquitin ligase, NEDL2, stabilizes p73 and enhances its transcriptional activity. Biochem Biophys Res Commun *308*, 106-113.

Moll, U. M., and Slade, N. (2004). p63 and p73: roles in development and tumor formation. Mol Cancer Res *2*, 371-386.

Momand, J., Zambetti, G. P., Olson, D. C., George, D., and Levine, A. J. (1992). The mdm-2 oncogene product forms a complex with the p53 protein and inhibits p53-mediated transactivation. Cell *69*, 1237-1245.

Murray-Zmijewski, F., Lane, D. P., and Bourdon, J. C. (2006). p53/p63/p73 isoforms: an orchestra of isoforms to harmonise cell differentiation and response to stress. Cell Death Differ *13*, 962-972.

Nakagawa, T., Takahashi, M., Ozaki, T., Watanabe Ki, K., Todo, S., Mizuguchi, H., Hayakawa, T., and Nakagawara, A. (2002). Autoinhibitory regulation of p73 by Delta Np73 to modulate cell survival and death through a p73-specific target element within the Delta Np73 promoter. Mol Cell Biol *22*, 2575-2585.

Nakano, K., Balint, E., Ashcroft, M., and Vousden, K. H. (2000). A ribonucleotide reductase gene is a transcriptional target of p53 and p73. Oncogene *19*, 4283-4289.

Ng, S. W., Yiu, G. K., Liu, Y., Huang, L. W., Palnati, M., Jun, S. H., Berkowitz, R. S., and Mok, S. C. (2000). Analysis of p73 in human borderline and invasive ovarian tumor. Oncogene *19*, 1885-1890.

Nomoto, S., Haruki, N., Kondo, M., Konishi, H., and Takahashi, T. (1998). Search for mutations and examination of allelic expression imbalance of the p73 gene at 1p36.33 in human lung cancers. Cancer Res *58*, 1380-1383.

Ongkeko, W. M., Wang, X. Q., Siu, W. Y., Lau, A. W., Yamashita, K., Harris, A. L., Cox, L. S., and Poon, R. Y. (1999). MDM2 and MDMX bind and stabilize the p53-related protein p73. Curr Biol *9*, 829-832.

Osada, M., Ohba, M., Kawahara, C., Ishioka, C., Kanamaru, R., Katoh, I., Ikawa, Y., Nimura, Y., Nakagawara, A., Obinata, M., and Ikawa, S. (1998). Cloning and functional analysis of human p51, which structurally and functionally resembles p53. Nat Med *4*, 839-843.

Ozaki, T., Naka, M., Takada, N., Tada, M., Sakiyama, S., and Nakagawara, A. (1999). Deletion of the COOH-terminal region of p73alpha enhances both its transactivation function and DNA-binding activity but inhibits induction of apoptosis in mammalian cells. Cancer Res *59*, 5902-5907.

Park, B. J., Lee, S. J., Kim, J. I., Lee, C. H., Chang, S. G., Park, J. H., and Chi, S. G. (2000). Frequent alteration of p63 expression in human primary bladder carcinomas. Cancer Res *60*, 3370-3374.

Pozniak, C. D., Radinovic, S., Yang, A., McKeon, F., Kaplan, D. R., and Miller, F. D. (2000). An anti-apoptotic role for the p53 family member, p73, during developmental neuron death. Science *289*, 304-306.

Prabhu, N. S., Somasundaram, K., Satyamoorthy, K., Herlyn, M., and El-Deiry, W. S. (1998). p73beta, unlike p53, suppresses growth and induces apoptosis of human papillomavirus E6-expressing cancer cells. Int J Oncol *13*, 5-9.

Ratovitski, E. A., Patturajan, M., Hibi, K., Trink, B., Yamaguchi, K., and Sidransky, D. (2001). p53 associates with and targets Delta Np63 into a protein degradation pathway. Proc Natl Acad Sci U S A *98*, 1817-1822.

Reis-Filho, J. S., Milanezi, F., Amendoeira, I., Albergaria, A., and Schmitt, F. C. (2003a). Distribution of p63, a novel myoepithelial marker, in fine-needle aspiration biopsies of the breast: an analysis of 82 samples. Cancer *99*, 172-179.

Reis-Filho, J. S., Simpson, P. T., Martins, A., Preto, A., Gartner, F., and Schmitt, F. C. (2003b). Distribution of p63, cytokeratins 5/6 and cytokeratin 14 in 51 normal and 400 neoplastic human tissue samples using TARP-4 multi-tumor tissue microarray. Virchows Arch *443*, 122-132.

Ribeiro-Silva, A., Zambelli Ramalho, L. N., Britto Garcia, S., and Zucoloto, S. (2003). The relationship between p63 and p53 expression in normal and neoplastic breast tissue. Arch Pathol Lab Med *127*, 336-340.

Rocco, J. W., Leong, C. O., Kuperwasser, N., DeYoung, M. P., and Ellisen, L. W. (2006). p63 mediates survival in squamous cell carcinoma by suppression of p73-dependent apoptosis. Cancer Cell *9*, 45-56.

Rodriguez, M. S., Dargemont, C., and Hay, R. T. (2001). SUMO-1 conjugation in vivo requires both a consensus modification motif and nuclear targeting. J Biol Chem *276*, 12654-12659.

Rosenbluth, J. M., Mays, D. J., Pino, M. F., Tang, L. J., and Pietenpol, J. A. (2008). A gene signature-based approach identifies mTOR as a regulator of p73. Mol Cell Biol *28*, 5951-5964.

Rosenbluth, J. M., and Pietenpol, J. A. (2008). The jury is in: p73 is a tumor suppressor after all. Genes Dev *22*, 2591-2595.

Roth, J., and Dobbelstein, M. (1999). Failure of viral oncoproteins to target the p53-homologue p51A. J Gen Virol *80 (Pt 12)*, 3251-3255.

Roth, J., Konig, C., Wienzek, S., Weigel, S., Ristea, S., and Dobbelstein, M. (1998). Inactivation of p53 but not p73 by adenovirus type 5 E1B 55-kilodalton and E4 34-kilodalton oncoproteins. J Virol *72*, 8510-8516.

Samuels-Lev, Y., O'Connor, D. J., Bergamaschi, D., Trigiante, G., Hsieh, J. K., Zhong, S., Campargue, I., Naumovski, L., Crook, T., and Lu, X. (2001). ASPP proteins specifically stimulate the apoptotic function of p53. Mol Cell *8*, 781-794.

Sarnow, P., Ho, Y. S., Williams, J., and Levine, A. J. (1982). Adenovirus E1b-58kd tumor antigen and SV40 large tumor antigen are physically associated with the same 54 kd cellular protein in transformed cells. Cell *28*, 387-394.

Schmale, H., and Bamberger, C. (1997). A novel protein with strong homology to the tumor suppressor p53. Oncogene *15*, 1363-1367.

Senoo, M., Pinto, F., Crum, C. P., and McKeon, F. (2007). p63 Is essential for the proliferative potential of stem cells in stratified epithelia. Cell *129*, 523-536.

Senoo, M., Seki, N., Ohira, M., Sugano, S., Watanabe, M., Inuzuka, S., Okamoto, T., Tachibana, M., Tanaka, T., Shinkai, Y., and Kato, H. (1998). A second p53-related protein, p73L, with high homology to p73. Biochem Biophys Res Commun *248*, 603-607.

Shangary, S., and Wang, S. (2008). Targeting the MDM2-p53 interaction for cancer therapy. Clin Cancer Res *14*, 5318-5324.

Shaul, Y. (2000). c-Abl: activation and nuclear targets. Cell Death Differ *7*, 10-16.

Shaulsky, G., Goldfinger, N., and Rotter, V. (1991). Alterations in tumor development in vivo mediated by expression of wild type or mutant p53 proteins. Cancer Res *51*, 5232-5237.

Steegenga, W. T., Shvarts, A., Riteco, N., Bos, J. L., and Jochemsen, A. G. (1999). Distinct regulation of p53 and p73 activity by adenovirus E1A, E1B, and E4orf6 proteins. Mol Cell Biol *19*, 3885-3894.

Stiewe, T. (2007). The p53 family in differentiation and tumorigenesis. Nat Rev Cancer *7*, 165-168.

Stiewe, T., and Putzer, B. M. (2000). Role of the p53-homologue p73 in E2F1-induced apoptosis. Nat Genet *26*, 464-469.

Stiewe, T., and Putzer, B. M. (2002). Role of p73 in malignancy: tumor suppressor or oncogene? Cell Death Differ *9*, 237-245.

Stiewe, T., Stanelle, J., Theseling, C. C., Pollmeier, B., Beitzinger, M., and Putzer, B. M. (2003). Inactivation of retinoblastoma (RB) tumor suppressor by oncogenic isoforms of the p53 family member p73. J Biol Chem *278*, 14230-14236.

Stiewe, T., Theseling, C. C., and Putzer, B. M. (2002a). Transactivation-deficient Delta TA-p73 inhibits p53 by direct competition for DNA binding: implications for tumorigenesis. J Biol Chem *277*, 14177-14185.

Stiewe, T., Zimmermann, S., Frilling, A., Esche, H., and Putzer, B. M. (2002b). Transactivation-deficient DeltaTA-p73 acts as an oncogene. Cancer Res *62*, 3598-3602.

Strano, S., Munarriz, E., Rossi, M., Cristofanelli, B., Shaul, Y., Castagnoli, L., Levine, A. J., Sacchi, A., Cesareni, G., Oren, M., and Blandino, G. (2000). Physical and functional interaction between p53 mutants and different isoforms of p73. J Biol Chem *275*, 29503-29512.

Sun, X. F. (2002). p73 overexpression is a prognostic factor in patients with colorectal adenocarcinoma. Clin Cancer Res *8*, 165-170.

Sunahara, M., Ichimiya, S., Nimura, Y., Takada, N., Sakiyama, S., Sato, Y., Todo, S., Adachi, W., Amano, J., and Nakagawara, A. (1998). Mutational analysis of the p73 gene localized at chromosome 1p36.3 in colorectal carcinomas. Int J Oncol *13*, 319-323.

Tannapfel, A., Engeland, K., Weinans, L., Katalinic, A., Hauss, J., Mossner, J., and Wittekind, C. (1999a). Expression of p73, a novel protein related to the p53 tumour suppressor p53, and apoptosis in cholangiocellular carcinoma of the liver. Br J Cancer *80*, 1069-1074.

Tannapfel, A., Wasner, M., Krause, K., Geissler, F., Katalinic, A., Hauss, J., Mossner, J., Engeland, K., and Wittekind, C. (1999b). Expression of p73 and its relation to histopathology and prognosis in hepatocellular carcinoma. J Natl Cancer Inst *91*, 1154-1158.

Tokuchi, Y., Hashimoto, T., Kobayashi, Y., Hayashi, M., Nishida, K., Hayashi, S., Imai, K., Nakachi, K., Ishikawa, Y., Nakagawa, K., *et al.* (1999). The expression of p73 is increased in lung cancer, independent of p53 gene alteration. Br J Cancer *80*, 1623-1629.

Trink, B., Okami, K., Wu, L., Sriuranpong, V., Jen, J., and Sidransky, D. (1998). A new human p53 homologue. Nat Med *4*, 747-748.

Tsai, K. K., and Yuan, Z. M. (2003). c-Abl stabilizes p73 by a phosphorylation-augmented interaction. Cancer Res *63*, 3418-3424.

Tsao, H., Zhang, X., Majewski, P., and Haluska, F. G. (1999). Mutational and expression analysis of the p73 gene in melanoma cell lines. Cancer Res *59*, 172-174.

Ueda, Y., Hijikata, M., Takagi, S., Chiba, T., and Shimotohno, K. (1999). New p73 variants with altered C-terminal structures have varied transcriptional activities. Oncogene *18*, 4993-4998.

Ueda, Y., Hijikata, M., Takagi, S., Chiba, T., and Shimotohno, K. (2001). Transcriptional activities of p73 splicing variants are regulated by inter-variant association. Biochem J *356*, 859-866.

Unger, T., Nau, M. M., Segal, S., and Minna, J. D. (1992). p53: a transdominant regulator of transcription whose function is ablated by mutations occurring in human cancer. EMBO J *11*, 1383-1390.

van Bokhoven, H., Hamel, B. C., Bamshad, M., Sangiorgi, E., Gurrieri, F., Duijf, P. H., Vanmolkot, K. R., van Beusekom, E., van Beersum, S. E., Celli, J., *et al.* (2001). p63 Gene mutations in eec syndrome, limb-mammary syndrome, and isolated split hand-split foot malformation suggest a genotype-phenotype correlation. Am J Hum Genet *69*, 481-492.

Vikhanskaya, F., D'Incalci, M., and Broggini, M. (2000). p73 competes with p53 and attenuates its response in a human ovarian cancer cell line. Nucleic Acids Res *28*, 513-519.

Vikhanskaya, F., Marchini, S., Marabese, M., Galliera, E., and Broggini, M. (2001). P73a overexpression is associated with resistance to treatment with DNA-damaging agents in a human ovarian cancer cell line. Cancer Res *61*, 935-938.

Vossio, S., Palescandolo, E., Pediconi, N., Moretti, F., Balsano, C., Levrero, M., and Costanzo, A. (2002). DN-p73 is activated after DNA damage in a p53-dependent manner to regulate p53-induced cell cycle arrest. Oncogene *21*, 3796-3803.

Waltermann, A., Kartasheva, N. N., and Dobbelstein, M. (2003). Differential regulation of p63 and p73 expression. Oncogene 22, 5686-5693.

Wang, X., Arooz, T., Siu, W. Y., Chiu, C. H., Lau, A., Yamashita, K., and Poon, R. Y. (2001a). MDM2 and MDMX can interact differently with ARF and members of the p53 family. FEBS Lett *490*, 202-208.

Wang, X. Q., Ongkeko, W. M., Lau, A. W., Leung, K. M., and Poon, R. Y. (2001b). A possible role of p73 on the modulation of p53 level through MDM2. Cancer Res *61*, 1598-1603.

Weber, A., Bellmann, U., Bootz, F., Wittekind, C., and Tannapfel, A. (2002). Expression of p53 and its homologues in primary and recurrent squamous cell carcinomas of the head and neck. Int J Cancer *99*, 22-28.

Westfall, M. D., and Pietenpol, J. A. (2004). p63: Molecular complexity in development and cancer. Carcinogenesis *25*, 857-864.

Wiman, K. G. (2006). Strategies for therapeutic targeting of the p53 pathway in cancer. Cell Death Differ *13*, 921-926.

Wong, S. W., Tiong, K. H., Kong, W. Y., Yue, Y. C., Chua, C. H., Lim, J. Y., Lee, C. Y., Quah, S. I., Fow, C., Chung, C., *et al.* (2010). Rapamycin synergizes cisplatin sensitivity in basal-like breast cancer cells through up-regulation of p73. Breast Cancer Res Treat.

Wu, G., Nomoto, S., Hoque, M. O., Dracheva, T., Osada, M., Lee, C. C., Dong, S. M., Guo, Z., Benoit, N., Cohen, Y., *et al.* (2003). DeltaNp63alpha and TAp63alpha regulate transcription of genes with distinct biological functions in cancer and development. Cancer Res *63*, 2351-2357.

Yamaguchi, K., Wu, L., Caballero, O. L., Hibi, K., Trink, B., Resto, V., Cairns, P., Okami, K., Koch, W. M., Sidransky, D., and Jen, J. (2000). Frequent gain of the p40/p51/p63 gene locus in primary head and neck squamous cell carcinoma. Int J Cancer *86*, 684-689.

Yang, A., Kaghad, M., Wang, Y., Gillett, E., Fleming, M. D., Dotsch, V., Andrews, N. C., Caput, D., and McKeon, F. (1998). p63, a p53 homolog at 3q27-29, encodes multiple products with transactivating, death-inducing, and dominant-negative activities. Mol Cell 2, 305-316.

Yang, A., Schweitzer, R., Sun, D., Kaghad, M., Walker, N., Bronson, R. T., Tabin, C., Sharpe, A., Caput, D., Crum, C., and McKeon, F. (1999). p63 is essential for regenerative proliferation in limb, craniofacial and epithelial development. Nature *398*, 714-718.

Yang, A., Walker, N., Bronson, R., Kaghad, M., Oosterwegel, M., Bonnin, J., Vagner, C., Bonnet, H., Dikkes, P., Sharpe, A., *et al.* (2000). p73-deficient mice have neurological, pheromonal and inflammatory defects but lack spontaneous tumours. Nature *404*, 99-103.

Yew, P. R., and Berk, A. J. (1992). Inhibition of p53 transactivation required for transformation by adenovirus early 1B protein. Nature *357*, 82-85.

Yokomizo, A., Mai, M., Tindall, D. J., Cheng, L., Bostwick, D. G., Naito, S., Smith, D. I., and Liu, W. (1999). Overexpression of the wild type p73 gene in human bladder cancer. Oncogene *18*, 1629-1633.

Yu, J., Zhang, L., Hwang, P. M., Rago, C., Kinzler, K. W., and Vogelstein, B. (1999). Identification and classification of p53-regulated genes. Proc Natl Acad Sci U S A *96*, 14517-14522.

Yuan, Z. M., Shioya, H., Ishiko, T., Sun, X., Gu, J., Huang, Y. Y., Lu, H., Kharbanda, S., Weichselbaum, R., and Kufe, D. (1999). p73 is regulated by tyrosine kinase c-Abl in the apoptotic response to DNA damage. Nature *399*, 814-817.

Zaika, A., Irwin, M., Sansome, C., and Moll, U. M. (2001). Oncogenes induce and activate endogenous p73 protein. J Biol Chem *276*, 11310-11316.

Zaika, A. I., and El-Rifai, W. (2006). The role of p53 protein family in gastrointestinal malignancies. Cell Death Differ *13*, 935-940.

Zaika, A. I., Kovalev, S., Marchenko, N. D., and Moll, U. M. (1999). Overexpression of the wild type p73 gene in breast cancer tissues and cell lines. Cancer Res *59*, 3257-3263.

Zaika, A. I., Slade, N., Erster, S. H., Sansome, C., Joseph, T. W., Pearl, M., Chalas, E., and Moll, U. M. (2002). DeltaNp73, a dominant-negative inhibitor of wild-type p53 and TAp73, is up-regulated in human tumors. J Exp Med *196*, 765-780.

Zeng, X., Chen, L., Jost, C. A., Maya, R., Keller, D., Wang, X., Kaelin, W. G., Jr., Oren, M., Chen, J., and Lu, H. (1999). MDM2 suppresses p73 function without promoting p73 degradation. Mol Cell Biol *19*, 3257-3266.

Zeng, X., Li, X., Miller, A., Yuan, Z., Yuan, W., Kwok, R. P., Goodman, R., and Lu, H. (2000). The N-terminal domain of p73 interacts with the CH1 domain of p300/CREB binding protein and mediates transcriptional activation and apoptosis. Mol Cell Biol *20*, 1299-1310.

Zheng, X., and Chen, X. (2001). Aquaporin 3, a glycerol and water transporter, is regulated by p73 of the p53 family. FEBS Lett *489*, 4-7.

Zhu, J., Jiang, J., Zhou, W., and Chen, X. (1998). The potential tumor suppressor p73 differentially regulates cellular p53 target genes. Cancer Res *58*, 5061-5065.

Zwahlen, D., Tschan, M. P., Grob, T. J., Peters, U. R., Fink, D., Haenggi, W., Altermatt, H. J., Cajot, J. F., Tobler, A., Fey, M. F., and Aebi, S. (2000). Differential expression of p73 splice variants and protein in benign and malignant ovarian tumours. Int J Cancer *88*, 66-70.

12

HER-2 Signaling in Human Breast Cancer

Kathleen M. Woods Ignatoski
University of Michigan,
USA

1. Introduction

1.1 *erb*B family

HER-2 is a member of the *erb*B family of receptor tyrosine kinases. Epidermal Growth Factor Receptor (EGFR) was first identified as the cellular homolog of the transduced oncogene of the avian retroviruses such as avian ERythroBlastosis virus, which causes erythroleukemia and fibrosarcoma and gives rise to the family name (erbB). EGFR, as its name implies, was shown by Stanley Cohen to induce the growth of epidermal cells (Todaro, DeLarco et al. 1976). The EGFR family consists of four members: *erb*B-1 (EGFR), *erb*B-2 (HER-2/neu), *erb*B-3 (HER-3), and *erb*B-4 (HER-4). Her-1, -2, and -3 have been associated with tumorigenesis (Suo, Emilsen et al. 1998). HER-4 has been implicated in development and tumor suppression, possibly by sequestration of the other *erb*B receptors in dimers. Ligand binding stabilizes dimer formation, leading to intracellular signaling. Each receptor consists of an extracellular domain that contains the ligand binding sites, an intracellular domain that contains the tyrosine kinase activity, and a cytoplasmic tail that is involved in cellular signaling. EGFR can be stimulated by an array of ligands, including EGF, transforming growth factor α (TGF-α), heparin-binding EGF (HB-EGF), and heregulins. HER-3 can bind heregulins (Holmes, Sliwkowski et al. 1992); although, it in and of itself does not have an active kinase domain. Heregulin binding to HER-3 facilitates dimerization with other *erb*B receptors which promote the phosphorylation of HER-3 and subsequent activation of downstream signals.

HER-2 does not have any known ligands; however, several intriguing papers have been published recently on this topic. The Calloway group has had a series of papers (Carraway, Carvajal et al. 1993; Carraway and Cantley 1994; Carraway, Sliwkowski et al. 1994; Carraway, Rossi et al. 1999; Komatsu, Jepson et al. 2001; Carraway and Carraway 2007; Kozloski, Carraway et al. 2010) showing that the extracellular domain of HER-2 can bind the intramembrane protein MUC4, suggesting that MUC4 was the ligand for HER-2. MUC4 appears to play a role in mammary gland development at the lactation step along with HER-2. In cancer, MUC 4 blocks apoptosis and stabilizes HER-2/HER-3 dimers. In normal epithelia, MUC 4 sequesters HER-2 to the apical surface, separating it from HER-3, which is on the lateral surface (Carraway and Carraway 2007). These data make a compelling argument for MUC4 as a ligand for HER-2.

More recently, Day, *et al.* (Najy, Day et al. 2008) showed that the extracellular domain of E-cadherin could activate HER-2 and EGFR. They have shown that the extracellular domain of E-cadherin is cleaved by the ADAM proteases. Since E-cadherin is normally present on epithelial cells and itself, or its sister protein N-cadherin, is present on cancer cells of epithelial origin, it is also a good candidate for a HER-2 ligand.

Pairings of the *erb*B receptors have been exquisitely elucidated by Josef Yarden and colleagues (Goldman, Benlevy et al. 1990; Karunagaran, Tzahar et al. 1996; Alroy and Yarden 1997). Yarden, *et al.* utilized the 32D cell line, an IL-3-independent murine myeloid cell line that does not express endogenous *erb*B receptors. They systematically expressed each family member separately and in pairs to determine which family members formed complexes. They found that each family member can homodimerize or heterodimerize with every other family member; although, certain heterodimers are preferred. Which dimer is present on the cell determines the biological phenotype of that cell. Although EGFR can homodimerize, it will pair with HER-2 when HER-2 is present and will only pair with itself when all of the HER-2 is paired or no HER-2 is present (Hendriks , Opresko et al. 2003).

EGFR dimerization results in the phosphorylation of tyrosine 1045 in the cytoplasmic domain. Phosphorylation of this tyrosine creates a docking site for the *cbl* protein (Yokouchi, Kondo et al. 1999). *Cbl* then recruits ubiquitin which targets the EGFR for degradation (Yokouchi, Kondo et al. 1999). Activation of HER-2 does not create a ubinquitin binding site, so HER-2 does not get degraded upon activation unless it is dimerized with EGFR. Over expression of HER-2 results in constitutive activation of both HER-2 and EGFR and in a decrease in degradation of both of the receptors.

Due to the fluidity of the plasma membrane, transient dimerization of the *erb*B receptors occurs. However, the transient dimers do not elicit a strong signal. Our model (*FIGURE 1*) (Woods Ignatoski, LaPointe et al. 1999) suggests that over expression of HER-2 leads to many transient homodimers. The transient homodimers lead to transphosphorylation of the receptor causing many small signals to be initiated. The overall effect is one of a strong, ligand-stabilized signal which results in constitutive activation of HER-2 and constitutive growth signals (*FIGURE 1C*). The type of HER-2 homo and heterodimerization, coupled with over expression, on mammary epithelial cells has consequences dealing with normal development, proliferation, and transformation.

2. HER-2 in development

HER-2 is expressed in almost all fetal tissues including the placenta, liver, kidney, mammary gland, brain, and lung (Kokai, Wada et al. 1988). On the basis of its expression pattern, HER-2 plays a role in general development. Although HER-2's role in tumorigenesis has been studied extensively, its role in normal mammary gland development has not. There are many articles about mammary gland development in HER-2 transgenic and knock-out mice, but since human and mouse mammary glands develop differently, the actual role of HER-2 in human mammary gland development is not fully understood. Mina Bissell and colleagues developed the three-dimensional *Matrigel* system to study mammary gland morphogenesis, discovering the role for integrins in anti-apoptotic signaling (Petersen, Ronnovjessen et al. 1992; Howlett, Bailey et al. 1995; Lochter, Galosy et al. 1997; Lochter, Navre et al. 1999). Joan Brugge and colleagues refined the *Matrigel* model to identify HER-2 as a modulator of the lumen compartment, by working through Bim-1 to regulate apoptosis of the pre-lumenal cells (Muthuswamy, Li et al. 2001). One caveat to the Brugge group's work is the use of a chimeric molecule that has an NGF extracellular domain and a HER-2 cytoplasmic domain that can be crosslinked to give a constitutive signal. While their work leads to important insight into the role of HER-2 in development, the system they use is not

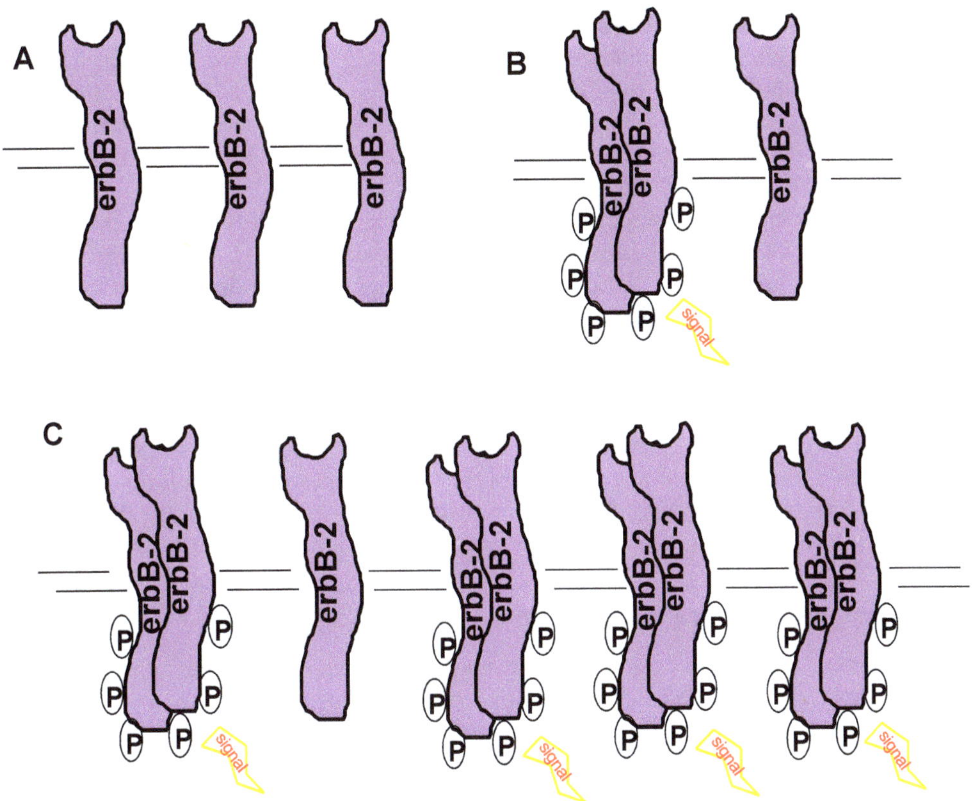

Fig. 1. Schematic of signaling from HER-2 during normal conditions and during over expression. (A) HER-2 is normally present as single molecules in the plasma membrane. (B) Due to the fluid nature of the membrane, random, transient dimers form producing weak signals that cannot elicit a response from the cell. (C) During over expression, many transient dimers produce a signal strong enough to elicit a response from the cell.

physiological, since HER-2 is not activated by a ligand but rather by the amount of protein, and constitutive HER-2 activation is not done by cross-linking the cytoplasmic domains.

Recently, we have developed a system that is more physiological than the one used by Brugge and colleagues (manuscript submitted). We used human mammary epithelial (HME) cells, obtained from reduction mammoplasties, plated in *Matrigel* to study the role of HER-2 in branching morphogenesis. We observed that HME cells form branching structures when plated in the 3D matrix *Matrigel* and determined that HER-2 is up-regulated at the time of branching. Using HER-2 over expressing HME cells (Woods Ignatoski, LaPointe et al. 1999) we showed that constitutive activation of HER-2 was necessary and sufficient to form the branches. By using genetic and chemical activators and inhibitors, we showed that AKT activation mediated the HER-2-facilitated branching morphogenesis. Our data imply that HER-2's role in mammary gland development is to facilitate ductal formation.

Korkaya, *et al.* (Korkaya, Paulson et al. 2008) and Magnifico, *et al.* (Magnifico, Albano et al. 2009) have shown that an increase in HER-2 in human mammary stem cells causes an increase in mammosphere formation and an increase in ductal structures when the cells are placed in animals. Both groups have also shown a reciprocal relationship between over expression of HER-2 and the expression of the developmental gene Notch. Their published data suggest that HER-2-mediated AKT activation is necessary for self-renewal leading to the ductal structures in their mouse models. Our data show that HER-2-mediated AKT activation is necessary for branching morphogenesis and is concordant with the data presented by Korkaya, *et al.* (Korkaya, Paulson et al. 2008) and Magnifico, *et al.* (Magnifico, Albano et al. 2009).

Since we have previously shown that HME cells in *Matrigel* and HER-2 over expressing cells have an increase in Focal Adhesion Kinase (FAK) phosphorylation (Woods Ignatoski and Ethier 1999), an implication of these data is that signaling from integrin binding to extracellular matrix may also play a role in this developmental phenotype. Indeed, Bissell, *et al.* (Petersen, Ronnovjessen et al. 1992; Howlett, Petersen et al. 1994; Howlett, Bailey et al. 1995; Gudjonsson, Ronnov-Jessen et al. 2002), has shown that β1 integrin is important in mammary cell morphology change. β1 integrins bind to and activate FAK (Zachary and Rozengurt 1992). FAK was shown to maintain the mammary gland stem cell pool (Nagy, Wei et al. 2007). Since HER-2 has recently been shown to play a role in human mammary stem cells (Korkaya, Paulson et al. 2008; Korkaya and Wicha 2009), the idea that FAK may be downstream of HER-2 to maintain the stem cell population is intriguing.

3. HER-2 signaling in transformation

HER-2 uses a variety of signaling pathways to elicit phenotypes associated with transformation and tumorigenesis. We and others used various *in vitro* methods in conjunction with constitutively active and dominantly negative mutants and chemical inhibitors to elucidate the multiple pathways HER-2 uses to transform cells (*FIGURE* 2).

Growth factor independence: One hallmark of a transformed cell is growth factor independence. Ram, *et al.* (Ram, Kokeny et al. 1995; Ram, Dilts et al. 1996) showed that human breast cancer (HBC) cells with increasing amounts of HER-2 had increasing degrees of growth factor independence. H16N2 cells, which are non-transformed, immortalized HME, have normal levels of HER-2 and required both insulin-like growth factor (IGF) and epidermal growth factor (EGF) to survive. 21MT-2 cells with an slight over expression of HER-2 still required EGF, but 21MT-1 cells with a clinically relevant HER-2 over expression did not require either IGF or EGF for growth. To determine the contribution of HER-2 over expression to growth factor independence without the other genetic abnormalities associated with HBC, we developed HME cell lines that over expressed HER-2 less than the HPV16-immortalized HME cell line (H16N2).

The MCF-10HER-2 cells were unable to grow in the absence of IGF, showing that a slight over expression resulted in IGF independence and that over expression to levels seen in amplified HBC cells conferred both IGF and EGF independence to the H16N2 cells (Woods Ignatoski, LaPointe et al. 1999). Over expression of HER-2 resulted in progressively increasing levels of tyrosine-phosphorylated HER-3, without any significant changes in HER-3 protein levels (Woods Ignatoski, LaPointe et al. 1999).

Our studies, while demonstrating a direct relationship between the level of expression, the activation of HER-2, and the requirements for IGF and EGF, suggest that genetic alterations present in breast cancer cells, or mediated by HPV-16-induced alterations, can influence the expression level and activation status of HER-2 and, in turn, their degree of growth factor independence. To this end, we were intrigued by the differences between

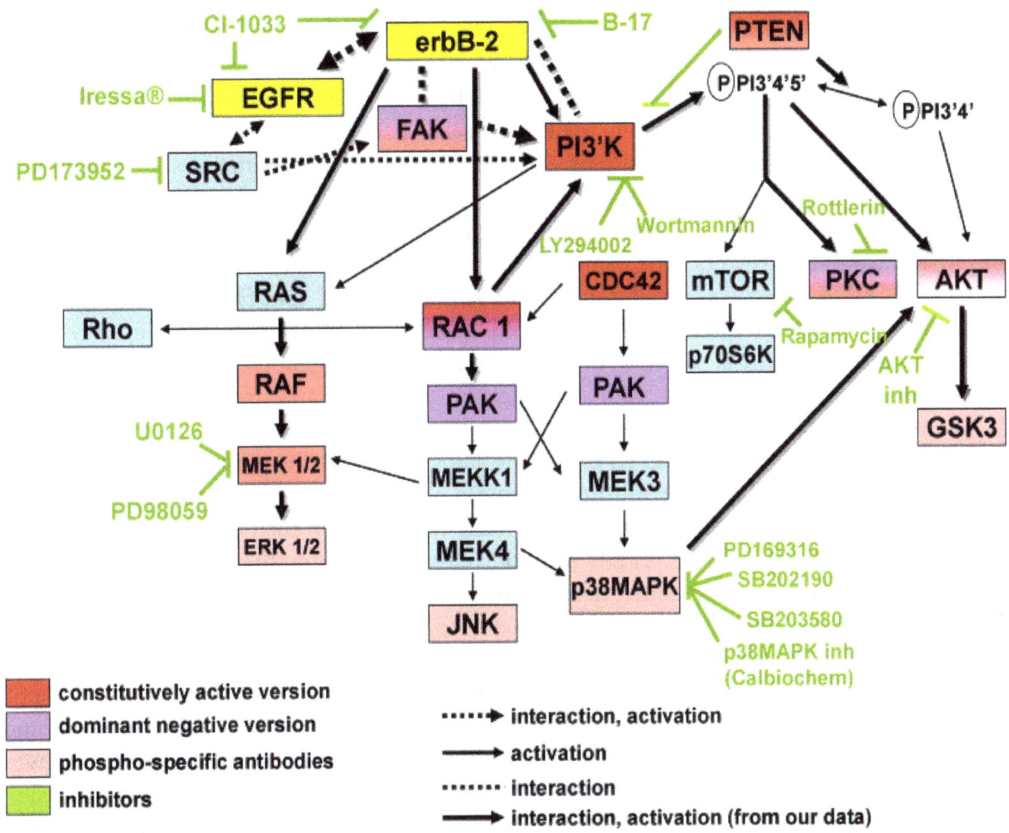

Fig. 2. The tools used to decipher HER-2 signaling. Various constitutively active and dominant negative constructs plus specific chemical inhibitors and phospho-specific antibodies were used to elucidate downstream signaling for HER-2 and associate them with transformed phenotypes.

the MCF-10A cell line and the H16N2 cell line in terms of their ability to over express HER-2 and their differences in growth factor independence. The biggest difference in the parental cell lines is the inclusion of the entire HPV16 genome in the H16N2 cells which is not in the MCF-10A cells. The HPV-16 genome produces the HPV E5, E6, and E7 oncogenes which have been shown to affect the tumor suppressors Rb and p53, among other proteins. To discern if the HPV genes played a role in HER-2-mediated transformation, we co-expressed E6, E7, or E6 and E7 with HER-2 in MCF-10A cells and tested for transformed phenotypes (Woods Ignatoski, Dziubinski et al. 2005). Co-expression of HER-2 with the HPV-16 oncoproteins E6 and E7 resulted in the emergence of fully EGF-independent cells that expressed very high levels of constitutively activated HER-2. Interestingly, co-expression of E7 with HER-2 resulted in cells that were EGF-independent for growth but which did not express HER-2 to higher levels than control MCF-10HER-2 cells. By contrast, co-expression of E6 with HER-2 resulted in cells expressing higher levels of HER-2 but which were still dependent on EGF for growth and survival. Examination of the expression and activation status of HER-1, -2 and -3 in the MCF-10HER-2 cells and their derivatives by immunoprecipitation/western blot analysis demonstrated that the EGF-independent MCF-10HER-2E7 cells and the HER-2/E6E7 cells exhibited constitutive EGF-independent activation of EGFR. Further, the constitutively active EGFR had a faster electrophoretic mobility than EGFR activated by exogenous growth factors. Exposure of MCF-10HER-2 cells and their derivatives as well as the HER-2 amplified SUM-225 breast cancer cell line to ZD1839 (IRESSA®) at concentrations specific for EGFR, eliminated EGFR tyrosine phosphorylation, blocked proliferation, but only modestly altered the levels of constitutively activated HER-2. By contrast, exposure of SUM-190 cells or MDA-351 cells, which have amplified HER-2 but express little or no EGFR, to these same concentrations of ZD1839 had little or no influence on cell proliferation. Our results showed that HER-2 over expression cooperates with EGFR and HPV-E7 to yield HME cells that are EGF-independent for growth. Together, HER-2, E6 and E7 cooperate with endogenous EGFR to yield fully transformed cells that express very high levels of HER-2 and that are growth factor autonomous for proliferation and survival.

Phophotidylinositol 3′ kinase (PI3′K) phosphorylates inositol in the plasma membrane at the 3′ position. Phosphorylation of inositol produces a docking site for the serine/threonine kinase AKT. Docking of AKT activates its kinase activity and elicits downstream signals. Activation of both HER-2 and HER-3 provide phosphotyrosines that can dock PI3′K and bring it to the membrane; therefore, activation of HER-2 mediates inositol phosphorylation and PI3′K signaling (Fedi, Pierce et al. 1994). Phospho-AKT remained detectable in HER-2 cells treated with the PI3′K inhibitor LY294002 or with expression of exogenous PTEN, a phosphatase that reverses the action of PI3′K, but was abolished by treatment with the p38 mitogen activated kinase (p38MAPK) inhibitor SB202190. Thus, both PI3K-dependent and p38MAPK-dependent pathways lead to activation of AKT. We also found that AKT was activated by p38MAPK in these cells, but this activation did not play a role in invasion (Woods Ignatoski, Livant et al. 2003). Since AKT has been shown in other systems to be a survival factor (Datta, Dudek et al. 1997; Brunet, Bonni et al. 1999; Hutchinson J, Jin J et al. 2001), we hypothesized that HER-2 mediated activation of AKT is necessary for growth factor independence. We found that, in the absence of EGF, p38MAPK-activated AKT is necessary for HER-2 over expressing cells to survive and to form colonies in soft agar (Woods Ignatoski, Livant et al. 2003). We showed that EGF works as a survival signal in the absence of p38MAPK-mediated activation of AKT and that HME cells expressing a constitutively active AKT did not require EGF for growth or colony formation in soft agar. Thus, our data indicate that AKT activation can compensate for EGF-mediated cell survival signals leading to growth factor-independence and anchorage-independent growth (Diehl, Grewal et al. 2007).

HER-2 in invasion: Using a model system for invasion that utilizes a naturally occurring membrane found in sea urchin embryos (Livant, Linn et al. 1995) in the configuration a cell would see upon extravasation (*FIGURE 3*), we determined that α5 integrin binding to the PHSRN sequence of fibronectin is necessary for invasion and that α4 integrin binding to the "LDV" sequence of fibronection abrogates invasion (Livant, Allen et al. 2000; Livant, Brabec et al. 2000; Woods Ignatoski, Maehama et al. 2000; Jia, Markwart et al. 2002) (*FIGURE 4*). Using this system, we showed that HER-2 requires PI3′K to drive invasion. With this same system we also showed that HER-2 mediates the down-regulation of α4 integrin from the cell surface to facilitate invasion via activation of p38MAPK (Woods Ignatoski, Maehama et al. 2000) (FIGURE 5).

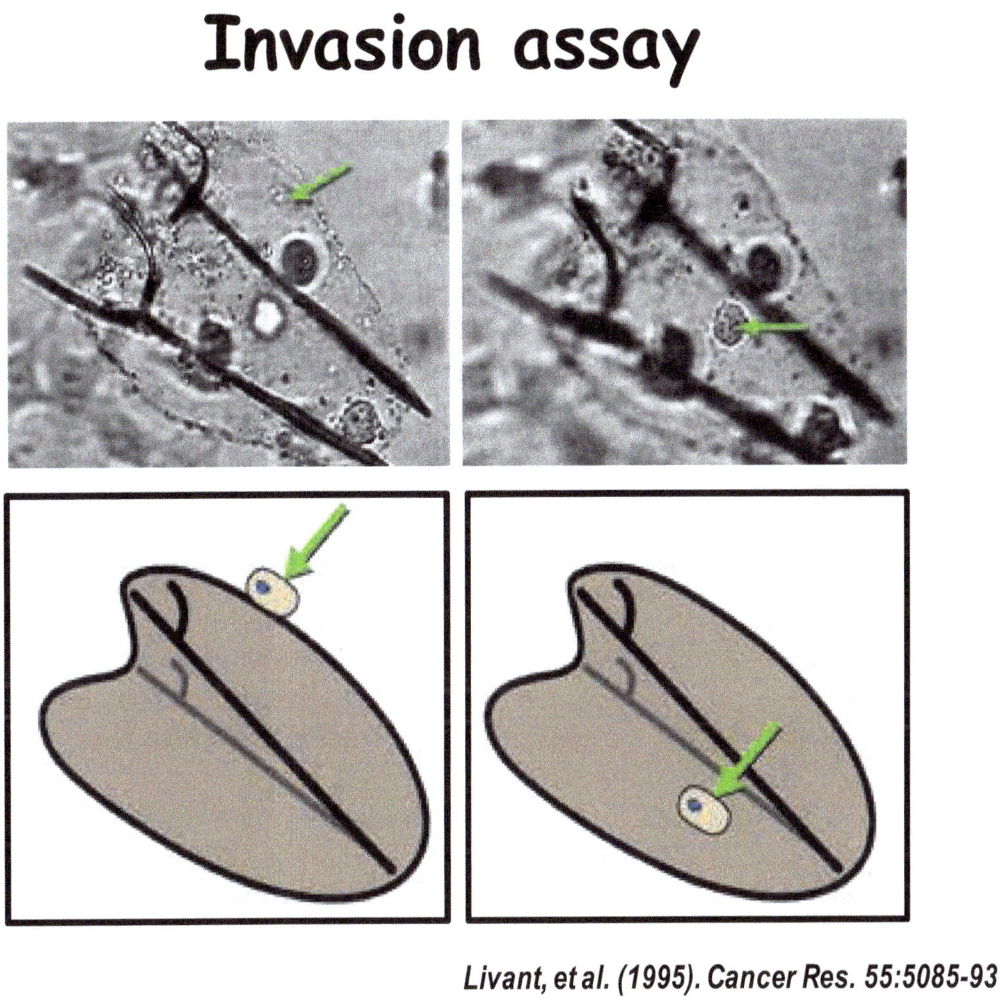

Fig. 3. Sea urchin embryo invasion assay. This assay utilizes the naturally occurring membrane found under a cell layer in sea urchin embryos. The outer cell layer is lysed and the cells are placed on top of the embryos. The number of cells that enter the embryo are blindly scored. Arrows point to cancer cells.

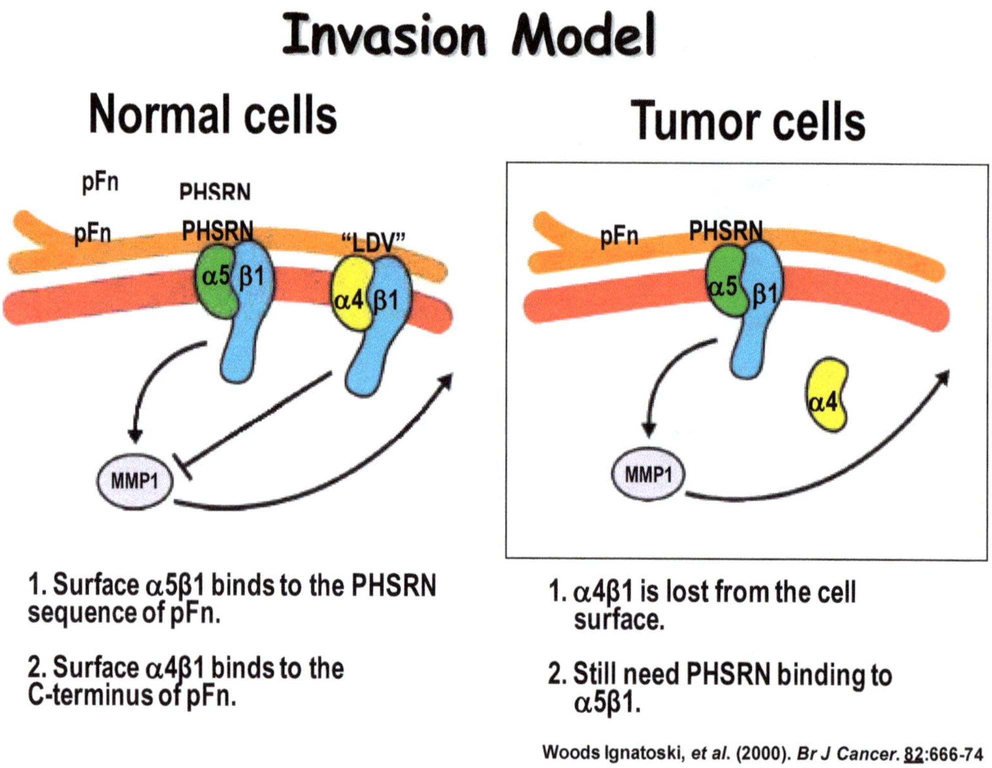

Fig. 4. Model of how cells are able to invade basement membranes. Fibronectin can bind α5 integrin through the PHSRN sequence. This binding drives the expression of MMP-1 and facilitates invasion. However, on normal cells, fibronectin binding to α4 integrin blocks MMP-1 release. On cancer cells, α4 integrin is not present on the cell surface, so invasion can proceed.

Utilizing a constitutively active form of PI3K, p110CAAX, we showed that PI3K can mediate most phenotypes observed in HER-2-overexpressing cells. PTEN expression blocked HER-2-mediated invasion. Down-regulated α4 integrin sequestered PTEN away from the surface, allowing PI3'K to activate PKCδ and facilitate the release of MMP-1 to drive invasion. These results led us to a model for HER-2-mediated invasion where the down-regulation of α4 integrin works in concert with the activation of PI3'K to facilitate the release of MMP-1 and drive invasion (*FIGURE 5*).

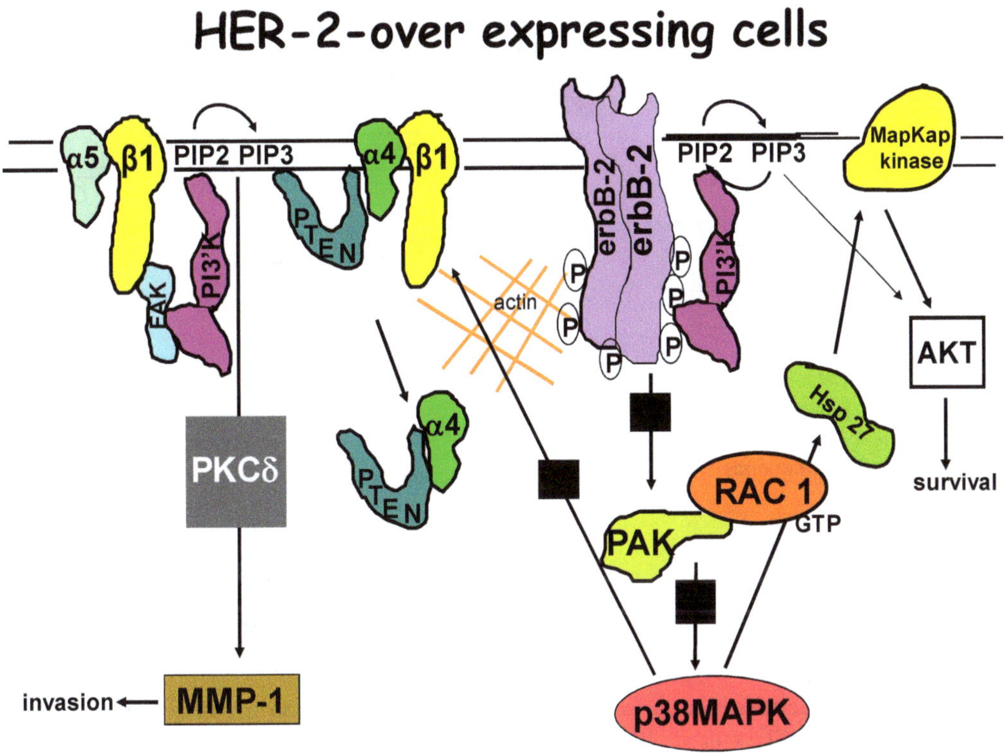

Fig. 5. Schematic of the signal pathways mediated by HER-2. HER-2 activates Rac 1 which activates p38MAPK. P38MAPK rearranges the actin cytoskeleton drawing α4 from the cell surface. It is hypothesized that PTEN is sequestered in the cytoplasm via its association with α4 (data not shown). Sequestration of PTEN allows PI3'K to activate PKCδ to release MMP-1 and facilitate invasion. P38MAPK also activates Hsp27 which activates MapKap kinase and, subsequently, AKT. AKT then facilitaes EGF-independent survival.

Using other *in vitro* transformation methods including anchorage-independent growth and cell motility assays, we were able to show that the PI3'K pathway can mediate most phenotypes observed when HER-2 is over expressed (Woods Ignatoski, Livant et al. 2003; Diehl, Woods Ignatoski et al. 2004). The HER-2-mediated signaling pathways are summarized in *FIGURE 6*.

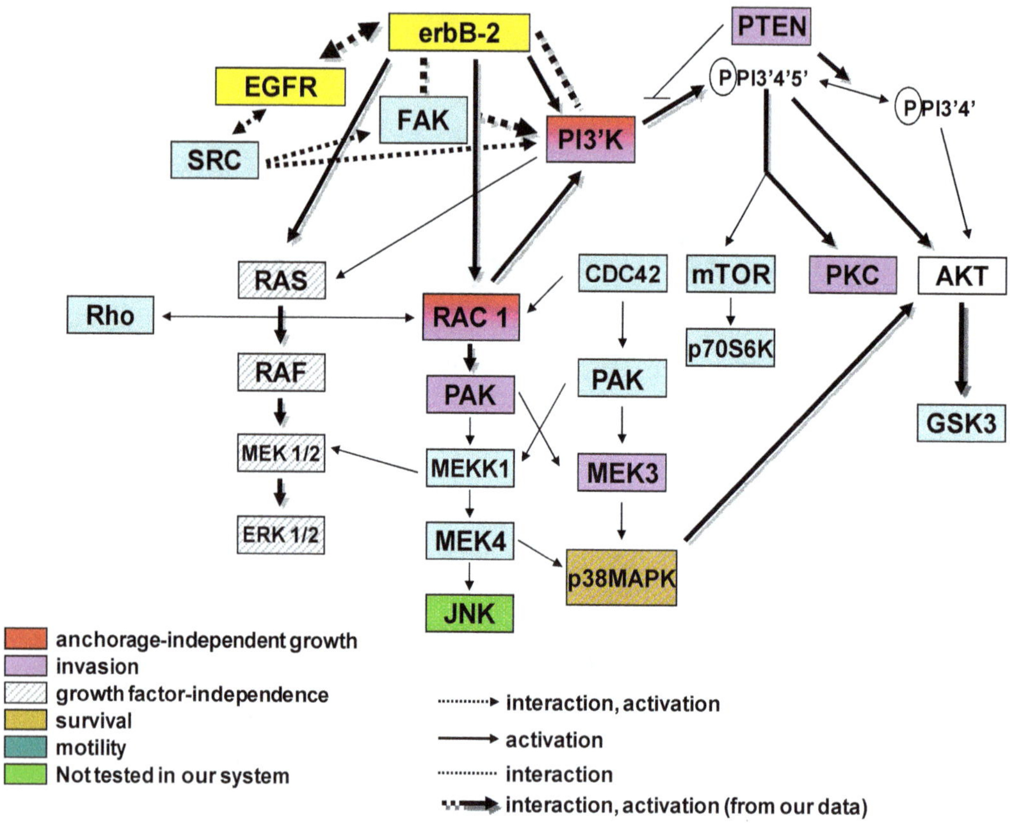

Fig. 6. Diagram of the HER-2-mediated signaling and designation of which pathways facilitate which transformed phenotypes.

Anti-HER-2 therapeutics: The presence of HER-2 over expression in HBC confers a poor prognosis (Slamon, Clark et al. 1987). Thus, the ultimate goal of the study of HER-2 is to offer women with HER-2 over expressing breast cancer an effective therapy. To this end, two relatively effective anti-HER-2 therapies have been FDA approved: trastuzumab (Herceptin®, *Genentech*) and lapatinib (Tykerb®, *Glaxo Smith-Kline*). Trastuzumab is a humanized anti-HER-2 antibody (Ewer, Gibbs et al. 1999; Palmieri, Powles et al. 2001; Rudlowski, Rath et al. 2001). The exact mode of action for trastuzumab is not known; however, trastuzumab is effective against 12-26% of HER-2-positive metastatic patients. Much of the resistance to trastuzumab has been shown to involve over activation of the PI3'K/ AKT pathway (O'Brien, Browne et al. 2010; Migliaccio I, Gutierrez et al. 2011). The survival advantage conferred upon a cell with an activated AKT overcomes the loss of HER-2 activity. Recently, Miller, *et al.* (Miller , Forbes et al. 2009) showed that trastuzumab in combination with rapamycin, which blocks the AKT pathway downstream of AKT at mTOR, could block HER-2 positive tumor growth in mice better than either treatment alone. Also, Zhang, *et al.* (Zhang, Huang et al. 2011) has shown that trastuzumab in combination with the *Src* inhibitor saracatinib can decrease HER-2 positive tumor growth in animals. *Src* is a non-receptor tyrosine kinase that has been shown to play a role in tumorigenesis. Zhang, *et al.* go on to show that *Src* activation is necessary for trastuzumab resistance and that all of the pathways that cause trastuzumab resistance, including different pathways that over activate AKT, originate from over active *Src*. Combination therapies, as the ones above, will be useful when using trastuzumab against HER-2 positive breast cancer.

Glaxo Smith-Kline has developed a small molecule EGFR/HER-2 dual inhibitor called lapatinib (Konecny, Pegram et al. 2006; Rusnak, Alligood et al. 2007; Molina, Kaufmann et al. 2008). Lapatinib has been shown to be a potent HER-2 inhibitor and a useful therapeutic against HER-2 positive breast cancer. Lapatinib, a 4-anilinoquinazoline kinase inhibitor of the intracellular tyrosine kinase domain of HER-2, is used with capecitabine for the treatment of advanced HER2-positive metastatic breast cancer (Molina, Kaufmann et al. 2008). Since response to lapatinib is predicted specifically by low levels of PTEN (Migliaccio I, Gutierrez et al. 2011) and resistance to trastuzumab is dependent on activation of the PI3'K pathway, studies showing the efficacy of a dual therapy using both lapatinib and trastuzumab will be very useful.

4. Conclusions

HER-2-mediated signaling is a convergence point that controls ductal development, the activity of the EGFR family of receptors, and many transformed phenotypes. Significantly abrogating the function of HER-2 is necessary to achieve prolonged survival for breast cancer patients.

5. References

Alroy, I. and Y. Yarden (1997). "The erbB signaling network in embryogenesis and oncogenesis: signal diversification through combinatorial ligand-receptor interactions." *FEBS Lett* 410: 83-86.

Brunet, A., A. Bonni, et al. (1999). "Akt promotes cell survival by phosphorylating and inhibiting a Forkhead transcription factor." *Cell* 96(6): 857-868.

Carraway, C. and K. Carraway (2007). "Sequestration and segregation of receptor kinases in epithelial cells: implications for ErbB2 oncogenesis." *Sci STKE* 2007(381): re3.

Carraway, C. A. C., M. E. Carvajal, et al. (1993). "Association of p185(neu) with Microfilaments via a Large Glycoprotein Complex in Mammary Carcinoma Microvilli - Evidence for a Microfilament-Associated Signal Transduction Particle." *J Biol Chem* 268(8): 5582-5587.

Carraway, K. L., 3rd, E. A. Rossi, et al. (1999). "An intramembrane modulator of the ErbB2 receptor tyrosine kinase that potentiates neuregulin signaling." *J Biol Chem* 274(9): 5263-5266.

Carraway, K. L. and L. C. Cantley (1994). "A neu acquaintance for ErbB3 and ErbB4: A role for receptor heterodimerization in growth signaling." *Cell* 78(1): 5-8.

Carraway, K. L., M. X. Sliwkowski, et al. (1994). "The erbB3 gene product is a receptor for heregulin." *J Biol Chem* 269(19): 14303-14306.

Datta, S. R., H. Dudek, et al. (1997). "Akt phosphorylation of BAD couples survival signals to the cell-intrinsic death machinery." *Cell* 91: 231-241.

Diehl, K. M., N. K. Grewal, et al. (2007). "p38MAPK-activated AKT in HER-2-over expressing human breast cancer cells acts as an EGF-independent survival signal." *Journal of Surgical Research* 142(1): 162-169.

Diehl, K. M., K. M. Woods Ignatoski, et al. (2004). "Signaling pathways in breast cancer cells influence the effects of the pan-erb-B kinase inhibitor CI-1033." *Proc. Am. Assoc. Cancer Res.* 45: 3683.

Ewer, M. S., H. R. Gibbs, et al. (1999). "Cardiotoxicity in patients receiving transtuzumab (Herceptin): primary toxicity, synergistic or sequential stress, or surveillance artifact? #1758." *Semin Oncol* 26(4 Suppl 12): 96-101.

Fedi, P., J. H. Pierce, et al. (1994). "Efficient Coupling with Phosphatidylinositol 3-Kinase, But Not Phospholipase C gamma or GTPase-Activating Protein, Distinguishes erbB-3 Signaling from That of Other erbB EGFr Family Members." *Mol Cell Biol* 14(1): 492-500.

Goldman, R., R. Benlevy, et al. (1990). "Heterodimerization of the erbB-1 and erbB-2 Receptors in Human Breast Carcinoma Cells - A Mechanism for Receptor Transregulation." *Biochemistry* 29(50): 11024-11028.

Gudjonsson, T., L. Ronnov-Jessen, et al. (2002). "Normal and tumor-derived myoepithelial cells differ in their ability to interact with luminal breast epithelial cells for polarity and basement membrane deposition." *J Cell Sci* 115(1): 39-50.

Hendriks , B. S., L. K. Opresko, et al. (2003). "Quantitative Analysis of HER2-mediated Effects on HER2 and Epidermal Growth Factor Receptor Endocytosis Distribution of Homo- AND Heterodimers Depends on Relative HER2 Levels." *J Biol Chem* 278(26): 23343-23351.

Holmes, W. E., M. X. Sliwkowski, et al. (1992). "Identification of heregulin, a specific activator of p185erb2 #636." *Science* 256: 1205-1210.

Howlett, A. R., N. Bailey, et al. (1995). "Cellular growth and survival are mediated by beta 1 integrins in normal human breast epithelium but not in breast carcinoma." *J Cell Sci* 108(Part 5): 1945-1957.

Howlett, A. R., O. W. Petersen, et al. (1994). "A novel function for the nm23-H1 gene: Overexpression in human breast carcinoma cells leads to the formation of basement membrane and growth arrest." *J Natl Cancer Inst* 86(24): 1838-1844.

Hutchinson J, Jin J, et al. (2001). "Activation of Akt (protein kinase B) in mammary epithelium provides a critical cell survival signal required for tumor progression." *Molecular and Cellular Biology* 21(6): 2203-2212.

Jia, Y., S. M. Markwart, et al. (2002). "Integrin receptors regulate MMP1 dependent invasion by breast cancer cells and by mammary epithelial cells." *Submitted to J Cell Biol.*

Karunagaran, D., E. Tzahar, et al. (1996). "ErbB-2 is a common auxiliary subunit of NDF and EGF receptors: Implications for breast cancer." *EMBO J* 15(2): 254-264.

Kokai, Y., T. Wada, et al. (1988). "The role of the neu oncogene product in cell transformation and normal development." *Princess Takamatsu Symp* 19: 45-57.

Komatsu, M., S. Jepson, et al. (2001). "Muc4/sialomucin complex, an intramembrane modulator of ErbB2/HER2/Neu, potentiates primary tumor growth and suppresses apoptosis in a xenotransplanted tumor." *Oncogene* 20(4): 461-470.

Konecny, G., M. Pegram, et al. (2006). "Activity of the dual kinase inhibitor lapatinib (GW572016) against HER-2-overexpressing and trastuzumab-treated breast cancer cells." *Cancer Research* 66(3): 1630-1639.

Korkaya, H., A. Paulson, et al. (2008). "HER2 regulates the mammary stem/progenitor cell population driving tumorigenesis and invasion." *Oncogene* 27(47): 6120-6130.

Korkaya, H. and M. Wicha (2009). "HER-2, notch, and breast cancer stem cells: targeting an axis of evil." *Clin Cancer Res* 15(6): 1845-1847.

Kozloski, G., C. Carraway, et al. (2010). "Mechanistic and signaling analysis of MUC4-ErbB2 signaling module: new insights into the mechanism of ligand-independent ErbB2 activity." *J Cell Physiol* 224(3): 649-657.

Livant, D. L., D. L. Allen, et al. (2000). "The PHSRN sequence induces extracellular matrix invasion and accelerates wound healing inobese diabetic mice." *J Clin Invest* 105(11): 1537-1545.

Livant, D. L., R. K. Brabec, et al. (2000). "Anti-invasive, antitumorigenic, and antimetastatic activities of the PHSCN sequence in prostate carcinoma." *Cancer Res* 60(2): 309-320.

Livant, D. L., S. Linn, et al. (1995). "Invasion of selectively permeable sea urchin embryo basement membranes by metastatic tumor cells, but not by their normal counterparts." *Cancer Res* 55: 5085-5093.

Lochter, A., S. Galosy, et al. (1997). "Matrix metalloproteinase stromelysin-1 triggers a cascade of molecular alterations that leads to stable epithelial-to-mesenchymal conversion and a premalignant phenotype in mammary epithelial cells." *J Cell Biol* 139(7): 1861-1872.

Lochter, A., M. Navre, et al. (1999). "alpha1 and alpha2 integrins mediate invasive activity of mouse mammary carcinoma cells through regulation of stromelysin-1 expression." *Mol Biol Cell* 10(2): 271-282.

Magnifico, A., L. Albano, et al. (2009). "Tumor-initiating cells of HER2-positive carcinoma cell lines express the highest oncoprotein levels and are sensitive to trastuzumab." *Clin Cancer Res* 15(6): 2010-2021.

Migliaccio I, D., M. Gutierrez, et al. (2011). "Loss of phosphatase and tensin homolog or phosphoinositol-3 kinase activation and response to trastuzumab or lapatinib in human epidermal growth factor receptor 2-overexpressing locally advanced breast cancers." *J Clin Oncol* 29(2): 166-173.

Miller , T., J. Forbes, et al. (2009). "Inhibition of mammalian target of rapamycin is required for optimal antitumor effect of HER2 inhibitors against HER2-overexpressing cancer cells." *Clin Cancer Res* 15(23): 7266-7276.

Molina, J., S. Kaufmann, et al. (2008). "Evaluation of Lapatinib andTopotecan CombinationTherapy:Tissue
Culture,Murine Xenograft, and Phase I ClinicalTrial Data." *Clin Cancer Res* 14(23): 7900-7908.

Muthuswamy, S., D. Li, et al. (2001). "ErbB2, but not ErbB1, reinitiates proliferation and induces luminal repopulation in epithelial acini." *Nat Cell Biol* 3(9): 785-792.

Nagy, T., H. Wei, et al. (2007). "Mammary epithelial-specific deletion of the focal adhesion kinase gene leads to severe lobulo-alveolar hypoplasia and secretory immaturity of the murine mammary gland." *J Biol Chem* 282(43): 1766-1776.

Najy, A., K. Day, et al. (2008). "The ectodomain shedding of E-cadherin by ADAM15 supports ErbB receptor activation." *J Biol Chem* 283(26): 18393-18401.

O'Brien, N., B. Browne, et al. (2010). "Activated phosphoinositide 3-kinase/AKT signaling confers resistance to trastuzumab but not to lapatinib." *Mol Cancer Ther* 9(6): 1489-1502.

Palmieri, C., T. Powles, et al. (2001). "Trastuzumab and breast cancer." *N Engl J Med* 345(13): 996-997.

Petersen, O. W., L. Ronnovjessen, et al. (1992). "Interaction with Basement Membrane Serves to Rapidly Distinguish Growth and Differentiation Pattern of Normal and Malignant Human Breast Epithelial Cells #713." *Proc Natl Acad Sci USA* 89(19): 9064-9068.

Ram, T. G., C. A. Dilts, et al. (1996). "Insulin-like growth factor and epidermal growth factor independence in human mammary carcinoma cells with c-erbB-2 gene amplification and progressively elevated levels of tyrosine phosphorylated erbB-2." *Mol. Carcinogen.* 15.: 227-238.

Ram, T. G., K. E. Kokeny, et al. (1995). "Mitogenic activity of neu differentiation factor/heregulin mimics that of epidermal growth factor and insulin-like growth factor-I in human mammary epithelial cells." *J. Cell. Physiol.* 163: 589-596.

Rudlowski, C., W. Rath, et al. (2001). "Trastuzumab and breast cancer." *N Engl J. Med* 345(13): 997-998.

Rusnak, D., K. Alligood, et al. (2007). "Assessment of epidermal growth factor receptor (EGFR, ErbB1) and HER2 (ErbB2) protein expression levels and response to lapatinib (Tykerb, GW572016) in an expanded panel of human normal and tumour cell lines." *Cell Prolif* 40(4): 580-594.

Slamon, D. J., G. M. Clark, et al. (1987). "Human breast cancer: Correlation of relapse and survival with amplification of the HER-2/neu oncogene." *Science* 235: 177-182.

Suo, Z., E. Emilsen, et al. (1998). "Type 1 protein tyrosine kinases in benign and malignant breast lesions #1767." *Histopathology* 33(6): 514-21.

Todaro, G. J., J. E. DeLarco, et al. (1976). "Transformation by murine and feline sarcoma viruses specifically blocks binding of epidermal growth factor to cells." *Nature* 264: 26-31.

Woods Ignatoski, K. and S. P. Ethier (1999). "Constitutive activation of pp 125fak in eleven newly isolated breast cancer cell lines." *Breast Cancer Res. and Treatment* 54: 173-182.

Woods Ignatoski, K. M., M. L. Dziubinski, et al. (2005). "Cooperative interactions of HER-2 and HPV-16 oncoproteins in the malignant transformation of human mammary epithelial cells." *Neoplasia* 7(8): 788-798.

Woods Ignatoski, K. M., A. J. LaPointe, et al. (1999). "ErbB-2 overexpression in human mammary epithelial cells confers growth factor independence." *Endocrinology* 140: 3615-3622.

Woods Ignatoski, K. M., D. L. Livant, et al. (2003). "The role of PI3'kinase and its downstream signals in erbB-2-mediated transformation." *Mol Cancer Res* 1(7): 551-560.

Woods Ignatoski, K. M., T. Maehama, et al. (2000). "ERBB-2 overexpression confers PI 3'-kinase-dependent invasion capacity on human mammary epithelial cells." *Br. J. Cancer* 82: 666-674.

Yokouchi, M., T. Kondo, et al. (1999). "Ligand-induced ubiquitination of the epidermal growth factor receptor involves the interaction of the c-Cbl RING finger and UbcH7." *J Biol Chem* 274(44): 31707-12.

Zachary, I. and E. Rozengurt (1992). "Focal Adhesion Kinase (p125(FAK)) - a Point of Convergence in the Action of Neuropeptides, Integrins, and Oncogenes." *Cell* 71(6): 891-894.

Zhang, S., W. Huang, et al. (2011). "Combating trastuzumab resistance by targeting SRC, a common node downstream of multiple resistance pathways." *Nat Med* 17(4): 461-469.

Permissions

All chapters in this book were first published by Springer; hereby published with permission under the Creative Commons Attribution License or equivalent. Every chapter published in this book has been scrutinized by our experts. Their significance has been extensively debated. The topics covered herein carry significant findings which will fuel the growth of the discipline. They may even be implemented as practical applications or may be referred to as a beginning point for another development.

The contributors of this book come from diverse backgrounds, making this book a truly international effort. This book will bring forth new frontiers with its revolutionizing research information and detailed analysis of the nascent developments around the world.

We would like to thank all the contributing authors for lending their expertise to make the book truly unique. They have played a crucial role in the development of this book. Without their invaluable contributions this book wouldn't have been possible. They have made vital efforts to compile up to date information on the varied aspects of this subject to make this book a valuable addition to the collection of many professionals and students.

This book was conceptualized with the vision of imparting up-to-date information and advanced data in this field. To ensure the same, a matchless editorial board was set up. Every individual on the board went through rigorous rounds of assessment to prove their worth. After which they invested a large part of their time researching and compiling the most relevant data for our readers.

The editorial board has been involved in producing this book since its inception. They have spent rigorous hours researching and exploring the diverse topics which have resulted in the successful publishing of this book. They have passed on their knowledge of decades through this book. To expedite this challenging task, the publisher supported the team at every step. A small team of assistant editors was also appointed to further simplify the editing procedure and attain best results for the readers.

Apart from the editorial board, the designing team has also invested a significant amount of their time in understanding the subject and creating the most relevant covers. They scrutinized every image to scout for the most suitable representation of the subject and create an appropriate cover for the book.

The publishing team has been an ardent support to the editorial, designing and production team. Their endless efforts to recruit the best for this project, has resulted in the accomplishment of this book. They are a veteran in the field of academics and their pool of knowledge is as vast as their experience in printing. Their expertise and guidance has proved useful at every step. Their uncompromising quality standards have made this book an exceptional effort. Their encouragement from time to time has been an inspiration for everyone.

The publisher and the editorial board hope that this book will prove to be a valuable piece of knowledge for researchers, students, practitioners and scholars across the globe.

List of Contributors

Graciela Cricco, Nora Mohamad, María Soledad Sáez and Elena Rivera
Laboratory of Radioisotopes, School of Pharmacy and Biochemistry, University of Buenos Aires, Argentina

Eduardo Valli and Gabriela Martín
Laboratory of Radioisotopes, School of Pharmacy and Biochemistry, University of Buenos Aires, Argentina
Scientific and Technical Research National Council (CONICET), Argentina

Van slambrouck Séverine and Steelant Wim
New Mexico Institute of Mining and Technology, St. Thomas University, USA

Pilar Roca, Jordi Oliver, Jorge Sastre-Serra and Mercedes Nadal-Serrano
Universitat de les Illes Balears, Spain

Mehmet Gunduz
Departments of Medical Genetics and Otolaryngology, Turkey

Esra Gunduz
Department of Medical Genetics, Turkey
Departments of Medical Genetics, School of Medicine, Fatih University, Ankara, Turkey

Ramazan Yigitoglu
Department of Medical Biochemistry, School of Medicine, Fatih University, Ankara, Turkey

Marianne Hauglid Flågeng, Ingvild S. Fenne and Jennifer Gjerde
Institute of Medicine, University of Bergen, Norway

Line L. Haugan Moi
Institute of Medicine, University of Bergen, Norway
Department of Clinical Pathology, University Hospital of North Norway, Norway

Ernst A. Lien and Gunnar Mellgren
Institute of Medicine, University of Bergen, Norway
The Hormone Laboratory, Haukeland University Hospital, Norway

Roisman Reuth, Klemm Ofer, Raphaeli Guy and Roisman Isaac
Carmel College, Haifa, Israel

Alex Beny
Rambam Medical Center, Haifa, Israel

Reznick Abraham Zeev
Rapapport Faculty of Medicine, Technion - Israel Institute of Technology, Haifa, Israel

M. Thill, S. Becker, D. Fischer and K. Diedrich
Department of Obstetrics and Gynecology, University Schleswig-Holstein, Campus Luebeck, Luebeck, Germany

D. Salehin and M. Friedrich
Department of Gynecology and Obstetrics, Helios Hospital Krefeld, Krefeld, Germany

Brian P. Ceresa
University of Oklahoma Health Sciences Center, United States of America

Mehmet Gunduz
Departments of Medical Genetics and Otolaryngology, School of Medicine, Fatih University, Ankara, Turkey

Bunyamin Isik
Department of Family Medicine, School of Medicine, Fatih University, Ankara, Turkey

Omer Faruk Hatipoglu
Department of Molecular Biology and Biochemistry, Graduate School of Medicine, Dentistry and Pharmaceutical Sciences, Okayama, Japan

Mikdat Bozer
Department of General Surgery-Surgical Oncology Section, Turkey

Christina T. Teng
Division of National Toxicology Program, National Institute of Environmental Health Sciences, National Institutes of Health, Durham, United States of America

Peggy R. Teng
Department of Experimental Pathology and Laboratory Medicine, Anderson School of Management, UCLA Alumnus, Los Angeles, United States of America

Chee-Onn Leong
International Medical University, Malaysia

Kathleen M. Woods Ignatoski
University of Michigan, USA

Index

Printed in the USA
CPSIA information can be obtained
at www.ICGtesting.com
LVHW082204201023
761596LV00009B/1566

9 781646 465965